Diseases and Management of

Breeding Stallions

Dickson D. Varner, DVM, MS

James Schumacher, DVM, MS

Terry L. Blanchard, DVM, MS

Larry Johnson, PhD

Book Editor: Paul W. Pratt, VMD

Production Manager and Cover Design: Elisabeth S. Stein

American Veterinary Publications

5782 Thornwood Dr, Goleta, CA 93117

Library of Congress Card Number: 90-085393
ISBN 0-939674-33-5

Printed in the United States of America

Authors

Dickson D. Varner, DVM, MS
Diplomate, American College of Theriogenologists
Assistant Professor
Department of Large Animal Medicine and Surgery
Texas Veterinary Medical Center
Texas A&M University
College Station, TX 77843

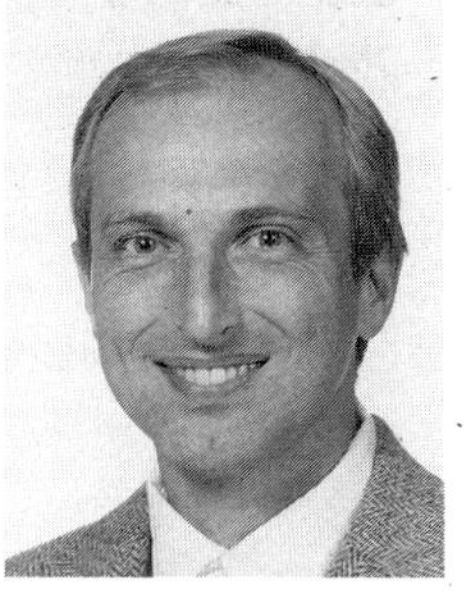

James Schumacher, DVM, MS
Diplomate, American College of Veterinary Surgeons
Associate Professor
Department of Large Animal Medicine and Surgery
Texas Veterinary Medical Center
Texas A&M University
College Station, TX 77843

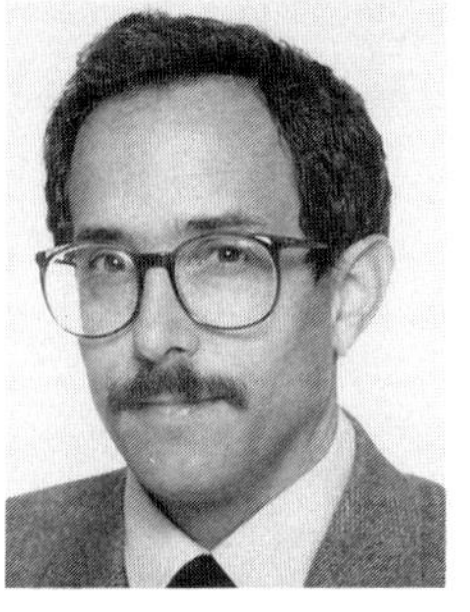

Terry L. Blanchard, DVM, MS
Diplomate, American College of Theriogenologists
Associate Professor
Department of Large Animal Medicine and Surgery
Texas Veterinary Medical Center
Texas A&M University
College Station, TX 77843

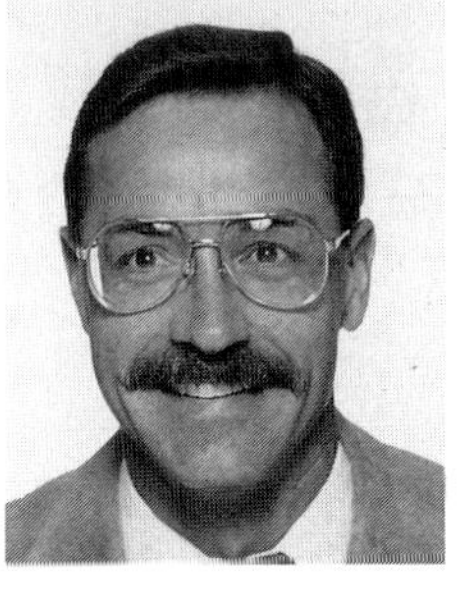

Larry Johnson, PhD
Associate Professor
Department of Veterinary Anatomy
Texas Veterinary Medical Center
Texas A&M University
College Station, TX 77843

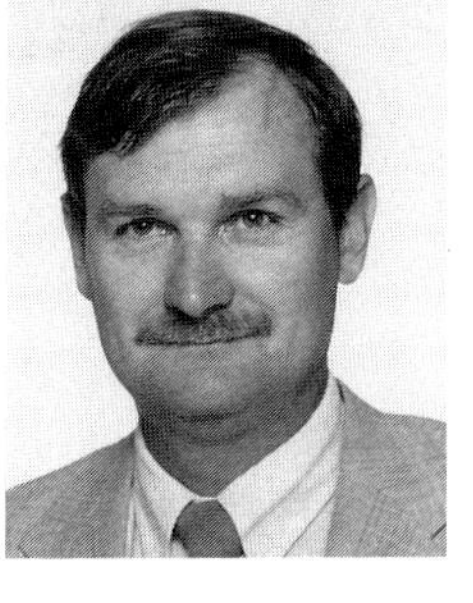

Contents

1

Reproductive Anatomy and Physiology

Genital Anatomy

The genital tract of the stallion consists of 2 testes and attached epididymides, contained within a scrotum; paired deferent ducts, which traverse the spermatic cord to enter the caudal abdomen, then penetrate the genital fold to terminate in the pelvic urethra; 4 distinct accessory genital glands; a musculocavernous penis; and its protective prepuce (Figs 1, 2).[1,2]

Scrotum

The scrotum of the stallion, situated high between the hind limbs, is slightly pendulous and has a globular shape (Fig 3). The distinct longitudinal indentation on its ventral midline is termed the scrotal raphe. This groove represents the most ventral part of the scrotal septum, which divides the scrotum into 2 distinct pouches. The scrotum invests and protects its contents (*eg,* the testes, epididymides, spermatic cords and cremaster muscles); and it also plays a vital role in testis/epididymis thermoregulation.

The wall of the scrotum is composed of 4 layers: skin, tunica dartos muscle, scrotal fascia, and the parietal layer of the vaginal tunic (from the outside inward). The scrotal skin is thin, pliable and relatively hairless, and contains numerous sweat and sebaceous glands (hence its smooth oily texture). Directly underlying

Figure 1. Anatomy of the stallion's reproductive tract: a. bulbourethral glands, b. prostate gland, c. left vesicular gland, d. left ampulla, e. bladder, f. left vaginal ring, g. left deferent duct, h. left spermatic cord, i. body of penis, j. glans penis, k. left epididymal head (caput), l. left testis, m. left epididymal tail (cauda), n. left epididymal body (corpus), o. urethra, p. retractor penis muscle.

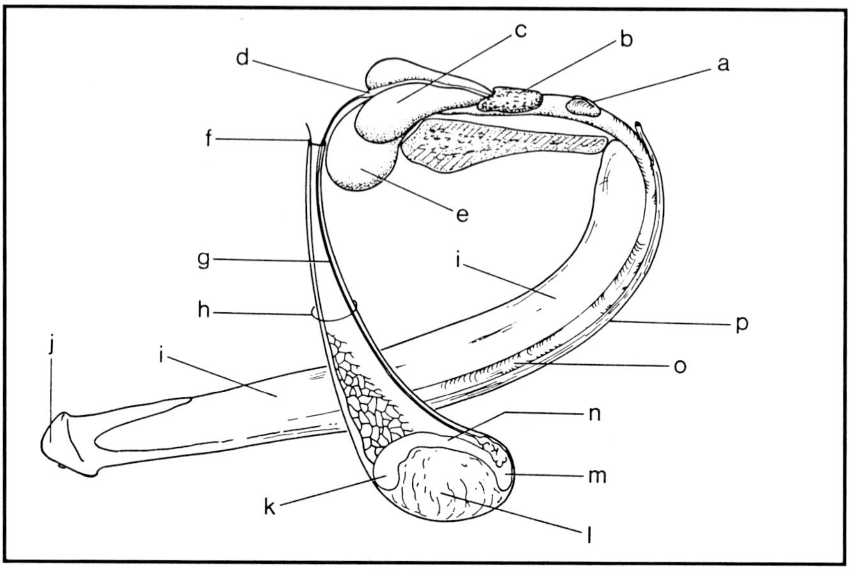

and adherent to the skin is the tunica dartos muscle. The smooth muscle and fibroelastic tissue of this layer bestow contractile properties to the scrotum, thereby permitting changes in its

Figure 2. Configuration of the stallion's prepuce and related structures.

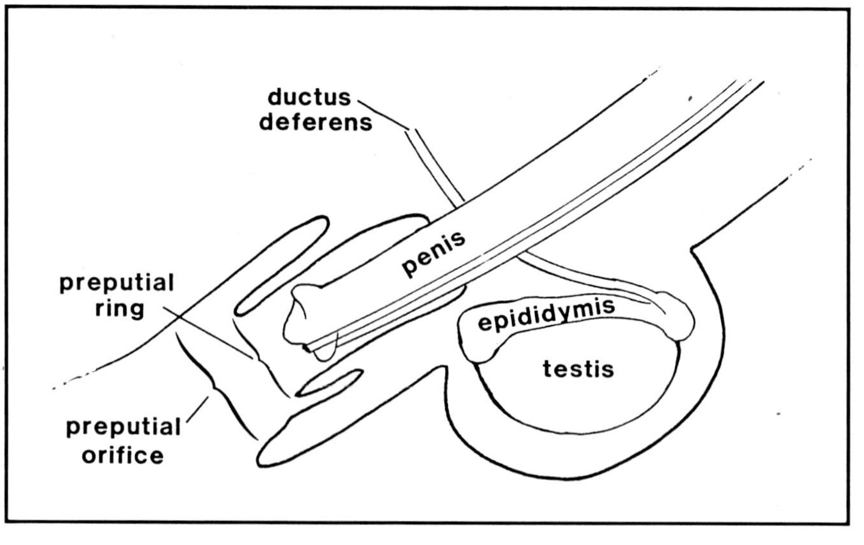

shape, size and position. The tunica dartos also forms the median partition of the scrotum (*ie*, the scrotal septum described above).

Scrotal fascia is interspersed between the tunica dartos and underlying parietal layer of the vaginal tunic. The loose architectural design of this fascia permits considerable movement of the testis within the scrotum. The parietal layer of the vaginal tunic is a membranous sac continuous with the parietal peritoneum at the level of the vaginal rings. It arises as an outpouching of the parietal peritoneum during testicular descent into the scrotum. The parietal layer of the vaginal tunic is lightly adhered to the overlying scrotal fascia.

Testes

The paired testes are situated in the scrotum, with their long axis directed horizontally. Testes perform both exocrine and endocrine functions. The exocrine role is spermatogenesis or production of male gametes. The testes also produce hormones that are important in spermatogenesis, sexual differentiation, and development of secondary sexual characteristics and sex drive (libido).

Figure 3. Slightly pendulous scrotum of a stallion, with a distinct longitudinal indentation on its ventral midline (scrotal raphe), and containing 2 testes along with their attached excurrent ducts.

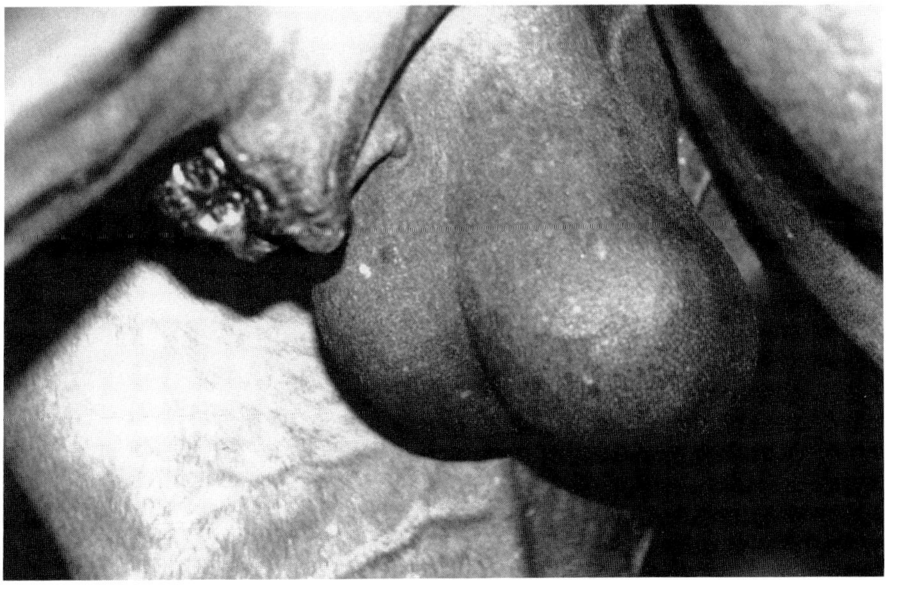

The testes are composed of testicular parenchyma encapsulated by the thick fibrous tunica albuginea (Fig 4). Extensions of the tunica albuginea penetrate the underlying testicular parenchyma, dividing it into numerous lobules. The tunica albuginea is composed of collagen and elastic fibers, myoid cells, and a network of blood vessels. The outermost portion of the capsule is intimately adhered to a serous membrane, the visceral layer of the vaginal tunic. The visceral and parietal layers of the vaginal tunic are separated by a narrow space (called the vaginal cavity, space or canal) that communicates directly with the peritoneal cavity. The vaginal cavity normally contains a small amount of serous fluid, and permits limited movement of the testes and attached epididymides within the sac of the parietal vaginal tunic.

Testicular parenchyma occupies nearly 90% of the total testis mass in adult horses but tends to decrease slightly in older adult horses (Table 1).[3] Over 70% of the testicular parenchyma is occupied by seminiferous tubules (Figs 4, 5).[4] The interstitial component of the testis is located between seminiferous tubules and occupies the remainder of the parenchyma. As a component of the interstitium, Leydig cells comprise 12-18% of the testicular parenchyma; other interstitial cells, such as fibroblasts, lymphocytes and mast cells, comprise 1%; noncellular components, 5-10%; blood vessels, 3-4%; and lymphatic vessels, 1%. Nerves are rarely seen in the testicular interstitium.

Seminiferous tubules are composed of a lumen surrounded by seminiferous epithelium (Sertoli cells and germ cells) that, in turn, is surrounded by myoid cells in boundary tissue. Testicular germ cells (spermatogonia, spermatocytes, spermatids) are discussed in the section on Spermatogenesis. Myoid cells form a single layer around the seminiferous tubules in the stallion. Myoid cells with the attached extracellular tissue maintain the integrity of seminiferous tubules. These cells have fine cytoplasmic filaments believed to be actin and thought to be involved in rhythmic contractions of seminiferous tubules. Myoid cells may assist in propulsive movements of spermatozoa and fluid from seminiferous tubules. Myoid-cell secretions stimulate secretion of important Sertoli-cell proteins, such as transferrin and androgen-binding protein, but may inhibit production of other proteins (*eg*, plasminogen activator protein) by Sertoli cells.[5,6]

Leydig Cells: Leydig cells support spermatogenesis, maintenance of secondary sex characteristics and sex drive. Leydig cells are stimulated by luteinizing hormone to produce testosterone, and are located in the interstitium adjacent to the seminiferous tubules (Figs 4, 5). This structural relationship enables Leydig cells to maintain a high concentration of testosterone within

Table 1. Age-related changes in testicular measurements, testicular composition, Leydig-cell and Sertoli-cell populations, seminiferous tubules and daily sperm production in horses 2-20 years of age.[3,4]

	Age (years)		
	2-3	4-5	13-20
Weight (g)			
Testicular	117 ± 5^{a}	161 ± 13^{b}	213 ± 11^{c}
Parenchymal	105 ± 4^{a}	$146 \pm 13^{b,e}$	184 ± 10^{f}
Tunica albuginea	12.2 ± 0.6^{e}	$14.8 \pm 0.9^{a,f}$	28.8 ± 1.8^{b}
Parenchymal pigmentation score	1.5 ± 0.1^{a}	2.5 ± 0.2^{b}	4.4 ± 0.3^{c}
Testicular composition (%)			
Leydig cells	6.0 ± 0.5^{a}	12.2 ± 1.1^{b}	18 ± 0.9^{c}
Nuclei of Leydig cells	0.54 ± 0.04^{a}	$0.87 \pm 0.7^{b,e}$	1.09 ± 0.05^{f}
Noncellular components	15.8 ± 0.9^{a}	9.8 ± 0.8^{b}	4.5 ± 0.8^{c}
Other interstitial cells	1.9 ± 0.1^{a}	1.2 ± 0.1^{b}	1.1 ± 0.1^{b}
Blood vessels	3.9 ± 0.3	3.7 ± 0.2	3.1 ± 0.4
Lymph vessels	0.7 ± 0.1	1.1 ± 0.1	0.8 ± 0.2
Seminiferous tubules	71.7 ± 1.2	72 ± 1.3	72.4 ± 0.6
Leydig-cell population			
Volume/testis (ml)	5.9 ± 0.4^{a}	17.8 ± 2.5^{b}	31.8 ± 2.5^{c}
Volume/g parenchyma (μl)	58 ± 5^{a}	117 ± 11^{b}	173 ± 8^{c}
Nuclear volume/testis (ml)	0.49 ± 0.04^{a}	1.14 ± 0.14^{b}	1.76 ± 0.14^{c}
Diameter of nucleus (μ)	8.7 ± 0.1	8.9 ± 0.1	9 ± 0.1
Volume of nucleus (fl)	344 ± 7	371 ± 14	381 ± 16
Number/testis (10^{9})	1.41 ± 0.11^{a}	3.06 ± 0.38^{b}	4.66 ± 0.42^{c}
Number/g parenchyma (10^{6})	13.6 ± 1.0^{a}	20.9 ± 2.0^{b}	25.2 ± 1.5^{b}
Volume of single cells (pl)	4.3 ± 0.2^{a}	5.8 ± 0.5^{b}	7.0 ± 0.6^{b}
Sertoli-cell population			
Number/g parenchyma (10^{6})	33.7 ± 3.9	128.9 ± 2.1	23.1 ± 1.6
Number/testis (10^{9})	2.77 ± 0.28	3.7 ± 0.44	3.59 ± 0.27
Number elongated spermatids/ Sertoli cell	3.5 ± 0.6	5.4 ± 0.8	7 ± 0.4
Seminiferous tubules			
Volume/testis (ml)	72 ± 3^{a}	$101 \pm 9^{b,e}$	127 ± 8^{f}
Diameter (μ)	212 ± 4^{a}	230 ± 3^{b}	242 ± 3^{b}
Length/testis (km)	2.04 ± 0.09^{e}	$2.39 \pm 0.19^{e,f}$	2.79 ± 0.21^{f}
Length/g parenchyma (m)	19.5 ± 0.64^{a}	16.6 ± 0.5^{b}	15.1 ± 0.4^{b}
Daily sperm production			
DSP/testis (10^{9})	1.27 ± 0.19^{a}	2.67 ± 0.26^{b}	3.18 ± 0.50^{b}
DSP/g parenchyma (10^{6})	11.4 ± 1.4^{a}	18.8 ± 1.6^{b}	17 ± 2.4^{b}

a, b, c – Means in rows with different superscripts differ ($P < 0.01$).
e, f – Means in rows with different superscripts differ ($P < 0.05$).

seminiferous tubules (70 mg/g parenchyma) as compared to peripheral blood (about 400 pg/ml serum).[7] Equine Leydig cell cytoplasm contains an abundance of smooth endoplasmic reticulum (about 80% v/v, Fig 6, Table 2) and 10% mitochondria (v/v).[7,8] Smooth endoplasmic reticulum is the organelle in which cholesterol, the substrate for testosterone, is synthesized and pregnenolone is rapidly metabolized to testosterone. Mitochondria contain the rate-limiting cholesterol side-chain cleavage step in the pathway for testosterone synthesis.[9] Individual Leydig cells are approximately 6 pl in volume.[7]

Figure 4.The equine testis viewed in a gross cross section (a) in a low-magnification histologic section (b) and a higher-magnification histologic section (c). a. The testis is composed of the tunica albuginea (capsule; TA) and testicular parenchyma (TP). The central vein (CV) has associated connective tissue. b. The testicular parenchyma contains numerous tightly coiled seminiferous tubules (ST). c. The interstitium between seminiferous tubules (ST) contains numerous Leydig cells (LC), blood vessels (BV) and lymphatic vessels (LV). Bar lengths equal 10 mm in (a), 1 mm in (b) and 30 μ in (c).[4,26]

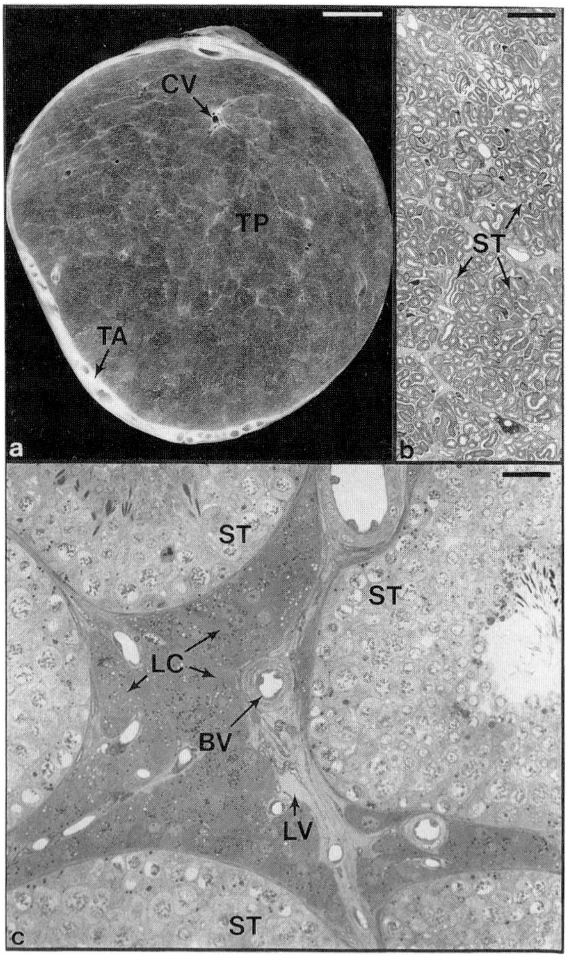

behind at spermiation. Sertoli cells also secrete luminal fluid and proteins (including inhibin and androgen-binding protein), form the blood-testis barrier, and participate in cell-to-cell communication.[10-12] In addition, Sertoli cells secrete lactate as a germ cell energy source, and mitogenic polypeptide that may function to stimulate germ cell or Sertoli cell proliferation, and stimulate RNA and DNA synthesis of germ cells.[13-15] All of these functions appear to be important to support of spermatogenesis; however, the precise role of Sertoli cells in spermatogenesis remains unclear.

Figure 10. Transmission electron micrograph of Leydig cells in adult (4-5 yr) (a) and older horses (13-20 yr) (b).[4] In both cases, Leydig cells contain an abundance of smooth endoplasmic reticulum (SER) and mitochondria (M). In older horses (b), Leydig cells may have an accumulation of lipofuscin (Lf). Bar length equals 1 μ.

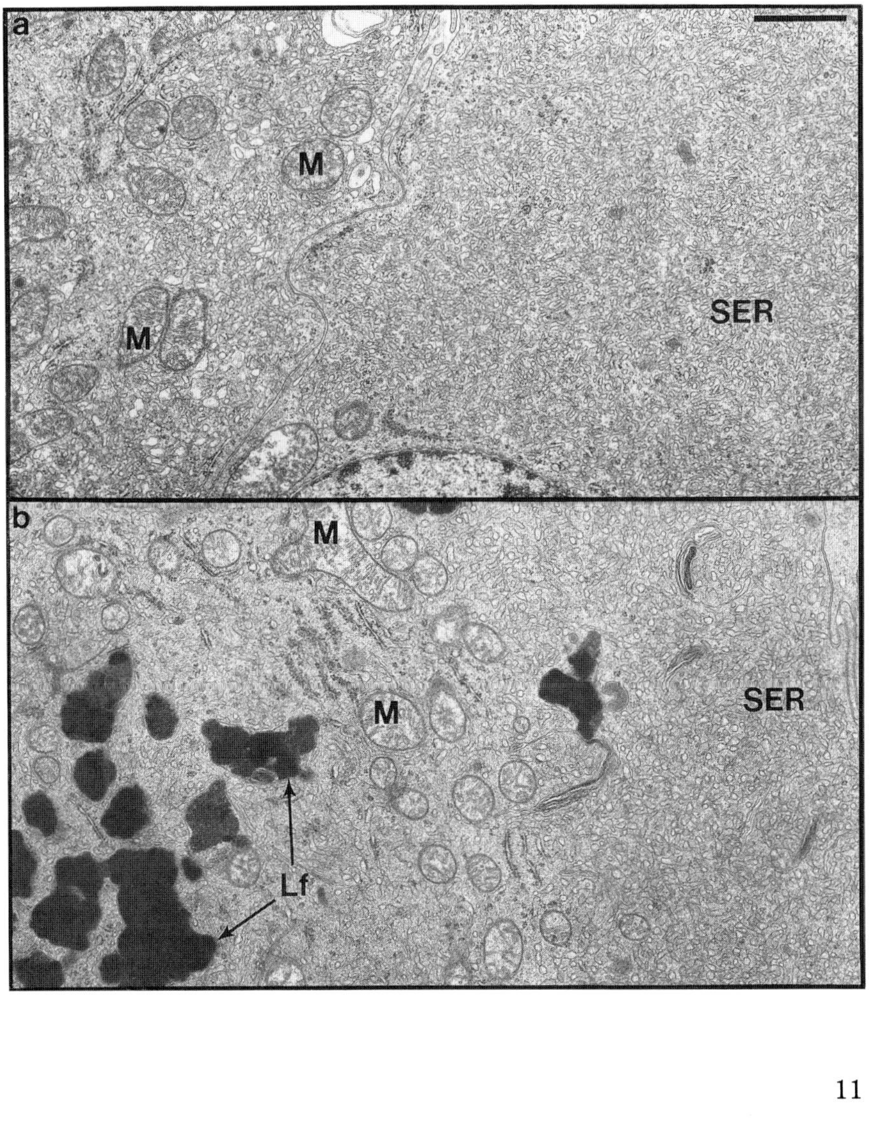

Junctional complexes between adjacent Sertoli cells form the blood-testis barrier and separate the seminiferous epithelium into basal and luminal compartments (Fig 12).[16,17] The blood-testis barrier isolates more advanced germ cells (spermatocytes and spermatids) from serum enzymes and high-molecular-weight components, and constitutes an immunologic barrier that allows these germ cells to develop normally. The blood-testis barrier does not affect incorporation of radioactive amino acids by germ cells inside the blood-testis barrier, indicating that it is not an absolute barrier to substances extraneous to the adluminal compartment.[18]

Figure 11. High-voltage electron micrographs of germ cells and Sertoli cells.[72,110] The Sertoli cell (a) basal and (b) apical regions are illustrated. a. The close association between Sertoli cells and germ cells representing different developmental steps is evident. Extending from the main body of a Sertoli cell and between germ cells are laminar processes (LP). One forms a rim of Sertoli-cell cytoplasm from the main body of the Sertoli cell to the site of an intercellular bridge (IB) between 2 primary spermatocytes (PS). The main body cytoplasm is characterized by long slender mitochondria (arrows) oriented with the long axis of the Sertoli cell. Numerous dense lipofuscin and lipid granules are present in the basal cytoplasm. Germ-cell mitochondria (M) are contrasted with those of Sertoli cells, which are long and slender. The cytoplasm of germ cells contains rough endoplasmic reticulum (RER). The highly indented nature of the nuclear surface is depicted by portions of Sertoli-cell nuclei (N). A Sertoli cell and an A spermatogonium (AS) share intercellular space (IS). The developing flagellum (F), formed from the centrioles (Ct) of a Golgi-phase spermatid (Sa), can be seen within the cytoplasm of such a spermatid. b. This profile reveals the apical region of a Sertoli cell with long slender mitochondria (M), along with 4 embedded Sd_1 spermatids. A nuclear portion and 3 Sa spermatic (Sa) mitochondria are present. Sertoli-cell cytoplasm is located between each spermatid as revealed by following the Sertoli-cell cytoplasm separated by intercellular space (IS) between the Sertoli cell and the Sd_1 spermatids. The Sd_1 spermatids are embedded in the Sertoli-cell apex via tubular indentations in the cell plasma membrane. The manchette (Mn), mitochondria (M) and the annulus (An) of the Sd_1 spermatids are shown. The space between the developing flagellum and manchette is the flagellar canal (FC). It is produced when the plasma membrane unfolds from the spermatid cell body surface. The manchette provides structural support to the flagellar canal. Bar lengths equal 2 μ (a) and 1 μ (b).

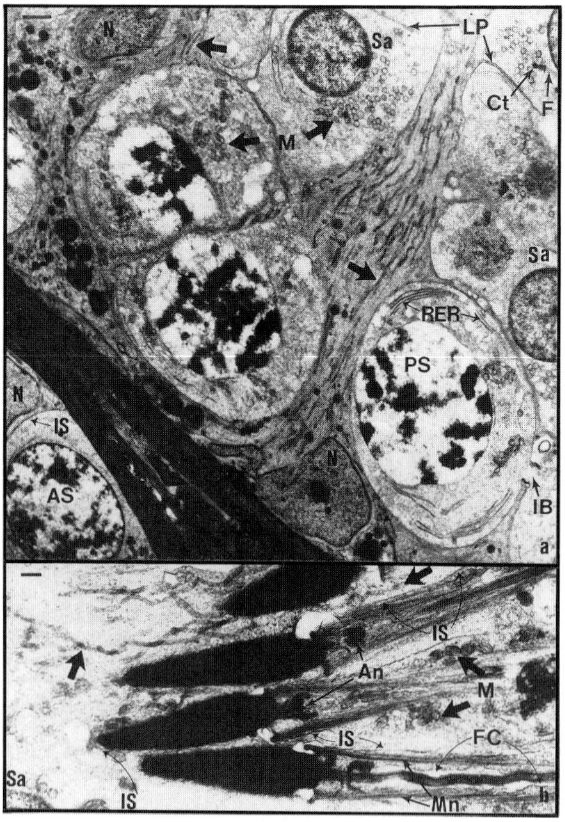

The number of Sertoli cells within the testis is important to spermatogenesis. Sertoli cell numbers closely relate to spermatogonial and spermatid numbers in the testis and spermatozoan production rates of rams, bulls, men and horses.[19-23] The number of Sertoli cells in testes of stallions is influenced by age and season (Fig 13).[3] The number of Sertoli cells per testis increases with age until 4-5 years, then remains at this level through 20 years of age or longer. Sertoli cell numbers in testes of adult horses are greater during the breeding season (summer) than in the nonbreeding season (winter).[3,22]

Figure 12. Transmission electron micrograph of Sertoli cells and germ cells and Sertoli cell-Sertoli cell junctional complexes (inset). Junctional complexes (JC) between adjacent Sertoli cells (SC) separate the basal compartment containing spermatogonia (Sg) from the adluminal compartment containing primary spermatocytes (PS) and spermatids (St). Junctional complexes between adjacent Sertoli cells in the stallion are similar to those of other mammals. These include fusion (F) of outer leaflets of the plasma membranes of 2 Sertoli cells and the presence of juxtaposed endoplasmic reticulum (ER) and bundles of fine filaments (BF). Bar lengths equal μ and 2μ (inset).

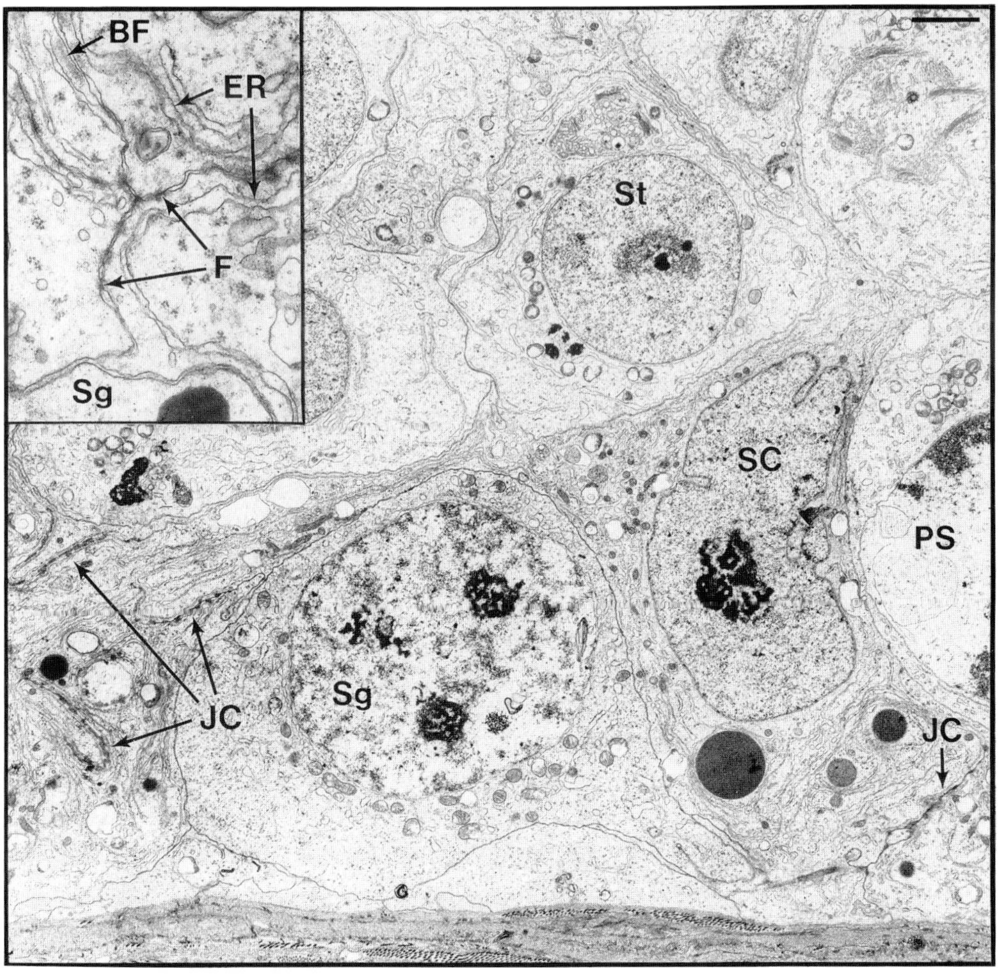

Figure 13. Graphic representation of the effect of season on the numbers of A spermatogonia (A), B Spermatogonia (B), preleptotene and leptotene plus zygotene primary spermatocytes (YP), Leydig cells (LC) and Sertoli cells (SC) per testis in 13-17 adult (4-20 years old) stallions each month.[24] In the breeding season, numbers of A and B spermatogonia are twice their values in the nonbreeding season. However, monthly differences in numbers of cells are seen in each cell type. There is no obvious trend for increases in a given cell type to precede increases in another cell type as the breeding season approaches. However, A spermatogonia numbers increase at a higher rate than do those of other cell types.

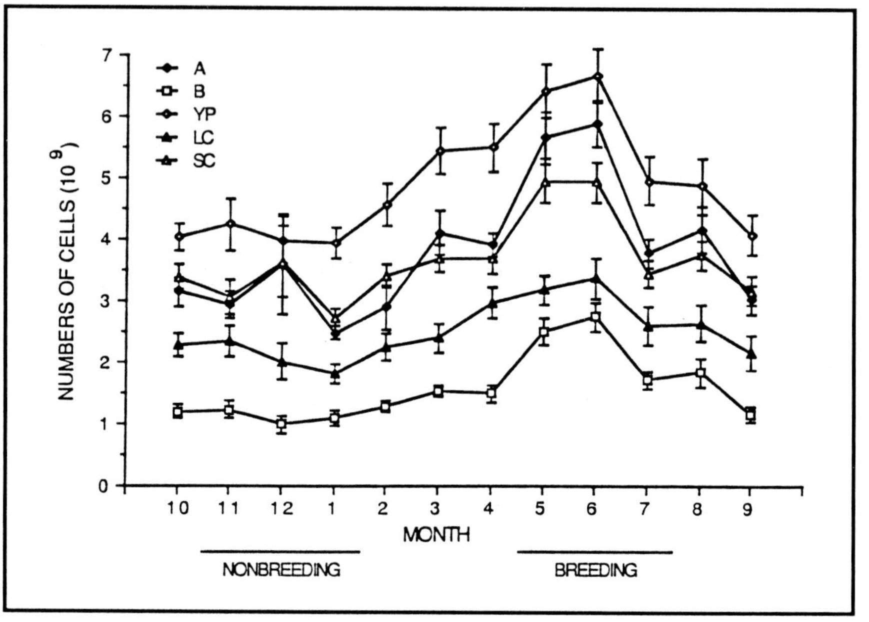

The temporal changes in Sertoli-cell, Leydig-cell and germ-cell numbers throughout the year were evaluated to determine whether changes in Sertoli-cell or Leydig-cell numbers preceded the seasonally increased daily sperm production of stallions (Fig 13).[24] The seasonal stimulus responsible for modulating equine spermatogenesis was not mediated through changes in Leydig-cell or Sertoli-cell numbers. In fact, the change in A spermatogonia numbers preceded and exceeded the magnitude of change in Sertoli-cell numbers, and may therefore influence seasonal changes in Sertoli-cell numbers in stallion testes.

The seminiferous tubules produce spermatozoa (Fig 14), which are then transported via the tubule lumina to the rete testis (Fig 15). Spermatozoa are produced in the convoluted portion of the seminiferous tubules, which is characterized by stratified epithelium (layers of cells on top of each other). As the seminiferous tubules approach the rete testis, their lumina become lined by a single layer of Sertoli cells only (called the transition zone), then end as tubules lined by simple cuboidal epithelium before connecting with tubules of the rete testis (Fig

Figure 14. Scanning electron micrograph of the equine testicular intertitium and seminiferous tubule. Clusters of Leydig cells (LC) are seen in the interstitium between seminiferous tubules (ST). One seminiferous tubule contains spermatids (Spermatids) with spherical nuclei and those whose tails already project into the lumen. Spermatozoa (Sperm) in transit are seen in the lumen. The open arrows mark the height of seminiferous epithelium. Bar length equals 20 μ.

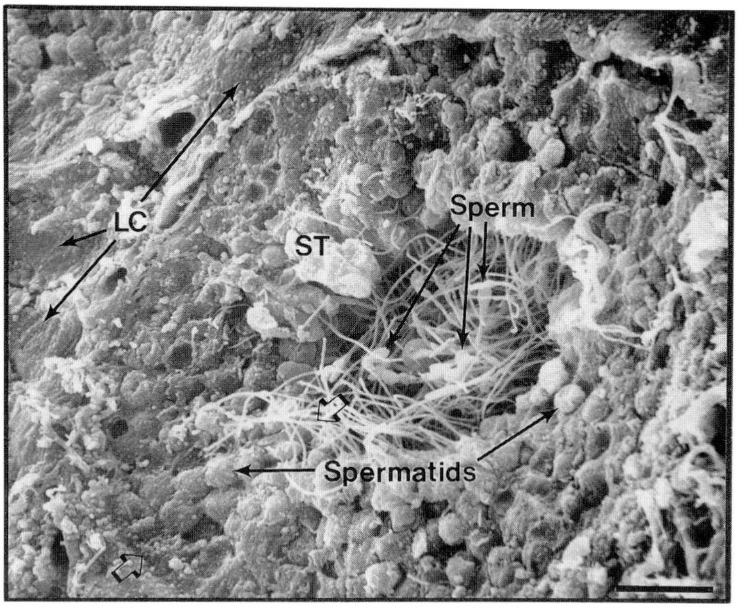

Figure 15. Scanning electron micrograph of a straight rete testis tubule that carries spermatozoa from the seminiferous tubule to the complex of anastomoses of several rete testis tubules near the central vein (see Figure 16).[26] This duct is lined by cuboidal epithelial cells (arrow) covered by microvilli and a single cilium. Bar length equals 20 μ.

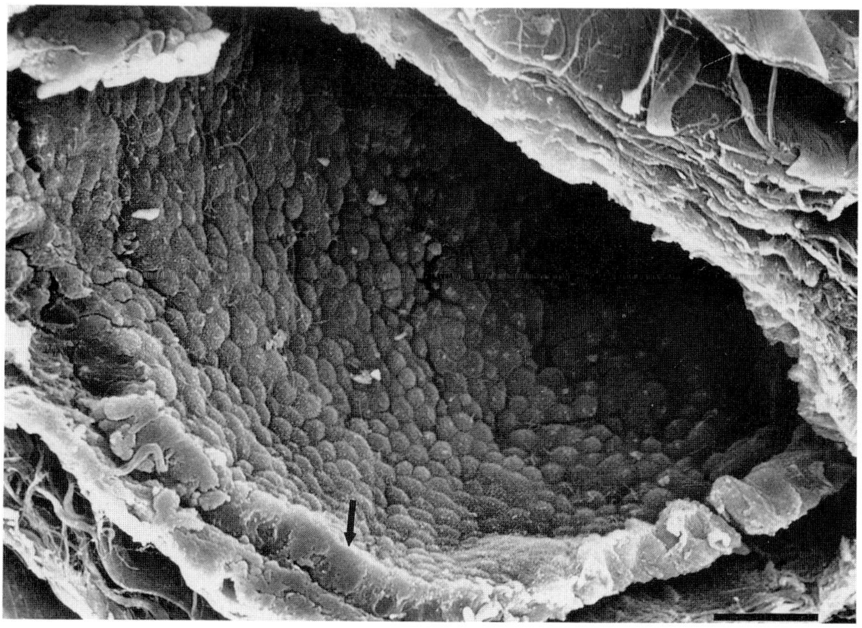

15). Individual rete testis tubules that collect spermatozoa from seminiferous tubules can be found throughout the equine testis. However, many seminiferous tubules converge directly with the network of the rete testis located near the central vein of the testis (Fig 16). The tubules of the rete testis serve to transport spermatozoa and seminiferous tubular fluid to the epididymis via the efferent ducts. Tubules of the rete testis typically pass through the tunica albuginea of the testis at its cranial pole to connect with the efferent ducts of the excurrent duct system (Fig 17);[25] however, an occasional seminiferous tubule can be found outside the testis in the region of the efferent ducts.[26]

Figure 16. Scanning electron micrograph of the rete testis complex (RTC) housed in the connective tissue around the central vein (CV) of the equine testis (a), and a cross support within the complex (b).[26] a. Seminiferous tubules (ST) are juxtaposed to the connective tissue around the rete testis complex. b. The epithelium of the rete testis tubules surrounds the cross support, and testicular spermatozoa have attached to this epithelium. Bar lengths equal 500 μ (a) and 4.6 μ (b).

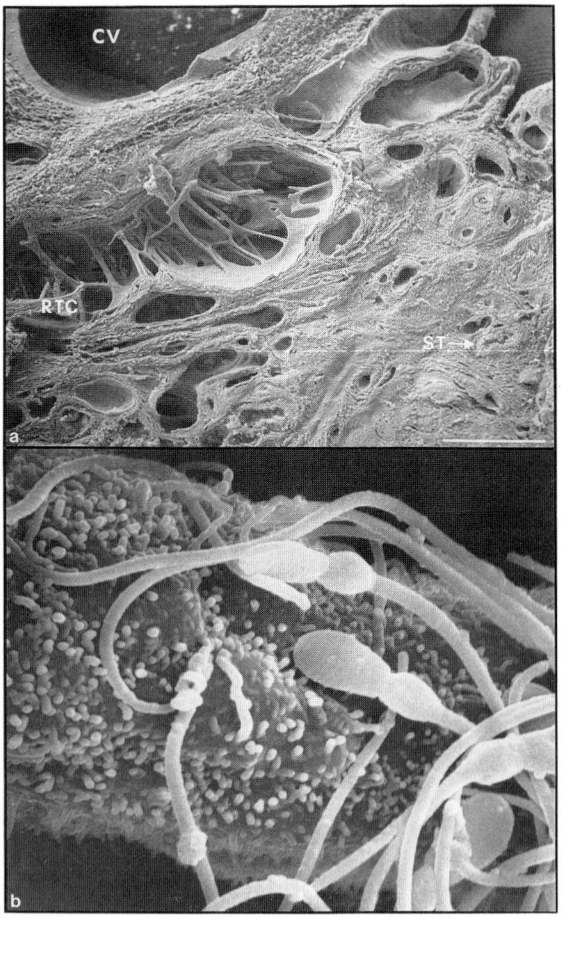

Figure 17. Scanning electron micrograph of an extratesticular rete testis tubule.[25] A cross support (CS) extends across the lumen of the duct, and spermatozoa (open arrow) can be seen on the microvilli-covered surface of the cuboidal epithelium. The single cilium on each individual cell can be seen (solid arrow). Bar length equals 10 μ.

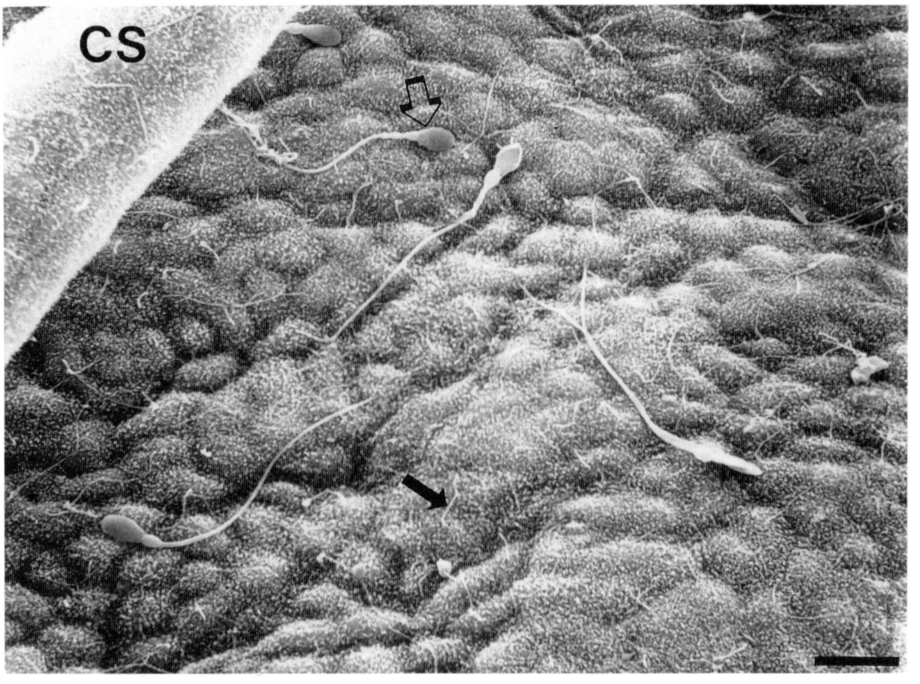

Epididymides

Each epididymis is an unbranched tortuous duct that spans 70-80 meters in the stallion.[2,27] It is formed from the 13-15 converging efferent ductules (Figs 13, 19) and terminates as the deferent duct. The epididymis is divided anatomically into a caput or head, corpus or body, and cauda or tail (Fig 20). The caput is closely applied to the cranial pole of the testis, the corpus courses over the dorsolateral surface of the testis, and the bulbous cauda is attached loosely to the caudal pole of the testis via the proper ligament of the testis.

The epididymis not only serves as a conduit for spermatozoa, but absorbs fluids within the epididymal lumen to concentrate the spermatozoa, and provides a special milieu that enables spermatozoa to mature and achieve fertilizing capacity. Spermatozoa entering the epididymis are incapable of fertilization; they acquire this capacity only after transit through the epididymis (at least through the caput and corpus segments of the epididymis). The caput epididymidis, which contains the distal segments of the efferent ductules along with the proximal epididymal duct, is primarily involved in absorption of luminal fluids and solutes to concentrate the spermatozoa. The efferent ducts are lined by pseudostratified columnar epithelium containing both ciliated and nonciliated cells (Fig 18). Multivesicular bodies in this epithelium are considered important for absorption of luminal fluids and proteins. The ductus epididymidis is lined by slender columnar, principal cells whose luminal borders are covered by very long microvilli called steriocilia (Fig 21).[25] Organelles of the principal cells in the caput epididymidis are compartmentalized with abundant rough endoplasmic reticulum at the basal region and large Golgi in the supranuclear region. These characteristics are suggestive of a secretory func-

Figure 18. Transmission (a,b) and scanning (c,d) electron microscopic views of the efferent ducts.[25] a,b. Cells lining the efferent ducts are composed of pseudostratified columnar epithelial cells and basal cells (BC). Ciliated cells (CC) provide a mechanism to move the spermatozoa through the duct, while nonciliated cells (NcC) contain microvilli that enhance absorption of fluid by endocytosis and pinocytosis. Vesicles (V) located at the apex of the cells near the lumen are evidence of the cells' absorptive functions. c,d. Spermatozoa in the efferent ducts still have proximal droplets characteristic of spermatozoa in the testis and efferent ducts. Bar lengths equal 4.7 μ (a), 1.33 μ (b), 5 μ (c) and 2.2 μ (d).

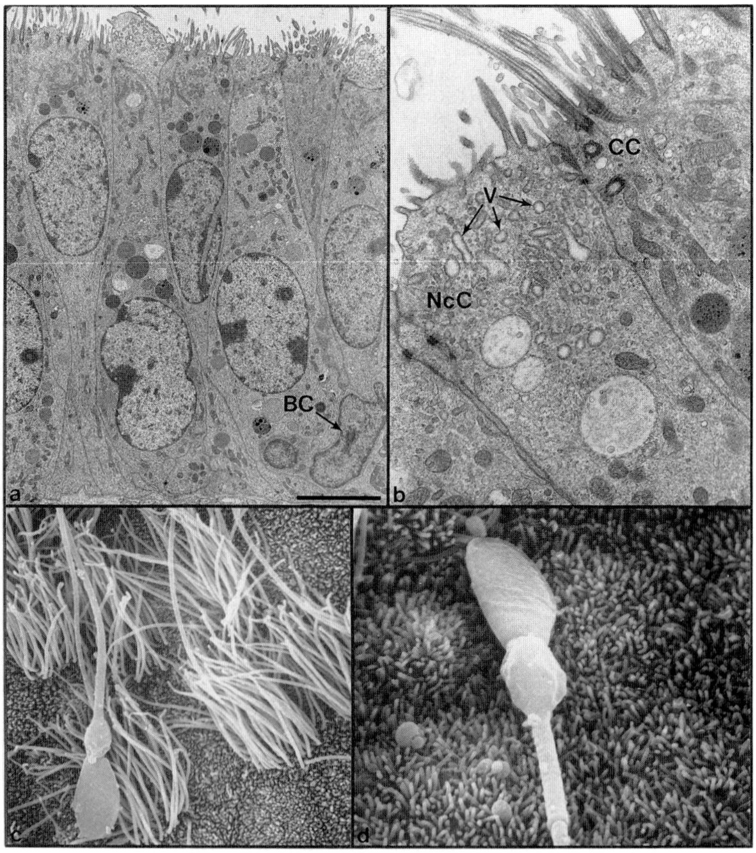

tion; however, the secretions have not been well characterized in the horse. Endocytotic invaginations of the apical cell membrane are consistent with an absorptive function.

Maturational changes in spermatozoa occur predominantly within the corpus epididymidis, which has specific absorptive and secretory activities. Within this maturational segment of the epididymis, regional differences exist in both biochemical composition of luminal fluid and epithelial morphology. This varying microenvironment within the corpus (and distal caput) suggests that these different regions function in different aspects of spermatozoal maturation.[28,29] Specific maturational changes that occur in spermatozoa during epididymal transit include: capacity for progressive motility, morphologic modifications (*eg*, translocation and shedding of the cytoplasmic drop-

Figure 19. Low-magnification scanning electron micrographs of an efferent duct (a) and the various profiles of the same single duct in the caput epididymidis (b).[25] b. A cluster of spematozoa (arrow) is seen filling the lumen of one cross section of this duct. Little smooth muscle surrounds the efferent ducts (a) or caput epididymidis (b). Bar lengths equal 10 μ (a) and 112 μ (b).

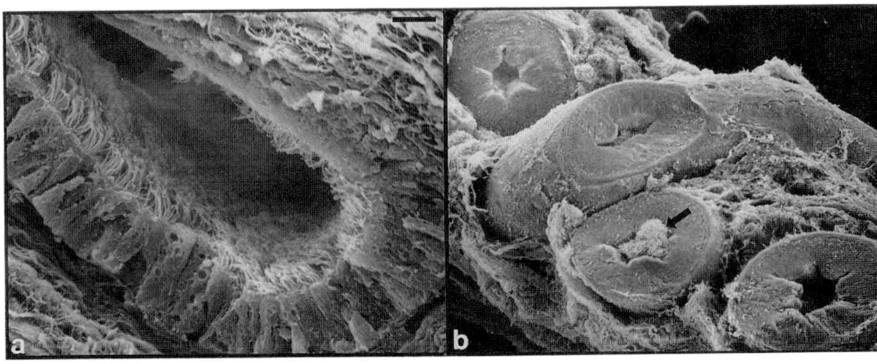

Figure 20. Gross view of the equine epididymis and proximal ductus deferens.[31] The efferent ducts (ED) are housed in the most proximal portion. The ductus epididymidis can be divided into the caput (head), corpus (body) or cauda (tail) epididymidis. The proximal ductus deferens (DD) is straight and thick walled. Bar length equals 10 mm.

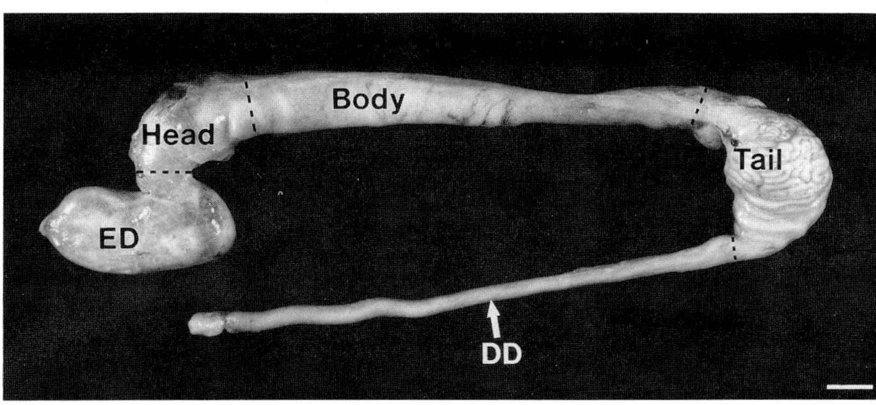

let, Figs 18, 22); ultrastructural and biochemical changes in the plasma and acrosomal membranes; increased structural stability of the nucleus (Fig 23); and changes in spermatozoal metabolism.[25,28-32]

Spermatozoa in the lumen of the caput epididymidis appear structurally similar to those in the efferent ducts in that the cytoplasmic droplet is still located in a proximal position near the neck of the middle piece (Fig 22). A few spermatozoa have bent middle pieces associated with translocation of the cytoplasmic droplet and spermatozoan maturation. When spermatozoa reach the proximal cauda epididymidis, most have completed translocation of the cytoplasmic droplet, as noted by droplets located near the junction of the middle piece and the principal piece (Fig 24). Few ejaculated spermatozoa have cytoplasmic droplets (Fig 24). Spermatozoa with cytoplasmic droplets are found throughout the ductus epididymidis and in the ejaculate; however, most spermatozoa have proximal droplets in the rete testis, efferent ducts and caput epididymidis, translocating droplets in the corpus epididymides, distal droplets in the cauda epididymidis, and few droplets in the ejaculate.[25]

Regional variation in epithelial morphology along the ductus epididymidis includes shortening of the principal epithelial height, shortening of stereocilia on the luminal surface of the principal cells, enfolding of the underlying connective tissue, and thickening of smooth muscle surrounding the duct.[25] The principal cells and steriocilia are the tallest in the caput epididymidis (Fig 21). Epithelial height varies in the corpus epi-

Figure 21. Scanning (a) and transmission (b) electron micrographs of the epithelium of the caput epididymidis.[25] Tall columnar cells are lined with stereocilia (extremely long microvilli; Sc). a. The cytoplasm (C) and luminal surface of these cells are revealed. b. Section through the apex of these cells reveals forming vesicles (FV) in the process of endocytosis. Bar lengths equal 10 μ (a) and 2 μ (b).

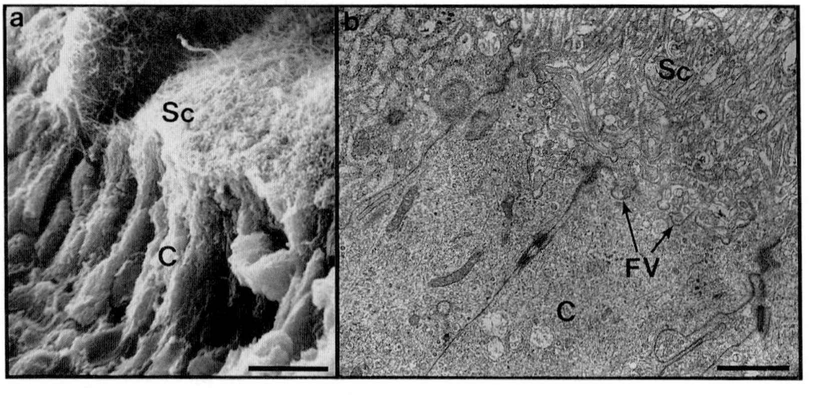

didymidis, creating undulations in the luminal surface of the duct (Fig 22). In the proximal cauda epididymidis, the luminal surface is greatly undulated with papillae of enfolded connective tissue (lamina propria and submucosa) surrounded by shortened principal cells (Figs 22, 24). The papillae are larger in the distal cauda epididymidis. The epididymis has a coat of smooth muscle (containing both longitudinal and circular fibers) that increases in thickness in a caput-to-cauda direction. The efferent ducts and caput have one or no smooth muscle layers, the corpus has few, the proximal cauda has many, and the distal cauda has the most smooth muscle layers. The highly muscular wall of the distal cauda epididymidis aids rapid removal of spermatozoa from its lumen at ejaculation.

The cauda epididymidis serves as a storage depot for mature spermatozoa. In sexually rested adult stallions (5-16 years old), the combined caudae epididymides typically contain $\geq$50 billion

Figure 22. Scanning electron micrographs of spermatozoa in the caput epididymidis with their proximally located cytoplasmic droplets (CD) (a), epithelium of the corpus epididymidis with its tall columnar cells with shorter stereocilia than found in the caput (b), corpus epididymidis spermatozoa undergoing translocation of the cytoplasmic droplet (c), and epithelium and thick smooth muscle (SM) wall of the proximal cauda epididymidis (d).[25] c. The corpus epididymidis is the site of droplet translocation from the proximal to the distal position by bending (arrow) the tail around the droplet and straightening it again. Bar lengths equal 10 μ (a), 45 μ (b), 10 μ (c) and 240 μ (d).

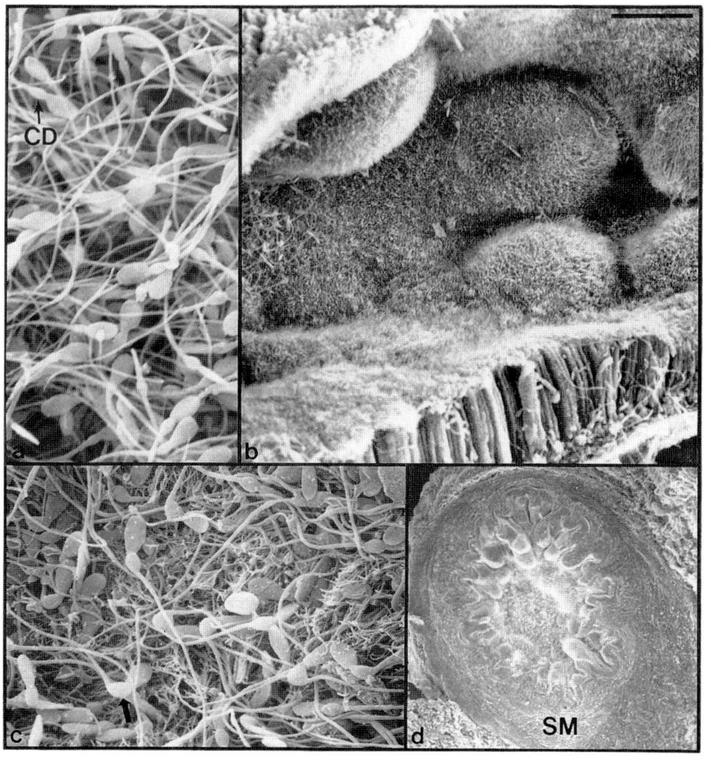

spermatozoa, or >60% of extragonadal spermatozoal reserves.[33] Though the relative percentage of spermatozoa contained within the caudae epididymides is similar in younger stallions (2-4 years old), the actual spermatozoal number tends to be lower than for adult stallions. Spermatozoa that are not removed from the caudae epididymides by ejaculation are thought to be emitted intermittently into the urethra and voided during urination. Resorption of spermatozoa within the excurrent duct system is not thought to occur under normal circumstances, so the fate of all epididymal spermatozoa is considered to be departure through the urethra.[1]

Spermatozoa are transported through the epididymis primarily by contractions of the smooth muscle within the epididymal wall, though luminal hydrostatic pressure and ciliary action of the luminal epithelium play supportive roles. Spermatozoal transit time through the caput and corpus segments of the epididymis is constant at 4.0-4.1 days in stallions.[1,34] Peristaltic epididymal contractions and speed of spermatozoal transit within the caput and corpus are apparently unaffected by extrinsic factors, such as frequency of ejaculation, age or season. The

Figure 23. Transmission electron micrographs of spermatozoa treated with the ionic detergent, sodium dodecyl sulfate, from the proximal corpus epididymidis (a) and distal corpus epididymidis (b).[31] a. Spermatozoa from the testis to the proximal corpus epididymidis have little resistance to detergent treatment, as noted by loss of all tail components and membranes and the decondensation of the nulceus (DN). b. Spermatozoa from the distal corpus epididymidis, through the epididymis and in the ejaculate have acquired some resistance to this detergent treatment during maturation in the epididymis as noted by the presence of the outer membrane of mitochondria (OM), dense fibers (DF) of the tail, and nucleus (N) that has not decondensed. Bar lengths equal 0.6 μ (a) and 1 μ (b).

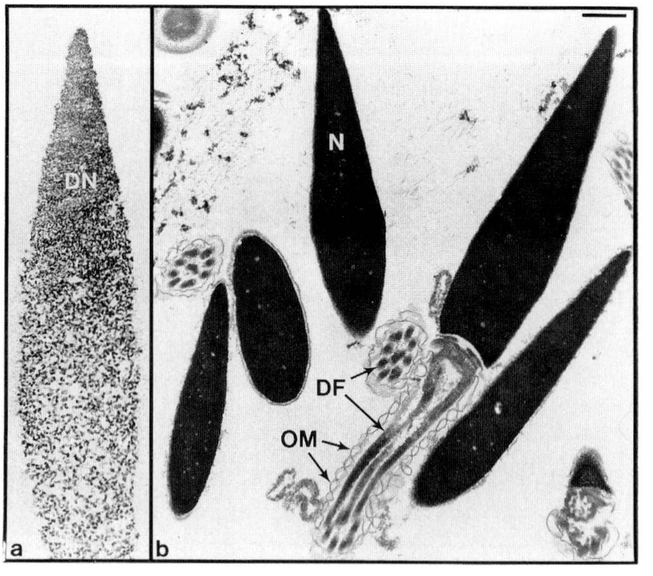

cauda epididymidis serves as a storage reservoir; hence, rate of spermatozoal passage through this epididymal segment is variable and a function of ejaculation frequency. Spermatozoal transit time through the cauda epididymidis is constant at about 10 days in sexually rested stallions but is reduced by 2-3 days in stallions that are sexually active.[1,34]

Spermatozoa tend to accumulate in the distal segment of the cauda epididymidis and attached ductus deferens until smooth muscle in the wall contracts in association with ejaculation, or spontaneous spermatozoal emission. The time that spermatozoa can be retained in the cauda epididymidis without developing senescent changes has not been determined in stallions. Experimental studies involving other animal species has revealed that spermatozoa may remain viable for several weeks following ligation of the ductus deferens.[30] Prolonged spermatozoal retention in the caudae epididymides (and ductus deferens), as occurs with "sperm accumulators," leads to marked

Figure 24. Scanning electron micrographs of epithelium and part of the smooth muscle (SM) wall of the proximal cauda epididymidis (a), spermatozoa of the cauda epididymidis (b), cross section of the distal cauda epididymidis with its unfolded mucosa of epithelium, supportive connective tissue, and thick smooth muscle (SM) wall (c), and ejaculated spermatozoa, most of which have lost their cytoplasmic droplets (d).[25] Bar lengths equal 50 μ (a), 10.8 μ (b), 556 μ (c) and 4.5 μ (d).

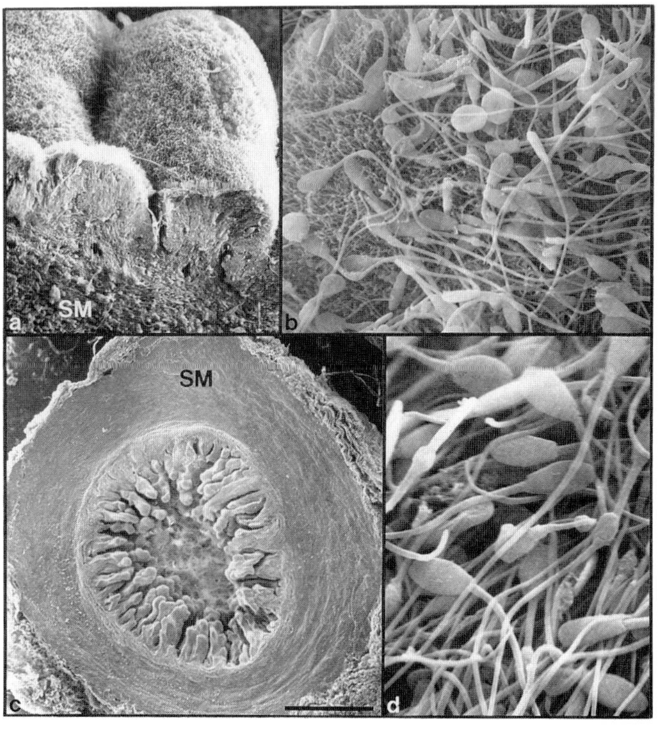

senescent changes in the spermatozoa, represented by morphologic alterations, as well as lowered motility and fertilizing capacity (see Spermiostasis in Chapter 9).

Deferent Ducts (Ductus Deferens)

The 2 deferent ducts serve as a passageway for mature spermatozoa, by connecting the tail of the epididymis with the pelvic portion of the urethra. These long, highly muscular ducts ascend through their respective spermatic cords to emerge via the vaginal rings into the abdominal cavity. They then pass caudally through the genital fold (peritoneum) to enter the pelvic cavity and terminate as slit-like openings in a small protuberence, the seminal colliculus, situated on the dorsal surface of the pelvic urethra.

Spermatic Cord

The 2 spermatic cords extend from the vaginal rings to the attached border of the associated testes. Each spermatic cord is enclosed by the parietal layer of the vaginal tunic. The parietal tunic is connected via the mesofuniculum to the mesorchium, or visceral tunic. The mesorchium is reflected around the contents of the spermatic cord, enveloping the testicular artery, testicular veins (pampiniform plexus), lymphatic vessels, nerves, small bundles of smooth muscle, and a deferent duct with its associated nutrient vessels. The cremaster muscle, a striated muscle that originates from the abdominal wall (*ie,* the internal abdominal oblique muscle), attaches to the lateral and caudal borders of each spermatic cord.

Accessory Genital Glands

Ejaculated semen is comprised primarily of secretions from the accessory glands. Aside from providing a vehicle for transport of spermatozoa from the male to the female reproductive tract during mating, the exact functions of the secretory products from the different accessory glands remain obscure. Accessory glands in stallions include the paired ampullae and vesicular glands (or seminal vesicles), a bilobed prostate gland, paired bulbourethral glands and disseminate urethral glands (Figs 1, 25).

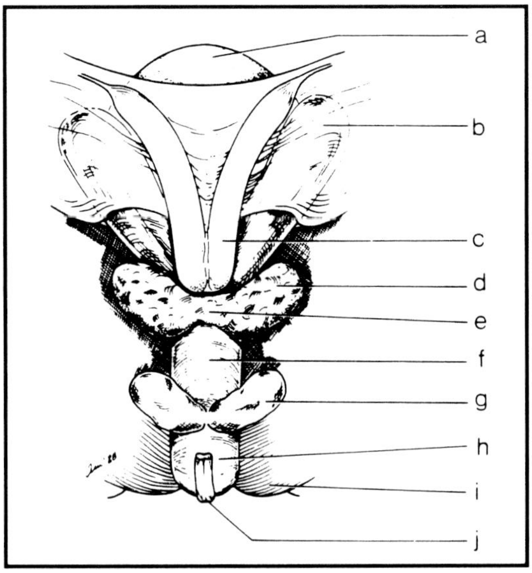

Figure 25. Accessory genital glands of the stallion (dorsal view): a. bladder, b. right vesicular gland, c. right ampulla, d. right lobe of prostate gland, e. isthmus of prostate gland, f. urethralis muscle, g. right bulbourethral gland, h. bulbospongiosus muscle, i. right ischiocavernosus muscle, j. retractor penis muscle.

Each ampulla is evident as a prominent 1- to 2-cm (diameter) circumferential enlargement in the distal 10- to 15-cm (terminal) segment of the deferent duct, located at or near the midline of the pelvic floor. The paired vesicular glands are thin-walled, elongated, slightly pyriform sacs that lie lateral to the ampullae. The base (fundus) of each vesicular gland lies within the abdominal cavity and is covered by the genital fold (peritoneum). Each vesicular gland expands greatly during sexual stimulation due to secretory products emitted into its lumen. These glands can reach 15-20 cm in length and 5 cm in diameter when fully distended. The duct of each vesicular gland converges with the ipsilateral deferent duct to form a common ejaculatory duct that enters the lumen of the pelvic urethra through the seminal colliculus.

The prostate gland of the stallion is a bilobed structure with a connecting isthmus. The lobes are situated lateral to the pelvic urethra and caudal to the corresponding vesicular glands. Each lobe is 5-8 cm long, 2-3 cm wide and 1-2 cm thick. The isthmus is a thin transverse band that courses over the dorsum of the pelvic urethra at the level of the seminal colliculus. The prostate gland has several ducts that enter the urethral lumen lateral to the seminal colliculus.

The paired bulbourethral glands lie 6-8 cm caudal to the prostate gland and are situated on the dorsolateral surface of the pelvic urethra near the ischial arch. These ovoid glands are 3-4 cm long and 2-2.5 cm wide. Each bulbourethral gland has several excretory ducts that enter the urethral lumen distal to the seminal colliculus and near the dorsal midline. The disseminate urethral glands of the stallion have not been well described but appear to be located along the distal pelvic urethra and proximal penile urethra, as evidenced by small papillae of the excretory ducts entering the urethral lumen.

The vaginal rings, paired ampullae, and lobes of the prostate gland can be identified consistently by palpation per rectum. The vesicular glands evade identification because of their thin wall, but usually can be detected by palpation per rectum when distended through sexual stimulation. The walls of the vesicular glands sometimes become thickened following vesicular adenitis (seminal vesiculitis), improving their identification by palpation per rectum, even when the affected stallion is not sexually stimulated. The bulbourethral glands usually are not palpable per rectum because they are covered by thick musculature.

Urethra

The urethra is a membranous canal that extends from the bladder to the distal end of the penis and serves as a passageway for both urine and semen. The pelvic portion of the urethra is surrounded by a layer of erectile tissue, the stratum cavernosum, which itself is enveloped by the thick striated urethralis muscle. The extrapelvic or penile portion of the urethra begins at the penile attachment to the ischial arch, then courses along the penis in the ventral groove of the corpus cavernosum penis to terminate as the urethral process at the tip of the penis.

Penis

This erectile copulatory organ is well developed in stallions (Figs 1, 26). It consists of a root (radix penis), body (corpus penis) and glans penis. The root of the penis is securely attached to the ischial arch by 2 strong ligamentous crura containing erectile lumina. These crura fuse in the root of the penis and extend distally to occupy the body of the penis as the expansive corpus cavernosum penis. The sizable glans penis is located distal to the body, capping the free end of the penis. The cranial surface of the glans has a deep depression, the fossa glandis, from which the urethral process protrudes. The fossa glandis contains 2 ventrolateral recesses and a large dorsal diverticulum (urethral sinus).

The penis of the stallion is of the musculocavernous type, because the erectile tissue is made up predominantly of cavernous spaces rather than trabeculae of connective tissue. This is in contrast to the fibroelastic penis of male ruminants. The penis is composed of 3 cavernous bodies: the corpus cavernosum penis, corpus spongiosum penis and corpus spongiosum glandis. The corpus cavernosum penis spans the entire length of the penile body and is covered by a thick tunica albuginea. Precopulatory erection in the stallion is achieved through engorgement of the corpus cavernosum penis. A longitudinal groove on the ventral surface of the corpus cavernosum penis shields the penile urethra. The corpus spongiosum penis surrounds the penile urethra along its entire length. This cavernous tissue is an extension of the erectile stratum cavernosum surrounding the pelvic urethra. The corpus spongiosum penis enlarges at its proximal end at the ischial arch as the bulb of the penis. Also continuous with the cavernous spaces of the corpus spongiosum penis is the corpus spongiosum glandis, located in the glans penis. It is capable of great expansion and is responsible for the marked "belling" or "flowering" of the glans penis during coitus.

Prepuce

The prepuce shields the detumescent penis. Unlike that of other domestic species, the prepuce of the stallion telescopes around the nonerect penis to form 2 distinct folds, creating both an external and internal prepuce (Figs 2, 26). The external

Figure 26. Structures of the stallion's penis and prepuce: a. preputial ring, b. internal lamina of the internal prepuce, c. attachment of the internal lamina of the internal prepuce to the penis, d. corona glandis, e. glans penis, f. urethral process, g. collum glandis, h. free portion of the penile body, i. external lamina of the internal prepuce, j. preputial orifice, k. scrotum.

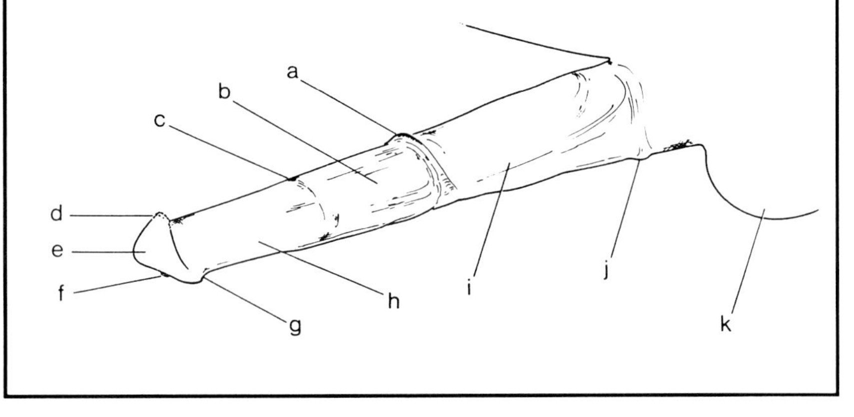

prepuce consists of external and internal laminae that meet at the preputial orifice. Only the external lamina of the external prepuce (sheath) is exposed when the penis is not extended.

The external prepuce of the stallion is similar to the entire prepuce of other domestic species; however, its internal lamina does not attach directly to the penis of the stallion, but continues as the internal prepuce, also with external and internal laminae that meet at a second orifice, the preputial ring. The internal prepuce separates the preputial cavity into 2 separate compartments, the external and internal preputial cavities (Fig 2). The internal lamina of the internal prepuce reflects onto the body of the penis at the fornix of the internal preputial cavity.

Semen

Semen is a composite of spermatozoa and secretions from the testes, excurrent duct system and accessory genital glands. Upon ejaculation, semen usually is contaminated with exfoliated epithelial cells and bacteria from the distal urethra and exterior of the penis. The liquid fraction of semen, termed seminal plasma, makes up the majority of seminal volume in an ejaculate. Though seminal plasma is known to consist of a number of physiologically active substances, its role in the fertilization process remains unclear, except as a vehicle for sperm transport to the female during coitus.

Spermatozoa are streamlined, highly specialized cells equipped to locate, fuse with and penetrate an oocyte at fertilization (Figs 27, 28).[35] The sperm head is an ovoid, elongated

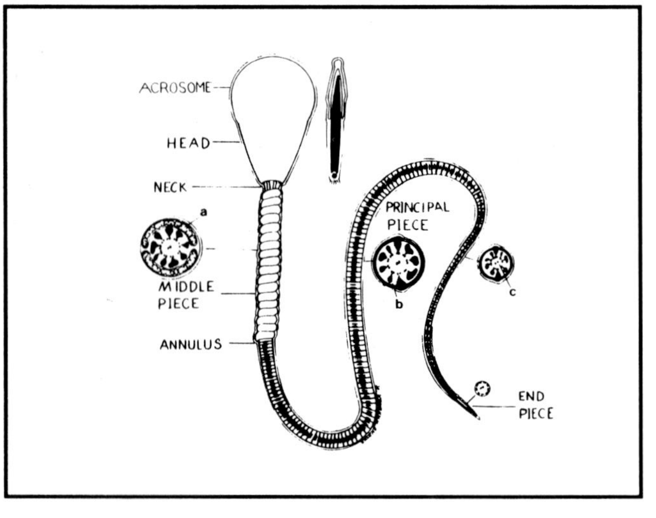

Figure 27. Anatomy of an equine spermatozoan: a. mitochondrial sheath, b. outer dense fibers, c. microtubules of the axoneme.

structure that is tapered dorsoventrally and composed primarily of a nucleus and overlying acrosomal cap. The nucleus contains a haploid complement of genetic material that unites with its female counterpart at fertilization to form a zygote. The acrosome, which is situated over the cranial aspect of the sperm nucleus like a bathing cap, is a specialized lysosome that contains enzymes considered necessary for penetration of the vestments of an egg at fertilization. These acrosomal contents are released from the acrosome's interior during the "acrosome reaction," elicited within the female reproductive tract. The tail (flagellum) of the spermatozoan connects to the head by a small neck, and is divided into a middle piece (or midpiece), principal piece and endpiece. The middle piece is composed of a core (consisting of an assembly of 9 microtubular doublets and a central pair of microtubules surrounded by 9 dense fibers) and an enveloping mitochondrial sheath (Figs 27, 28). The mitochondria supply the energy required for cellular processes, including initiation and maintenance of spermatozoal motility. The microtubular assembly and overlying fibrous sheath continue distally in the tail as the principal piece. The sliding microtubules and elastic properties of the fibrous sheath permit the characteristic pattern of tail beating required to propel the sperm through a viscous medium. Oyster spermatozoa, which need to swim only in sea water, do not have dense fibers in their flagellum. A spermatozoon is enclosed by a single plasma membrane.

The average volume of an ejaculate is 60-70 ml, but a considerable range (20-250 ml) is possible. Ejaculate volume is affected by several factors, including individual variation, frequency of ejaculation, intensity and length of precopulatory sexual stimulation, and season of the year. Spermatozoal concentration in ejaculated semen averages 120-180 million sperm/ml but is also subject to a large range of values (20-600 million sperm/ml). Spermatozoal concentration is inversely proportional to ejaculate volume; therefore, if a large seminal volume is encouraged through excessive sexual stimulation before copulation, spermatozoal concentration is decreased accordingly. The pH of ejaculated stallion semen normally ranges from 7.2 to 7.7 and is affected by frequency of ejaculation and season, increasing with successive ejaculates and during the nonbreeding season.[36,37]

Ejaculated semen is discharged from the penis in 5-10 successive "jets" that coincide with rhythmic contractions of the urethral and penile musculature. The composition of successive seminal jets is not constant; rather, the various contributions to semen are voided in sequence.[38] The first fraction emitted is clear and virtually sperm-free. This "presperm" fraction of an ejaculate originates from the urethral and/or bulbourethral glands. It is not discharged forcefully from the urethra, so it is not considered part of the seminal jets. Following are the seminal jets, beginning with a "sperm-rich" fraction that contains a high concentration of spermatozoa contained primarily in prostatic and ampullar secretions. The latter part of the ejaculate contains a "sperm-poor" fraction, which consists of a low con-

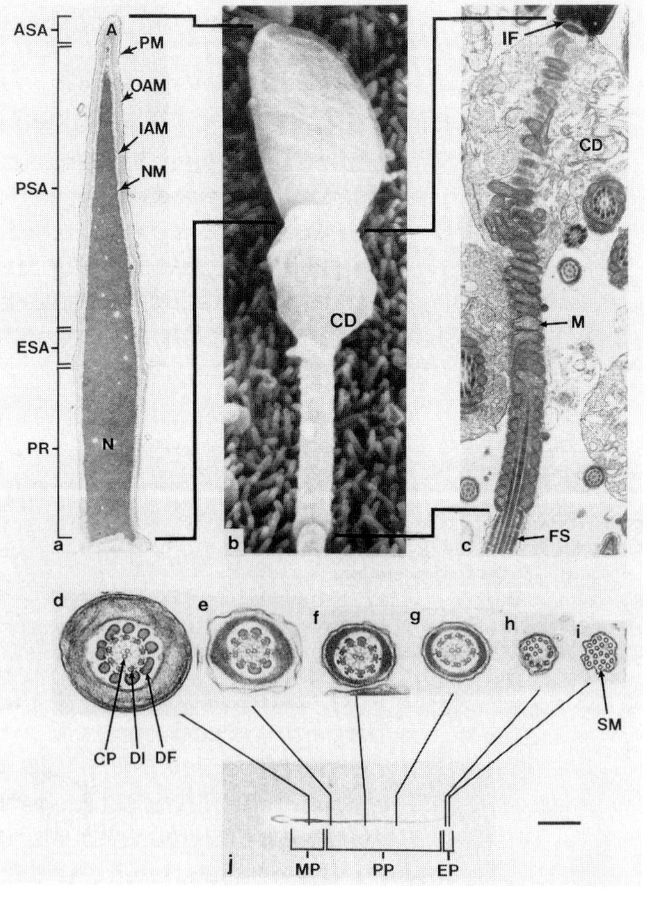

Figure 28. Composite of (a,c-i) transmission electron, (b) scanning electron, and (j) phase contrast micrographs of equine spermatozoa.[25,31,72] Attaching lines between (a) and (b) or (b) and (c) and between (d-i) and (j) reveal corresponding regions of the spermatozoa. a. The plasma membrane (PM) encloses the entire head and tail. The head is composed of the nucleus (N), overlying acrosome (A) and postacrosomal region (PR). The acrosome can be divided into the apical segment (ASA), principal segment (PSA) and equatorial segment (ESA). The inner acrosomal membrane (IAM) is in juxtaposition with the nuclear membrane (NM). The outer acrosomal membrane (OAM) fuses with the plasma membrane to discharge the acrosomal contents during the acrosome reaction. j. The tail is composed of the middle piece (MP), principal piece (PP) and end piece (EP). c. The tail attaches at the implantation fossa (IF), and contains mitochondria (M) in the middle piece and the fibrous sheath (FS) in the principal piece. d-i. The distal centriole is continuous with the outer 9 doublet microtubules (DI) of the axoneme, which also has the characteristic central pair (CP) of microtubules. The 9 dense fibers (DF) parallel the axoneme and extend to different lengths of the principal piece. In the end piece, the axonemal doublets become disorganized and ultimately separate into 20 single microtubules (SM), but they still are enclosed in the plasma membrane. The cytoplasmic droplet (CD) located at the proximal end of the middle piece of this spermatozoan from the equine efferent ducts is characteristic of spermatozoa that have not yet matured in the epididymis. Bar lengths equal 0.5 μ (a), 0.5 μ (b), 0.75 μ (c), 0.24 μ (d-i) and 1.28 μ (j).

centration of sperm suspended in secretions predominantly from the vesicular glands. A "tail-end" portion sometimes follows the "sperm-poor" fraction and contains little to no sperm and only scant secretions from the ampullae and vesicular glands. The first 3 jets of the sperm-rich fraction generally contain 75-80% of the spermatozoa in an ejaculate.

Reproductive Physiology

Testicular Descent

The testes develop embryologically in a retroperitoneal position near the caudal pole of the kidneys, then traverse the abdominal cavity with their attached epididymides, and descend through the inguinal canal to reach a final position within the scrotum by late fetal or early postnatal life (between 300 days of gestation and 10 days after birth, Fig 29). The mechanism controlling testicular descent is not well understood, but gonadotropin-induced androgen production by the developing testes plays a major role in the process.[40-44]

In male equine fetuses, the gonads differentiate into testes at approximately day 40 of gestation.[39] Transabdominal passage of the testes and attached epididymides to the inguinal rings is achieved via "traction" by the gubernaculum, a cord-like mesenchymal structure that anchors the caudal pole of each testis

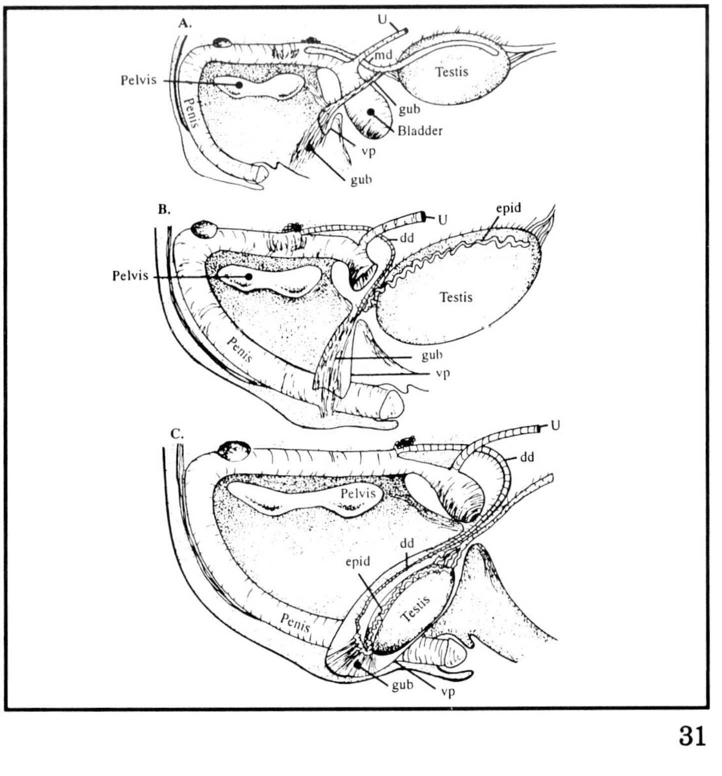

Figure 29. Stages of testicular descent into the scrotum of the horse fetus.[39] A. Fetus at 75 days of gestation, B. Fetus at 175 days of gestation, C. Fetus near term (330 days of gestation). Urethra (U), gubernaculum (gub), epididymis (epid), deferent duct (dd) and vaginal process (vp).

to the inguinal area. The gubernaculum actually consists of 2 distinct parts: an intraabdominal segment (or cord) that extends from the peritoneum overlying the eventual inguinal canal to the caudal pole of each testis; and an extraabdominal segment (or bulb) located outside the peritoneal cavity, coursing from the opening of each inguinal canal to the scrotum. Fibrous strands connect the distal tip of the gubernacular bulb to the wall of the developing scrotum.

Swelling of the extraabdominal portion of the gubernaculum and differential growth between the body and gubernaculum pull the intraabdominal portion of the gubernaculum, and attached gonad, toward the inguinal area. Inguinal passage of each testis/epididymis is preceded by formation of the vaginal process, an evagination of the parietal peritoneum that extends into the extraabdominal part of the gubernaculum. Elongation of the vaginal process, continued expansion of the extraabdominal gubernaculum, and intraabdominal pressure probably act collectively to mechanically pull/push each testis and attached epididymis through the inguinal canal and into a scrotal position.[45-47] The gubernaculum then gradually regresses to permit full development of the testes within the scrotum. The gubernaculum can be mistaken for a testis when palpating the scrotal contents of a newborn foal. A portion of the gubernaculum remains palpable in adult life as a small dense fibrous band called the scrotal ligament.

The fetal gonads (either testes or ovaries) become unusually large during gestation. They grow rapidly between days 100 and 200 (to 30-50g) to become larger than the gonads of the dam, then begin to decrease in size after day 250, such that their weight at birth is only about 10% of their maximal weight during gestation.[48] Inguinal passage of the testes does not begin until about 270-300 days of gestation, after the testes begin to diminish in size.[39] The vaginal ring constricts soon after birth. After this occurs it is very unlikely that an abdominal testis would subsequently descend into a scrotal position.[49] Though considered abnormal, descent of inguinal testes into the scrotum has been observed at up to 2-3 years of age in stallions.

Estrogen given to pregnant rats caused cryptorchidism in male progeny by preventing reduction in testicular size.[50] The effect was reversed when both human chorionic gonadotropin (HCG) and estrogen were given to pregnant rats at the same time. The gonadotropic effect may be mediated via secretion of testosterone, as testosterone alone causes testicular descent in immature monkeys and even causes descent of wax pellets substituted for testicles in rats.[51]

Puberty

Puberty in the male is the age when a it can first impregnate a female. Sexual desire, ability to copulate and presence of viable spermatozoa in the ejaculate are required to accomplish this feat. In experimental studies involving larger domestic animals (*eg,* horses, cattle, sheep, pigs), puberty in males has been defined, practically, as the age at which an ejaculate first contains 50 million spermatozoa, of which ≥10% are progressively motile.[10,52,53]

Age at puberty in stallions ranges from 12 to 24 months; breed, nutritional plane and season of birth may influence this process.[53-56] Rapid testicular growth and development of secondary sex characteristics are the most easily recognizable traits of the peripubertal period.

Puberty represents the culmination of a series of reproductive events initiated in early postnatal life. These events are under endocrine control, and the hypothalamus (gonadotropin-releasing hormone, GnRH) appears to be the principal mediator, with possible modulation by the testis.[10-57] In Quarter Horse colts, secretion of gonadotropins (follicle-stimulating hormone, FSH; luteinizing hormone, LH) is minimal during the first 8-10 months of life. A brief rise in gonadotropin secretion (lasting approximately 1 month) is followed by a decline, then a resurgence in the late prepubertal period.[23,53,58] In bulls and rams, the rise in plasma LH concentration is a result of increased frequency and amplitude of LH discharges from the pituitary gland.[59,60] Pulsatile release patterns of LH have not been investigated in peripubertal stallions, but a similar phenomenon is thought to occur. Increased secretion of LH stimulates differentiation of Leydig cells, followed by testicular production of testosterone, maturation of Sertoli cells, and initiation of spermatogenesis.[10]

Puberty in stallions should not be confused with sexual maturity, as spermatogenic potential and size of the testes continue to increase after puberty is attained. Efficiency of spermatogenesis (determined by daily spermatozoal production per gram of testicular parenchyma) reaches adult levels by 2.5-3 years of age, whereas daily spermatozoal production per testis and testicular weight continue to increase until 4-5 years of age.[3,23]

Spermatogenesis

Briefly, spermatogenesis is the series of germ-cell divisions and transformations within the testis that result in formation of spermatozoa. More specifically, spermatogenesis is a lengthy, chronologic process by which spermatogonial cell division maintains a normal stem-cell population, and cyclically produces primary spermatocytes that divide by meiosis to produce haploid spermatids, which, in turn, differentiate into spermatozoa. The process occurs in the convoluted portion of the seminiferous tubules, which constitute most (>70%) of the testicular parenchyma.[4]

Our current understanding of spermatogenesis is based on the insight of earlier scientists. Aristotle introduced castration as a means to study reproduction. Von Leuwenhoek (1679) invented the microscope and was the first to observe spermatozoa in semen. Von Kolliker (1841) identified germ cells in the testis that gave rise to spermatozoa, while Von Leydig (1857) and Sertoli (1865) described Leydig cells and Sertoli cells, respectively. Von Lavellette (1876) classified germ cells morphologically, and Von Ebner (1871) and Benda (1887) made possible comprehension of the orderly spermatogenic process. This comprehension led to the concept of the spermatogenic cycle.[61,62]

Spermatogenesis can be divided into 3 phases (spermatocytogenesis, meiosis, spermiogenesis), each encompassing the activity of 1 of the 3 major germ cell types (spermatogonia, spermatocytes, spermatids). Important but different functions are performed during these 3 phases of spermatogenesis. During spermatocytogenesis, stem-cell spermatogonia divide by mitosis to produce other stem cells and committed spermatogonia that begin proliferation to produce primary spermatocytes. Continued production of new stem cells during spermatocytogenesis is responsible for the continued lineage of spermatozoal production throughout the adult life of males. Exchange of genetic material between homologous chromosomes of primary spermatocytes in meiosis is followed by reduction division that results in short-lived secondary spermatocytes that immediately divide to produce haploid spermatids. Spermiogenesis encompasses differentiation of spermatids with spherical nuclei to mature spermatids with elongated nuclei, and the release of spermatids as spermatozoa at spermiation. Hence, spermatogonia divide to increase spermatozoal yield; spermatocytes exchange genetic material and divide to increase spermatozoal yield and produce haploid spermatids; spermatids undergo amazing cellular differentiation to form spermatozoa.

Spermatocytogenesis lasts for about one-third of the duration of spermatogenesis. During this phase of spermatogenesis, spermatogonia mitotically divide for stem-cell renewal, cyclically produce primary spermatocytes, and initiate the next phase of spermatogenesis, meiosis.

Five different subtypes of spermatogonia have been identified in stallions (Fig 30).[63] A_1 spermatogonia represent the most immature cells and possibly the stem cells. Division of B_2 spermatogonia, produced by division of A_1 to A_2, A_2 to A_3, A_3 to B_1, and B_1 to B_2, marks the end of spermatocytogenesis, with production of primary spermatocytes. Cyclic variations in numbers of different subtypes of spermatogonia illustrate changes associated with different stages of the spermatogenic cycle (Fig 31).

Meiosis I begins with production of preleptotene primary spermatocytes from the division of B_2 spermatogonia. Meiosis II ends with division of secondary spermatocytes to produce spermatids. Primary spermatocytes in meiosis I are categorically

Figure 30. Equine spermatogonia (Spermatogonia) and spermatocytes (Spermatocytes) in 5-μ methacrylate sections.[63,72] Spermatogonial subtypes are classified by nuclear profiles, including primitive cells with a small, oval or flattened nucleus (A_1), a pale center (A_2), a single large nucleolus (A_3), 2-3 nucleoli (A_3), or large nucleoli with fragmented chromatin flakes (B_1), or a small spherical nucleus (B_2). Spermatocytes Include preleptotene (Pl), leptotene (L), zygotene (Z), early pachytene (EP), late pachytene (LP), diplotene (D: open arrow), primary speratocytes, and secondary spermatocytes (SS; closed arrow). Arrows designate cells of interest. Bar length equals 10 μ.

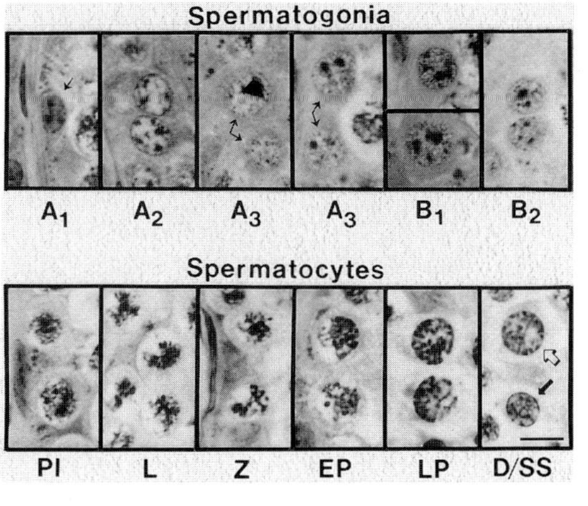

divided into phases called preleptotene, leptotene, zygotene, pachytene and diplotene (Fig 30). During these phases, chromosomes are duplicated and exchange of genetic material between paired homologous chromosomes occurs at the synaptonemal complex. Meiosis I ends with division of primary spermatocytes to produce secondary spermatocytes. Meiosis II does not include duplication of chromosomes, but does include rapid division of secondary spermatocytes to produce spermatids. One duplication of chromosomes followed by 2 divisions (one to separate paired homologous chromosomes and the second to separate sister chromatids) results in reduction of chromosomes to a haploid number. It is necessary for each of the 2 sexes to have haploid gametes to produce a diploid cell at fertilization.

Spermiogenesis, which follows meiosis, is the final phase of spermatogenesis. Spermiogenesis consists of the remarkable morphologic transformation from spherical spermatids with spherical nuclei to streamlined flagellum-equipped spermatozoa with a condensed elongated head and overlying acrosomal cap. Based largely on development of the acrosome, spermatid development can be divided into 4 phases of spermiogenesis (Golgi, cap, acrosomal and maturation phases). Sequential differentiation of spermatids during the various phases of spermiogenesis is illustrated by phase contrast microscopy (Fig 32) and transmission electron microscopy (Fig 33).

Figure 31. Effect of stage of the spermatogenic cycle on numbers of various subtypes of spermatogonia per 100 Sertoli cells.[63]

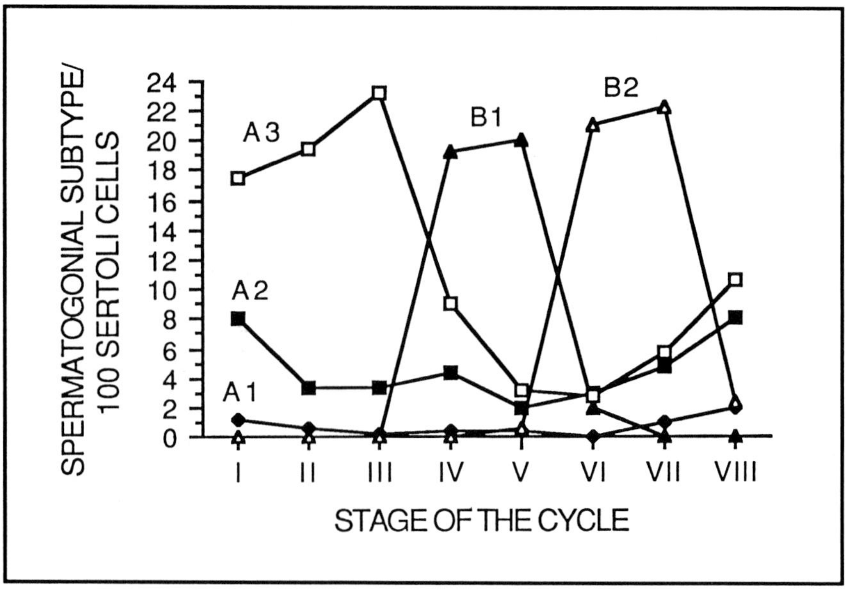

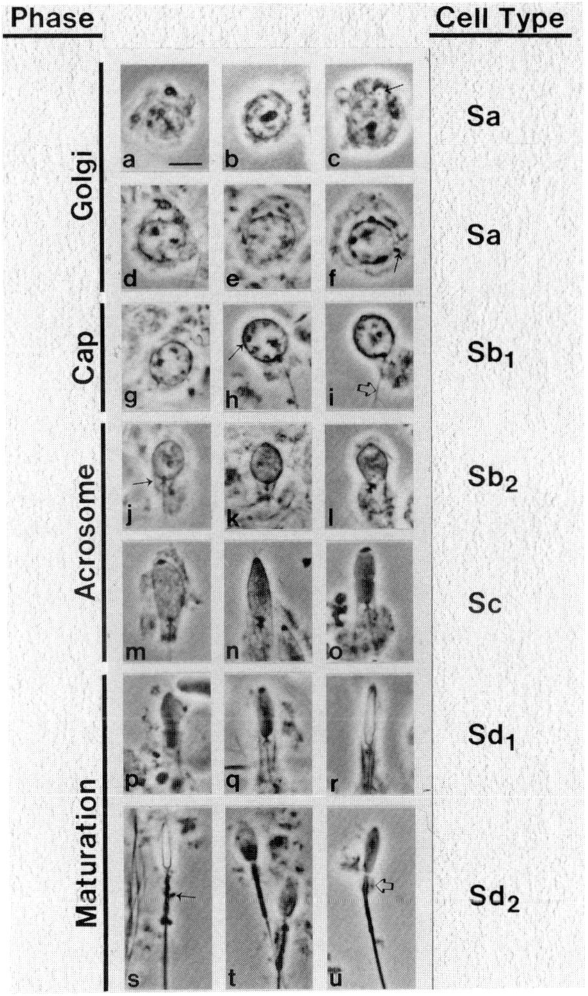

Figure 32. Phase contrast micrographs of different types of spermatids in testicular homogenates revealing different steps of development during spermiogenesis.[3,72] a-c. Nuclei of the newly formed Sa spermatids (Sa) are spherical and contain coarse and fine granules. a-f. Nuclei of early spermatids, like nuclei of all spermatids with spherical nuclei, are the smallest germinal-cell nuclei. Early spermatids may be characterized by a large, single centrally located nucleolus and lack of an acrosomal structure. c. However, later, the acrosomal vesicle with its granule (arrow) appears in the cytoplasm. d-f. Spherical nuclei of more developed spermatids reveal further signs of acrosomal development with the spherical acrosomal vesicle and granule present (d) or the flattened acrosomal vesicle attached to the nucleus (e). Formation and extension of the acrosomal cap over the nucleus and the first appearance of a distinct flagellum (arrow) attached to the side of the nucleus adjacent to the developing acrosome (f) characterize later development of Sa spermatids or early Sb_1 spermatids (Sb_1). g-i. The latest spermatids with spherical nuclei have acrosomal caps (arrow) and developing flagella (open arrow). Nuclei of these Sb_1 spermatids are essentially spherical. j-l. Nuclei of spermatids undergoing elongation are characterized by the first appearance of the manchette (arrow), which extends from the middle of the nucleus to a short distance down the flagellum. The developing flagellum with a distinct annulus just below the connection of the head with the nucleus characterizes Sb_2 spermatids (Sb_2). m-o. Nuclei of Sc spermatids (Sc) develop further by elongation without distinct chromatin condensation. The manchette extends further down the developing flagellum, and the dense acrosomal granule is still concentrated at the cranial tip of the nucleus. p-r. The manchette of the early Sd_1 spermatid (Sd_1) now encloses only about one-fourth of the nucleus and extends down the developing flagellum. The manchette is removed during Sd_1 spermatid development, and the nucleus has undergone condensation to take the shape of a typical equine spermatozoan. s-u. Sd_2 spermatids (Sd_2) have undergone further chromatin condensation and flagellar development. The annulus has migrated to its most distal location, and mitochondria (arrow) have surrounded the middle piece from the nucleus to the annulus. u. The cytoplasmic droplet (open arrow) located at the proximal position, next to where the flagellum attaches to the head, can be seen on flagella of the most advanced Sd_2 spermatids. Sa spermatids are classified as Golgi phase (Golgi), Sb_1 as cap phase (Cap), Sb_2 and Sc as acrosome phase (Acrosome), and Sd_1 and Sd_2 as maturation phase (Maturation). Bar length is 5 μ.

Figure 33. Transmission electron micrographs of equine spermatids representing different steps of development during spermiogenesis.[72] a-d. The Sa spermatid (sa) is characterized by a large Golgi apparatus (GA). These vesicles (V) fuse to form larger vesicles and ultimately to form the acrosomal vesicle (AV). The acrosomal vesicle indents the nuclear envelope and then flattens over the nucleus (arrows) (d). b. Developing flagella (F) from neighboring Sa spermatids extend away from the spermatid cell body into the extracellular space. Intercellular bridges (IB) connect adjacent spermatids. e. In the Sb_1 spermatids (Sb_1), the acrosome has formed a head cap over the nucleus (arrow). f. In the Sb_2 spermatids (Sb_2), the appearance of the manchette (Mn) coincides with the beginning of nuclear elongation. g,h. The Sc spermatid (Sc) has a distinct manchette (Mn), an elongating and condensing nucleus, an attached flagellum with a distinct annulus (AN), and a well-defined acrosome (A) over the cranial portion of the nucleus. i-j. The Sd_1 and Sd_2 spermatids have further condensation of their nuclei. The flagellum begins in the early Sa spermatid (b) and appears as a growing axoneme in Sb_1, Sb_2 (not shown), and Sc spermatids (g,h). i. The late Sd_1 spermatid is characterized by dense fibers (DF), a completed fibrous sheath (FS), and mitochondrial (M) migration around the flagellum. Before mitochondrial migration in the Sd_1 spermatid, the manchette is removed and the annulus (An) migrates to its permanent position at the distal end of the middle piece. Note the abaxial (off center of the head) attachment of the flagellum. j. The late Sd_2 spermatid is mostly extended into the tubular lumen (TL) and has complete migration of mitochondria (M) around the middle piece. Excess cytoplasm of the spermatid remains in the proximal region of the middle piece as a cytoplasmic droplet (CD). Bar length equals 2 μ.

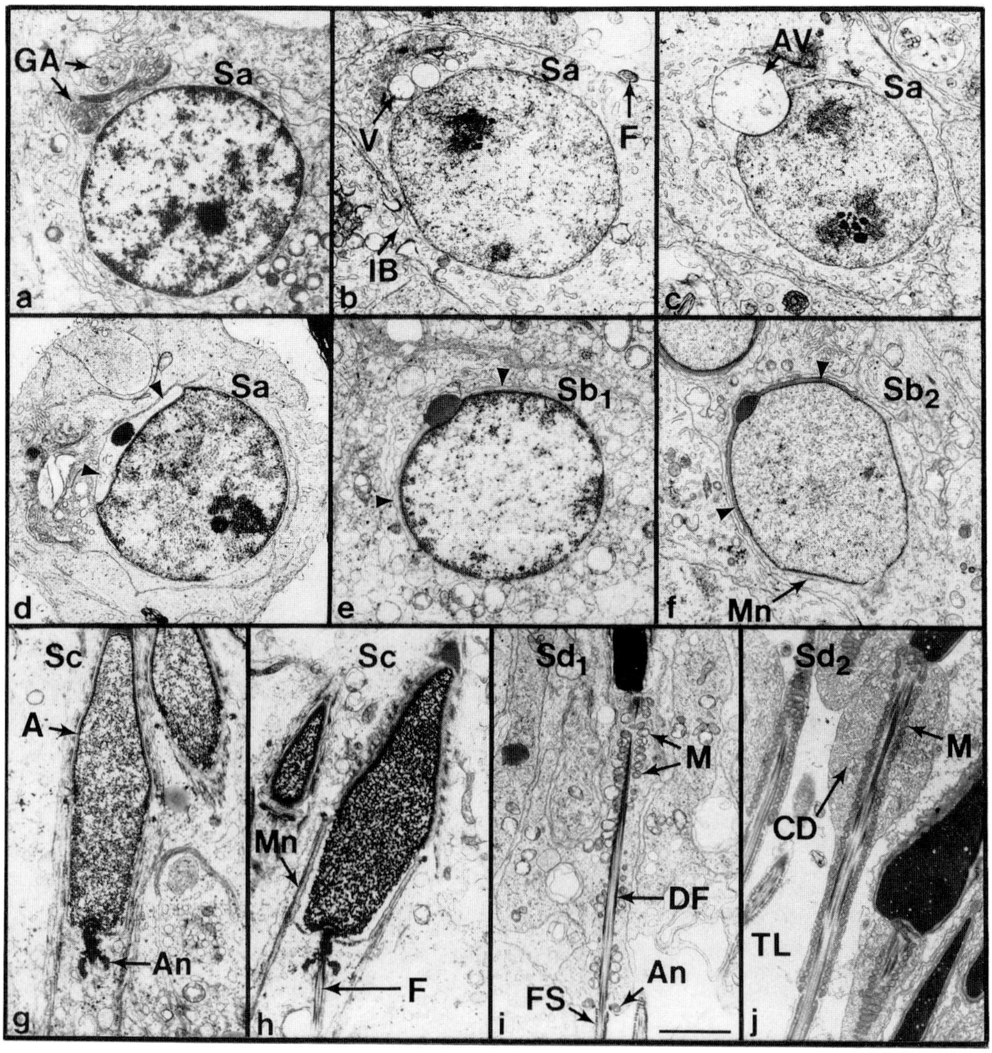

The Golgi apparatus of the newly formed Sa spermatids gives rise to the acrosome by producing enzyme-containing vesicles that fuse to form the acrosomal vesicle (Figs 32, 33). The vesicle flattens over the nucleus and forms the head cap of cap-phase Sb_1 spermatids. When the nuclei of Sb_1 spermatids elongate, they differentiate to Sb_2 spermatids of the acrosomal phase. Sc spermatids, also in the acrosomal phase, have further elongation of the nucleus with obvious chromatin condensation. The maturation phase (involving Sd_1 and Sd_2 spermatids) is the final phase of spermatid development. The dense fibers and fibrous sheath are produced, mitochondria move around the developing tail, nuclear condensation is completed, excess cytoplasm is removed, and spermiation occurs. The end product is a spermatozoon with a cytoplasmic droplet located in the proximal position of the middle piece, characteristic of spermatozoa in the rete testis, efferent ducts and caput epididymidis (Fig 33).

Superimposed on the 3 major phases of spermatogenesis (spermatocytogenesis, meiosis, spermiogenesis) is the spermatogenic cycle (Figs 34-36). The spermatogenic cycle, also called the cycle of the seminiferous epithelium, is "a series of changes in a given area (region) of seminiferous epithelium between 2 appearances of the same developmental stages."[64] In other words, the seminiferous cycle comprises all of the events that occur between 2 consecutive spermiations (release of spermatozoa) in a given region of the seminiferous epithelium. The cycle length (12.2 days in the stallion) is the time between 2 consecutive spermiations and is a fraction of the duration of spermatogenesis from newly formed, committed spermatogonia to spermiation (57 days in the stallion).[65] This results in multiple generations of germ cells (1-2 groups of spermatogonia, spermatocytes, spermatids) in the same region of the seminiferous tubule, producing a stratified epithelium composed of germ cells from sequential generations and Sertoli cells. The difference in developmental age between consecutive generations is one cycle length or 12.2 days in the horse. In a typical region of the seminiferous epithelium, multiple generations grouped together may consist of A_2 and B_2 spermatogonia, pachytene primary spermatocytes, Sa spermatids and Sd_2 spermatids whose developmental ages are 8.2, 20.4, 32.6, 44.8 and 57.0 days, respectively. This combination constitutes stage VII of the equine spermatogenic cycle.[72]

A stage of the spermatogenic cycle is defined as an association of 4 or 5 generations of germ cells in specific, chronologic developmental steps that differ in developmental age by a multiple of the cycle length plus a constant.[63,66] Germ-cell division and degeneration, and rate of new germ cells entering the process of spermatogenesis influence spermatozoal production. Given the number of cell divisions (mitosis and meiosis) that occur, each committed spermatogonium has the potential of producing 64 spermatozoa. However, germ-cell degeneration prevents this optimal yield of 64 spermatozoa per spermatogonium.

Age and season influence the rate of germ-cell degeneration and the specific types of germ cells that degenerate.[63,67] The interval between consecutive entry of committed spermatogonia into a given region determines the cycle length. However, production of newly produced, committed spermatogonia is not synchronized among tubules and not simultaneous along the length of the same tubule.

At each second, and in seminiferous epithelium somewhere in the testis, newly committed spermatogonia are entering into the process of spermatogenesis. Resulting from continued entry of spermatogonia into spermatogenesis, spermatozoa are continuously released. Continual release of spermatozoa helps ensure that male gametes will be available when needed to fertilize female gametes.

The spermatogenic cycle has been arbitrarily divided into groupings of the naturally occurring and continuously changing cellular associations or stages in a given region of the seminiferous tubule. In the stallion, 8 stages of the spermatogenic cycle have been defined (Figs 34-36).[65,68] Classification of stages of the spermatogenic cycle is based on the presence and location of specific germ cells and changes associated with acrosome development, nuclear elongation, location and release of spermatids.[64,69]

The frequency of appearance of individual stages (*ie,* number of tubules in a given stage/total tubules counted in all stages) is indicative of the duration of those stages. The duration of a given spermatogenic stage is calculated by multiplying the frequency times the cycle length for a given species. Stage frequency is similar for the same species, but different among species. The duration of different phases of spermiogenesis differs among species.[70]

The frequency of individual stages within a cross section of a seminiferous tubule indicates the size of the region occupied by that individual stage within the tubule. In the equine seminiferous tubule, more than one stage may be represented in a tubular cross section (Fig 35).[71]

The horse has a spermatogenic wave. The wave is a spatial, sequential order of stages along the tubular length at a given time (Fig 37), and results from a synchronized but a nonsimultaneous production of newly committed spermatogonia in adjacent tubular segments along the tubular length.[68] The function of the spermatogenic wave may be to: ensure continual release of spermatozoa; reduce competition among stages for hormones and metabolites; reduce congestion in tubular lumen by release of spermatozoa at different regions along the tubular length; ensure a constant flow of tubular fluid (needed to move and nurture spermatozoa and hormones for epididymal epithelium); and facilitate spermatozoal maturation in the epididymis by a constant entry of spermatozoa into the epididymis.[72]

Figure 34. Eight stages of the equine spermatogenic cycle observed by Nomarski optics in 20-μ Epon sections.[68] Structures identified include stage of the cycle (I-VIII), spermatogonia (B, AS), primary spermatocytes (Pl, L, Z, P), secondary spermatocytes (SS), spermatids (Sa, Sb_1, Sc, Sd_1, Sd_2), Sertoli cells (SC), myoid cells (MC), Leydig cells (LC), a newly developing flagellum (F), the annulus (An), manchette (Mn), meiotic figures (MF), cytoplasmic droplet (CD), middle piece (MP), residual body (RB), acrosomal granule (AG), acrosomal cap (AC), group of mitochondria (GM), Golgi apparatus (GA), chromatoid body (CB), and acrosomal vesicle (AV). Bar length equals 10 μ.

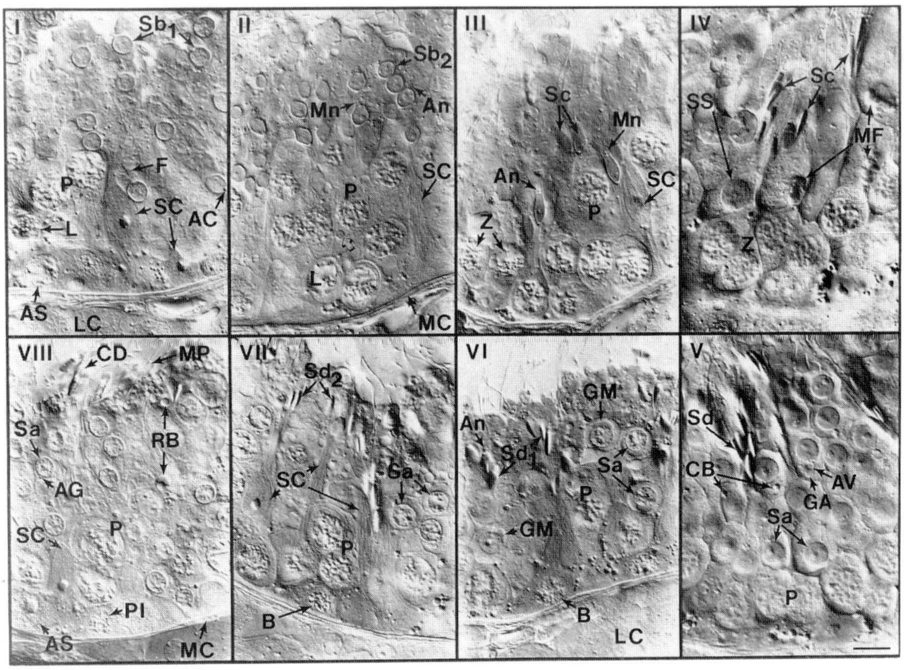

Figure 35. Bright-field light (a,c,e) and scanning electron (b,d,f) micrographs of different stages of the equine spermatogenic cycle.[71] a,b. Stages I and II are illustrated. c,d. Stages III, IV and V are represented. e,f. Stages VI and VII reveal changes in preparation of the release of spermatozoa in Stage VIII. Bar length equals 20 μ.

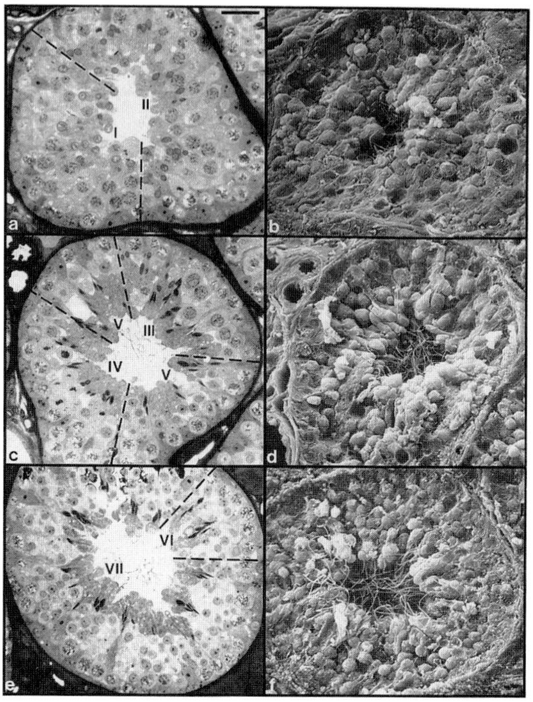

Figure 36. Scanning electron micrograph of stage-VII (a), early stage-VIII (b) and late stage-VIII tubules (c,d).[71] Spermatid tails project into the lumen in stages VII and VIII, but the entire spermatid projects in the lumen in late stage VIII, attached only by cytoplasmic stalks (CS). c,d. An enlarged luminal view of (c) is seen in (d). Maturation-phase spermatids are located in the lumen; however, tails (T) of Sa spermatids with round nuclei already project into the lumen. One luminal spermatozoan, recently released, has its characteristic cytoplasmic droplet (CD) in the proximal position where the middle piece attaches to the head. Bar lengths equal 10 μ (a,c), 5 μ (b) and 2.6 μ (d).

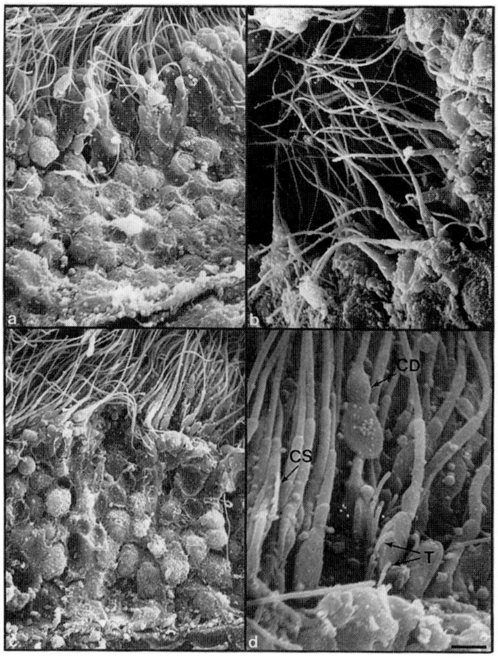

Stage-specific changes in the seminiferous epithelium has been revealed by the spermatogenic wave.[73] Stage-specific differences include preference for FSH and androgen, production of androgen-binding protein, and maximal secretion of plasminogen activator and meiosis-inducing substance. These studies were made possible by staging of live rat seminiferous tubules by transillumination.[74]

Equine seminiferous tubules are tightly bound by collagen and must undergo enzymatic dispersion before they can be staged.[68,75] Enzymatically isolated equine tubules can be staged successfully by transillumination, as is evident by preservation of ultrastructural features of Sertoli cells and by incorporation of ^{3}H thymidine in spermatogonia and early primary spermatocytes in isolated tubules.

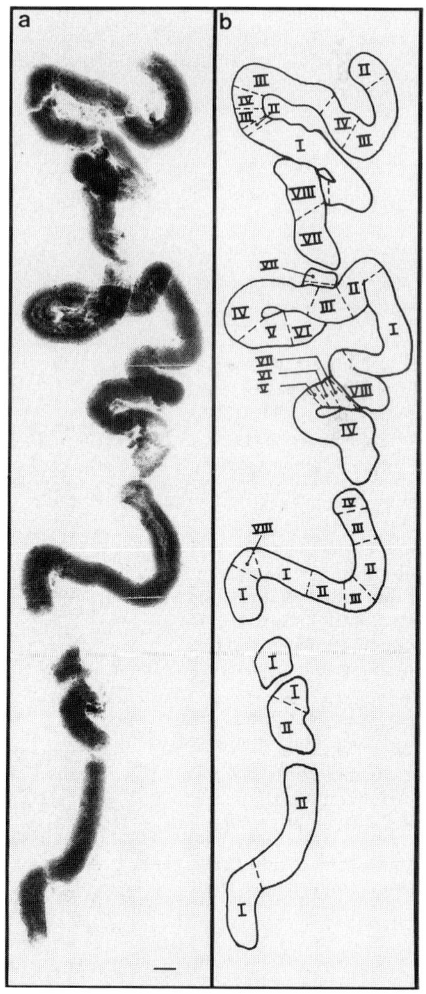

Figure 37. Spermtogenic wave in the equine seminiferous tubule revealed by a tubule mounted *in toto* (a) and observed by Nomarski optics (b).[68] The corresponding drawing (b) shows the consecutive stages (I-VIII) at the same time along the tubular length. Bar length equals 200 μ.

Throughout spermatogenesis, germ cells degenerate and reduce the yield of spermatozoa production.[72] In horses, the numerous different types of A spermatogonia per 100 Sertoli cells (Fig 31) indicate that divisions of subtypes of spermatogonia are not efficient.[63] However, there are seasonal differences in equine spermatogenesis. The 2-fold increase in numbers of type-A spermatogonia in the breeding season that results from a seasonal increase in yield of type-A_2 spermatogonial population is sufficient to override this degeneration.[67] In fact, the large number of type-B spermatogonia that degenerate in the breeding season is likely caused by overpopulation of type-A spermatogonia. This supports the notion that germ-cell degeneration may exist to reduce the number of spermatogonial progeny to that which can be sustained by the available Sertoli-cell population.[72]

There is a seasonal variation in the number of various types of germ cells that can be accommodated by a given Sertoli cell (Table 3).[77] Given that the number of type-A spermatogonia is doubled in the summer as compared to winter and there is no degeneration of type-B spermatogonia, each Sertoli cell would have to accommodate 44 instead of the typical 28 germ cells.[67]

Table 3. Effect of season on the volume density of Sertoli-cell nuclei, average volume of an individual Sertoli-cell nucleus, number of Sertoli cells and Sertoli cell:germ cell ratios.[22,27]

	Season		
	Nonbreeding	Breeding	% Increase in Breeding Season
Parenchymal volume (ml)	103.2 ± 7.6	144.1 ± 8.4	40[a]
Sertoli cell nuclei			
Volume density (%)	1.60 ± 0.08	1.77 ± 0.09	11
Volume in parenchyma (ml)	1.59 ± 0.12	2.59 ± 0.24	63[a]
Mean maximum diameter (μ)	11.8 ± 0.3	12.2 ± 0.2	3
Averaged volume (fl)	678 ± 71	693 ± 38	2
Number of Sertoli cells/g (10^6)	22.8 ± 1.2	24 ± 1.5	5
Number of Sertoli cells/testis (10^9)	2.37 ± 0.18	3.68 ± 0.34	55a
Number of germ cells accommodated by a single Sertoli cell in Stage VIII			
Type A spermatogonia	1.1 ± 0.1	1.5 ± 0.1	36[a]
Preleptotene and leptotene plus zygotene primary spermatocytes	2.9 ± 0.4	2.9 ± 0.2	0
Pachytene plus diplotene primary spermatocytes	2.6 ± 0.2	3 ± 0.2	15
Spermatids with round nuclei	8.1 ± 0.8	10.9 ± 0.8	35[b]
Spermatids with elongated nuclei	8 ± 0.8	10.2 ± 0.7	28[b]
All germ cell types combined	22.8 ± 2.1	28.5 ± 1.7	25[b]

a – Difference is significant at P <0.01.
b – Difference is significant at P <0.05.

This would be difficult with the restraints of limited testicular size, differences between season, and size of the seminiferous tubules.

Spermatogenesis in stallions is established over a long period (about 4 years) (Figs 38, 39). There is a large variation among horses regarding the age at which development is established. Before birth, primordial germ cells in the early embryo migrate from the yolk sac into the undifferentiated fetal gonads. The primordial germ cells divide several times to produce gonocytes found in the fetal male sex cords, along with darker-staining undifferentiated supporting cells that eventually differentiate into Sertoli cells. Before puberty, gonocytes divide and differentiate to yield spermatogonia. In colts as young as 12 months of age, gonocytes may have differentiated already to spermatogonia and some primary spermatocytes, while pre-Sertoli cells may have differentiated to Sertoli cells, revealing tubules associated with the formation of the tubular lumen. Spermatids with round

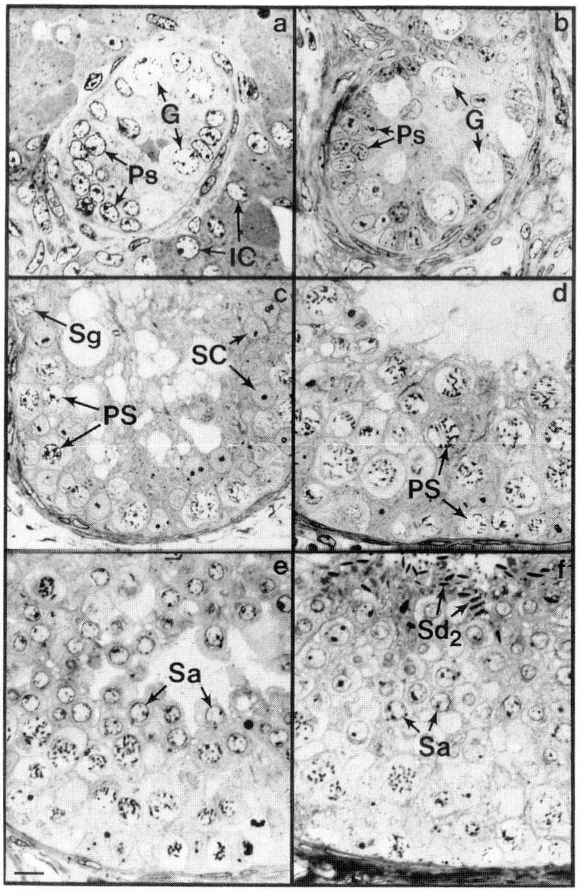

Figure 38. Establishment of spermatogenesis.[23,63,72] Steps in development of spermatogenesis from 270 days of gestation (a) through 10-12 months (b,c) and 16 months (d,e) to 36 months of age (f). a. Fetal male sex cords, scarce among a high density of robust interstitial cells (IC), are composed of darker-staining support cells or pre-Sertoli cells (Ps) and lighter-staining gonocytes. b. The seminiferous tubules at 10-12 months are similar to the fetal sex cords containing gonocytes (G); however, some nuclear maturation can be seen in pre-Sertoli cells with a larger number of pre-Sertoli cells located in the center of the tubule. c. Other 10- to 12-month-old colts exhibit considerable maturation of Sertoli cells (SC) whose apical regions extend toward the forming lumen. Gonocytes have matured into spermatogonia (Sg), and some primary spermatocytes (PS) are present. d. By 16 months, 2 generations of primary spermatocytes are present, and the lumen is completely formed. e. Also at 16 months, some seminferous tubules contain Sa spermatids with spherical nuclei (Sa) as the most advanced cell type. f. By 36 months, spermatogenesis has been completed, as is evident by numerous Sa (Sa) and Sd_2 (Sd_2) spermatids. Variation in the most advanced cell type present in the seminiferous epithelium exists among tubules of the same testis and among horses. Bar length equals 10 μ.

nuclei may be seen by 16 months and mature spermatids by 36 months (Fig 38). There is significant variation among stallions in the time when given germ cells appear.[23]

Establishment of spermatogenesis is associated with a large amount of germ-cell degeneration. However, once spermatogenesis is complete, the adult level of efficiency of spermatogenesis is reached before total production per testis has been reached (Fig 39).[23] Sexual maturation, has been measured by testicular weight, daily sperm production (DSP), number of Sertoli cells, number of elongated spermatids per Sertoli cell and serum hormonal concentrations. While adult values for the percentage of tubules containing spermatids with round nuclei or elongated nuclei, DSP/g and DSP/horse were statistically obtained by 3

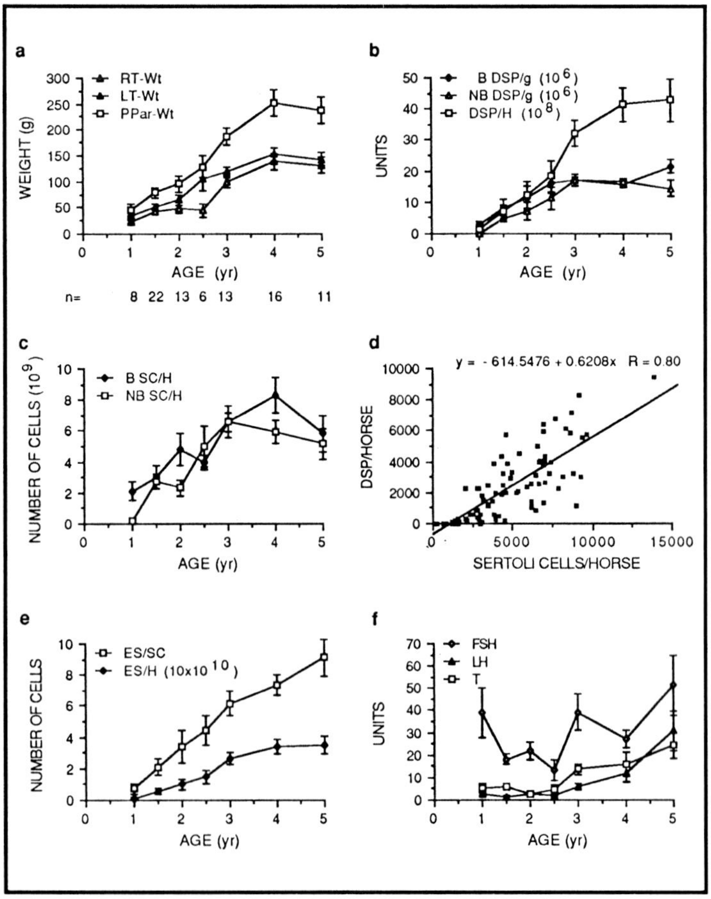

Figure 39. Sexual maturation measured by testicular weight, number of Sertoli cells, spermatids with elongated nuclei per Sertoli cell, daily sperm production (DSP), and serum hormonal concentration.[23] a. Number (n) of horses in each age group is indicated. Left testis weight (LT-Wt), right testis weight (RT-Wt) and paired parenchymal weight (PPar-Wt) increased ($P<0.01$) with sexual development. b. DSP/g testicular parenchyma in the summer (B DSP/g) and winter or nonbreeding season (NB DSP/g) and DSP per horse (DSP/H) increased ($P<0.01$) with age and reached adult levels by year 3. c. Sertoli-cell number per horse in the breeding season (B SC/H) or nonbreeding season (NB SC/H) increased with age to adult levels at 3 years of age. d. Though spermatogenesis was not complete in some younger horses, there was a significant relationship between the number of Sertoli cells per horse and DSP per horse. e. The number of elongated spermatids per horse (ES/H) increased to year 3 or 4, but the number of elongated spermatids per Sertoli cell (ES/SC) reached adult levels at 4 years with continued increase to year 5. f. Serum concentrations of follicle-stimulating hormone (FSH; pg/ml), luteinizing hormone (LH; ng/ml) and testosterone (T; 10 x pg/ml) were increased by age of maturation.

years of age, paired parenchymal weight increased to 4 years of age and serum hormonal concentrations increased to 5 years of age. In addition, DSP/horse tended to increase until 4 years of age.[77] Establishment of spermatogenesis is associated with increased numbers and volume of Leydig cells, Sertoli-cell numbers and germ cell:Sertoli cell ratio (Fig 39).[3,4,77-79]

Age and season influence testicular and hormone characteristics (Tables 1-3). Table 1 presents a composite of 2 studies on the effect of age on various testicular and hormonal characteristics. Tables 2 and 3 are a composite of studies using the same or similarly aged horses to illustrate the effect of season on hormones and various testicular characteristics in adult (4-20 years old) stallions. In horses aged 4-20 years, season appears to have a greater influence than does age.[72]

Thermoregulation of the Testis

The testes and epididymides of domestic mammals require a temperature below that of normal core body temperature to function properly. Elevated temperature in this portion of the reproductive tract impairs spermatogenesis and sperm-fertilizing capability. The combined actions of the scrotum, pampiniform plexus and cremaster muscle regulate gonadal temperature to provide a suitable environment for spermatozoal production.

The scrotum allows the testes and epididymides to assume a position outside the body proper. The scrotal wall is thin walled, with very little fat, and contains numerous sweat glands that help lower the temperature of its contents through evaporation of moisture. Temperature receptors also may be present in the scrotal skin and influence general body thermoregulatory mechanisms. In addition, the tunica dartos muscle in the wall of the scrotum relaxes in warm weather to produce a more pendulous scrotum and thereby provides more surface area for evaporative cooling.

The pampiniform plexus is formed by the testicular vein that leaves each testis and then divides to form many intercommunicating vessels that, in turn, intertwine with the highly coiled testicular artery en route to the testes. The temperature of blood in the superficial branches of the testicular vein is lower than body temperature because of the loss of heat by evaporation. The cooled venous blood enters the pampiniform plexus, which then serves as a countercurrent heat-exchange area. As the pampiniform plexus and testicular artery intertwine, heat is transferred from the warm testicular artery to the cooler pampiniform plexus, reducing the temperature of the arterial blood by several degrees as it leaves the area. More heat may be lost from the testicular artery as it passes over the testicular surface.

The cremaster muscles can contract to raise the testes nearer to the body wall, but only for short intervals. Complete relaxation of these muscles permits the testes to assume a more distal scrotal position, which facilitates cooling.

Endocrine Regulation of Testicular Function

Testicular function is governed primarily by the neuroendocrine system (termed endocrine regulation), with modulation by factors within specific regions of the testis parenchyma (termed paracrine or autocrine regulation).[80-82] Endocrine control of testicular function is very complex and relies on integrated patterns of hormonal secretion by the testes and hormone-secreting tissues extrinsic to the reproductive tract (*ie,* the hypothalamus, pituitary gland and, most probably, the pineal gland), and input from the central nervous system. Most data available on regulation of testicular function have been obtained using tissues of animals other than stallions, primarily laboratory and food-producing animals, and people). Therefore, much information regarding hormonal regulation of testicular function in stallions must be extrapolated from data on other species.

The hypothalamus is considered to be the principal orchestrator of testicular function.[10] Integrated input from neurotransmitters, neuropeptides and hormones secreted by the testes controls biosynthesis and release of gonadotropin-releasing hormone (GnRH) by hypothalamic neurons.[83] This decapeptide hormone is released episodically into the hypothalamic-hypophyseal portal vascular system, then travels to the anterior lobe of the pituitary gland, where it exerts its effect. The GnRH binds with high-affinity receptors of gonadotropin-producing cells in the anterior pituitary gland, initiating pulsatile release of 2 large glycoprotein hormones, luteinizing hormone (LH) and follicle-stimulating hormone (FSH).

The pulsatility of LH and FSH release in stallions is not as apparent as in other species studied, but short-term fluctuations in both LH and FSH can be detected in stallion serum.[84-86] In one study involving stallions, frequency of LH pulses ranged from about 3 to 6 per 24-hour period, and amplitude of the pulses ranged from about 5 to 10 ng/ml.[85] In stallions, the dependencies of LH and FSH on GnRH differ, with pituitary release of FSH being less dependent on GnRH input.[87,88] This dissimilarity has also been detected in mares.[88-90] One study, however, did report significant elevations in serum concentrations of both LH and FSH in stallions subsequent to GnRH injection.[91]

The gonadotropins, LH and FSH, have direct but differing effects on testicular function. Luteinizing hormone binds specifically with Leydig cells, whereas FSH binds with Sertoli cells and, possibly, spermatogonia.[83] In response to LH stimulation, Leydig cells synthesize and secrete androgens (*eg,* testosterone and dihydrotestosterone) and estrogens. These steroids then diffuse into the blood and lymph, which drain the testis, or into the seminiferous tubules and surrounding peritubular cells. This high local concentration of testosterone achieved within the testicular parenchyma is considered essential to normal spermatogenesis. The minimal local concentration of testosterone required for qualitatively and quantitatively normal spermatogenesis has not been determined, nor is the exact mechanism by which testosterone exerts its effect known.[82,92] Existing data suggest that testosterone acts specifically through Sertoli cells and peritubular cells to mediate spermatogenesis.[93]

Follicle-stimulating hormone is necessary for initiation of spermatogenesis at puberty, and, thereafter, its normal maintenance. In response to FSH, and possibly testosterone, Sertoli cells synthesize and secrete many substances important to normal testicular function, including androgen-binding protein (ABP), inhibin, activin, estrogen, several products that influence meiosis, maturation of spermatocytes, spermiation, and even Leydig-cell function, and a variety of proteins with unknown functions.[81,94,95] Androgen-binding protein traps testosterone and dihydrotestosterone within the seminiferous tubules to maintain a high androgen concentration within the seminiferous tubules in the presence of episodic release patterns by the Leydig cells. In addition, ABP assists in transport of androgens from the testis to the epididymis, where they influence spermatozoal maturation and epididymal transit.[94] Inhibin, activin and estrogen have putative roles in feedback control of FSH release. Secretory patterns of rat Sertoli cells *in vitro* vary in response to changes in the frequency and duration of FSH pulses, demonstrating the importance of FSH to Sertoli-cell function.[96] In turn, a positive correlation between Sertoli-cell numbers per testis and spermatogenic capability has been detected in rats, rams, bulls and stallions.[3,95]

Mechanisms that control the hypothalamic-pituitary-gonadal axis are not completely understood; however, the feedback loops that control LH or FSH release are known to differ. Androgens (testosterone and dihydrotestosterone) and estrogen are the key regulators of LH synthesis and secretion, imposing a negative feedback at either the hypothalamus or the anterior pituitary gland.[10,83] Inhibin appears to be the most potent inhibitor of FSH secretion, even though the gonadal steroids also suppress its release. Inhibin selectively suppresses secretion of FSH at the level of the anterior pituitary gland without affecting LH activity.[97] Sertoli-cell secretions contain a subunit dimer of inhibin, termed activin. Though the physiologic role of this peptide is presently unknown, it stimulates FSH secretion by pituitary cells *in vitro*.[94]

The mare typically exhibits seasonality by entering a state of reproductive hibernation during the winter, whereas the stallion produces fertile spermatozoa all year long.[48] The stallion, however, does display some annual regression and recrudescence of libido, seminal volume, testicular size and spermatozoal production/output.[3,98-101]

The circannual reproductive cycle of stallions is apparently established endogenously but can be modified by photoperiod.[101] The seasonal pattern of reproductive processes seems to be mediated through reduction and replenishment of LH content in the anterior pituitary gland.[87] Annual patterns have been detected in serum concentrations of LH and testosterone, and in intratesticular concentrations of testosterone, with highest levels being attained in the breeding season (summer).[3,7,85,100,102] The seasonal changes in serum FSH concentration are less consistent and, indeed, less pronounced than that for serum LH.[3,85,88,102] One study revealed no seasonal differences in pituitary or serum concentrations of FSH in stallions.[88] These workers also noted that LH concentration in the pituitary gland was doubled in the summer, as compared to the winter. The effect of season on pituitary concentrations of FSH and LH in stallions is similar to that reported for mares.[103,104] Thus, neuroendocrine control of seasonality may be similar between mares and stallions. Hypothalamic content of GnRH in mares is affected by season, with lowest concentrations detected in the winter.[104]

Seasonal suppression of GnRH synthesis and secretion is not well understood but probably involves a neural mechanism of GnRH inhibition.[105] Pinealectomized mares lose the ability to respond to photostimulation.[106] This finding suggests that the pineal gland, through melatonin production, may mediate changes in hypothalamic GnRH activity, photoperiodically.

Serum concentrations of LH, FSH and testosterone, and intratesticular concentration of testosterone increase with age in stallions.[3,77,79] Daily spermatozoal production per gram of testis, daily spermatozoal production per testis, number of Sertoli cells per testis, number of elongated spermatids per Sertoli cell, number of Leydig cells per testis, and volume of smooth endoplasmic reticulum (SER) per testis (SER is involved in testicular steroidogenesis) are all positively correlated with serum concentrations of LH and testosterone in stallions.[3,7] The relationship of serum FSH to the various testicular values is less consistent, but serum FSH concentration is positively correlated with the number of Sertoli cells per gram of testis parenchyma. Because gonadotropins and testosterone are correlated with many measures of spermatogenesis, the effect of age on spermatogenesis in stallions is likely to be mediated through variations in gonadotropin or testosterone secretion.

Erection and Ejaculation

Successful mating requires coordination of erection and ejaculation, both of which are under direct control by the nervous system. Erection appears to be primarily under the influence of the parasympathetic nervous system, whereas ejaculation is controlled principally by the sympathetic portion of the autonomic nervous system. Somatic innervation to the reproductive tract plays a supportive role in both these events.

The nonerect penis has a soft compressible texture because of its musculocavernous construction. Typically, it is retracted fully into the prepuce because of the collapsed cavernous spaces of the penis coupled with contraction of the paired retractor penis muscles. Sexual excitement initiates a series of hemodynamic and neuromuscular events that transform the penis into a rigid copulatory organ. Understanding the mechanism of erection and ejaculation requires knowledge of some key anatomic features.

Two different arterial branches supply the cavernous tissue of the equine penis. This vascular pattern is different from that of other domestic animals, which have a common arterial source for all erectile bodies. The obturator artery of stallions extends to the crura of the corpus cavernosum penis as the deep artery of the penis. It branches to penetrate the thick tunica albuginea and extends into the corpus cavernosum penis as coiled helicine arteries.[2] The corpus spongiosum penis and associated corpus spongiosum glandis are supplied by another vessel, the internal pudendal artery.

Extrinsic musculature vital to erection and ejaculation includes the paired ischiocavernosus and retractor penis muscles, bulbospongiosus muscle and urethralis muscle. The strong ischiocavernosus muscles extend from the ischium to the base of the penis, and cover the crura of the corpus cavernosum penis. The bulbospongiosus muscle is a thick, circular muscle (with a median septum) that covers the bulb of the penis and corpus spongiosum penis (and contained penile urethra). The bulbospongiosus muscle is continuous proximally with the urethralis muscle, which encircles the pelvic urethra. The bulbospongiosus muscle extends the entire length of the penis, terminating just proximal to the glans penis. The retractor penis muscles are composed of smooth muscle and connect the penis with the caudal vertebrae. They maintain the detumescent penis within the protective prepuce. The ischiourethralis muscle, which extends from the urethralis muscle to the ischium, also may contribute to the erection/ejaculation mechanism. A branch of this muscle, the bulboglandularis muscle, covers the bulbourethral glands and may aid expulsion of their luminal contents.

Exposure of a stallion to a mare in estrus or other stimulatory element causes the flaccid penis to drop from the prepuce through relaxation of the retractor penis muscles (Fig 40). Continued sexual stimulation produces relaxation of smooth muscle within the walls and trabeculae of the corpus cavernosum penis, vasodilation of the helicine arteries, and rhythmic contractions of the ischiocavernosus muscles. These combined effects lead to rapid engorgement of the corpus cavernosum penis and production of a rigid, elongated penis (Fig 41). Contractions of the ischiocavernosus muscles pump arterial blood into the corpus cavernosum penis but also press the dorsum of the penile root against the ischium to occlude venous outflow

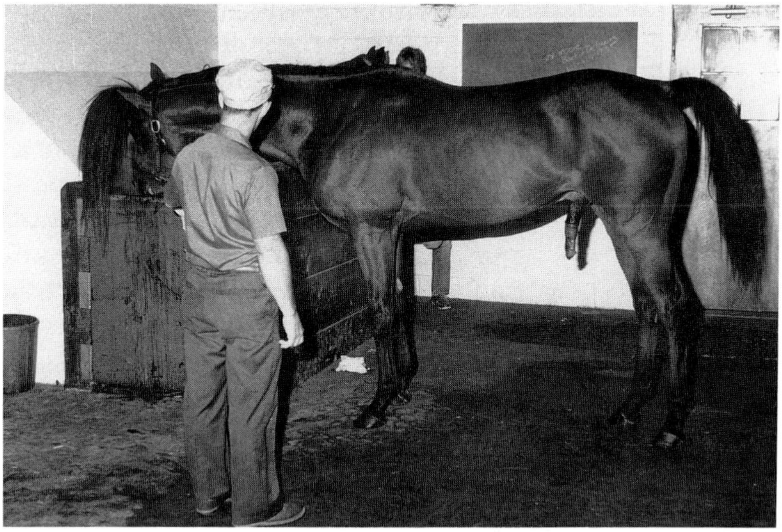

Figure 40. Stallion exposure to an estrous mare initially results in protrusion of the flaccid penis from the prepuce.

from this erectile body.[107] The closed system thus established results in a local blood pressure that far exceeds that of the systemic circulation.

With this precopulatory erection (*ie,* erection without "belling" of the glans penis), the stallion is prepared for intromission and copulation. After mounting a mare in estrus (or other mounting device), the stallion begins irregular thrusting motions with the pelvis while searching for the vulva with the erect penis. Once the sensitive glans penis is inserted in the vagina, the amplified sensation elicits penetrating intravaginal thrusts,

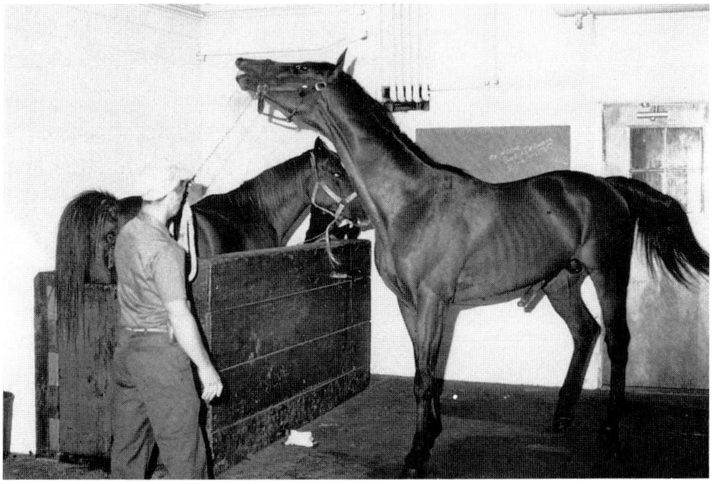

Figure 41. Continued stallion exposure to an estrous mare results in attainment of a rigid, erect penis.

vasodilation of vessels entering the corpus spongiosum penis, and a burst of rhythmic bulbospongiosus muscle contractions. The net effect of these changes is engorgement of the corpus spongiosum penis and connecting corpus spongiosum glandis, indicating maximal penile stimulation. Increased blood pressure in these erectile bodies results in the characteristic "belling" of the glans penis that precedes ejaculation (Fig 42). These 2 erectile bodies do not form a closed system, so the blood pressure in these tissues does not reach the magnitude of that in the corpus cavernosum penis during erection.[108]

Ejaculation is divided into 2 phases. The first involves emission of all seminal contributions from the various genital ducts into the urethra, generated by contraction of muscles within duct walls or overlying the glands. Emission is followed by forceful evacuation, or discharge of accumulated semen from the urethral lumen. Intense contractions of the urethralis, bulbospongiosus and ischiocavernosus muscles are necessary for effective ejection of semen from the urethra. The ejaculate is composed of several "jets" of semen released from the urethral orifice in rapid succession.[38,109] Ejaculation is noticeable externally by palpable pulsations of the bulbospongiosus muscle on the ventral aspect of the penis and a characteristic "flagging" motion of the stallion's tail. Following ejaculation, relaxation of the bulbospongiosus and ischiocavernosus muscles, contraction of smooth muscle of the cavernous trabeculae and retractor penis muscles, and vasoconstriction of arteries supplying cavernous tissue result in rapid evacuation of blood from the erectile bodies and penile withdrawal into the prepuce.

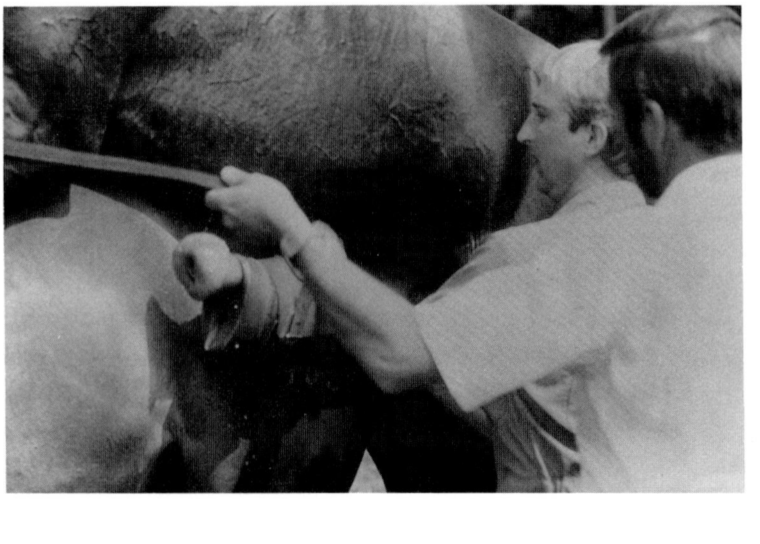

Figure 42. Characteristic "belling" of the glans penis indicates good penile stimulation during coitus.

References

1. Amann RP: A review of anatomy and physiology of the stallion. *J Equine Vet Sci* 1:83-105, 1981.

2. Nickel R *et al:The Viscera of Domestic Animals*. Springer-Verlag, New York, 1973. pp 303-349.

3. Johnson L and Thompson DL Jr: Age-related and seasonal variation in the Sertoli cell population daily sperm production and serum concentrations of follicle-stimulated hormone luteinizing hormone and testosterone in stallions. *Biol Reprod* 29:777-789, 1983.

4. Johnson L and Neaves WB: Age-related changes in the Leydig cell population, seminiferous tubules, and sperm production in the stallion. *Biol Reprod* 24:703-712, 1981.

5. Skinner MK and Fritz IB: Identification of a non-mitogenic paracrine factor involved in mesenchymal-epithelial cell interactions between testicular pertubulae cells and Sertoli cells. *Mol Cell Endocrinol* 44:85-97, 1986.

6. Hettle JA *et al:* Rat testicular peritubular cells in culture secrete on inhibitor of plasminogen activator activity. *Biol Reprod* 38:359-371, 1988.

7. Johnson L and Thompson DL Jr: Effect of seasonal changes in Leydig cell number on the volume of smooth endoplasmic reticulum in Leydig cells and intratesticular testosterone content in stallions. *J Reprod Fertil* 81: 227-237, 1987.

8. Johnson L and Thompson DL Jr: Seasonal variation in the total volume of Leydig cells in stallions is explained by variation in cell number rather than cell size. *Biol Reprod* 35:971-979, 1986.

9. Christensen AK, in Greep RO and Astwood EB: *Handbook of Physiology*. Vol V. American Physiological Society, Washington, DC, 1975. pp 57-94.

10. Amann RP and Schanbacher BD: Physiology of male reproduction. *J Anim Sci* (Suppl 2) 57:380-403, 1983.

11. Dym M and Raj HGM: Response of adult rat Sertoli cells and Leydig cells to depletion of luteininzing hormone and testosterone. *Biol Reprod* 17:676-696, 1977.

12. Ritzen EM *et al,* in Burger H and de Kretser D: *The Testis*. 2nd ed. Raven Press, New York, 1989. pp 269-302.

13. Jutte HPN *et al:* Regulation of survival of rat pachytene spermatocytes by lactate supply from Sertoli cells. *J Reprod Fertil* 65:431-438, 1982.

14. Feig LA *et al:* Sertoli cells contain a mitogenic polypeptide. *Proc Natl Acad Sci* 77:4774, 1980.

15. Rivarola MA *et al:* Stimulation of ribonucleic acid and deoxyribonucleic acid synthesis in spermatogenic cells by their coculture with Sertoli cells. *Endocrinology* 117:1796-1802, 1985.

16. Fawcett DW: The mammallian spermatozoon. *Dev Biol* 44:394-436, 1975.

17. Fawcett DW, in Greep RO and Astwood EB: *Handbook of Physiology*. Vol. V. American Physiological Society, Washington, DC, 1975. p 21.

18. Dadoune JP *et al: In vivo* and *in vitro* radioautographic investigation of amino acid incorporation into male germ cells. *Biol Reprod* 24:153-162, 1981.

19. Hochereau-de-Reviers MT and Courot M: Sertoli cells and development of seminiferous epithelium. *Ann Anim Biochem Biophys* 18:573-583, 1978.

20. Berndtson WE *et al:* Relationship of absolute numbers of Sertoli cells to testicular size and spermatogenesis in young beef bulls. *J Anim Sci* 64:241-246, 1987.

21. Johnson L *et al:* Quantification of the human Sertoli cell population: its distribution, relation to germ cell numbers, and age-related decline. *Biol Reprod* 31:785-795, 1984.

22. Johnson L and Nguyen HB: Annual cycle of the Sertoli cell population in adult stallions. *J Reprod Fertil* 76:311, 1986.

23. Johnson L *et al:* Establishment of adult levels of spermatogenesis in the horse. *J Reprod Fertil* (Suppl) (submitted 1990).

24. Johnson L and Tatum ME: Temporal appearance of seasonal changes in numbers of Sertoli cells, Leydig cells, and germ cells in stallions. *Biol Reprod* 40:994-999, 1989.

25. Johnson L *et al:* Scanning electron microscopy of the epithelium and spermatozoa in the equine excurrent duct system. *Am J Vet Res* 39:1428-1434, 1978.

26. Amann RP *et al:* Connection between the seminiferous tubules and the efferent duct in the stallion. *Am J Vet Res* 38:1571-1579, 1977.

27. Maneely RB: Epididymal structure and function: A historical and critical review. *Acta Zool* 42:2, 1959.

28. Amann RP: Function of the epididymis in bulls and rams. *J Reprod Fertil* 34:115-131, 1987.

29. Amann RP: Maturation of spermatozoa. *Proc Intl Cong Anim Reprod Artif Insem,* 1988. pp 321-328.

30. Ewing LL and Chang TSK, in: *Campbell's Urology.* 5th ed. Saunders, Philadelphia, 1986. pp 200-233.

31. Johnson L *et al:* Maturation of equine epididymal spermatozoa. *Am J Vet Res* 41:1190-1196, 1980.

32. Robaire B and Hermo L, in Knobil E and Neill J: *The Physiology of Reproduction.* Raven Press, New York, 1988. pp 999-1080.

33. Amann RP *et al:* Effects of age and frequency of ejaculation on sperm production and extragonadal sperm reserves in stallions. *J Reprod Fertil* (Suppl) 27:1-6, 1979.

34. Amann RP: A critical review of methods for evaluation of spermatogenesis from seminal characteristics. *J Androl* 2:37-58, 1981.

35. Fawcett DW: The mammalian spermatozoon. *Dev Biol* 44:394-436, 1975.

36. Kenney RM *et al: Manual for Clinical Fertility Evaluation of the Stallion.* Soc for Theriogenol, Hastings, NE, 1983.

37. Pickett BW *et al: Management of the Stallion for Maximum Reproductive Efficiency* - II. Colorado State University Exp Sta Anim Reprod Lab, Gen Series Bull 05, 1989. pp 39-120.

38. Mann T and Lutwak-Mann C: *Male Reproductive Function and Semen.* Springer-Verlag, New York, 1981. pp 1-37, 171-193.

39. Bergin WC *et al:* A developmental concept of equine cryptorchism. *Biol Reprod* 3:82-92, 1970.

40. Hamilton JB: The effect of male hormone upon descent of the testes. *Anat Record* 70:533-541, 1938.

41. Martins T: La testosterone peut provoquer la deescente de testicules artificiels de paraffine. *CR Soc Biol* (Paris) 131:299-302, 1939.

42. Backhouse KM: Development and descent of the testis. *Eur J Pediatr* 139:249-252, 1982.

43. Elder JS *et al:* Androgenic sensitivity of the gubernaculum testis: Evidence for hormonal/mechanical interactions in testicle descent. *J Urol* 127:170-176, 1982.

44. Rajfer J and Walsch CP: Hormonal regulation of testicular descent: experimental and clinical observations. *J Urol* 118:985-990, 1978.

45. Gier HT and Marion GB, in Johnson AD *et al: The Testis.* Vol 1. Academic Press, New York, 1970. pp 1-45.

46. Hadziselimovic F and Herzog B, in Hafez ESE: *Descended and Cryptorchid Testes.* Martinus Nijhoff, Boston, 1980. pp 138-147.

47. Wensing CJG *et al,* in Hafez ESE: *Descended and Cryptorchid Testes.* Martinus Nijhoff, Boston, 1980. pp 125-137.

48. Ginther OJ: *Reproductive Biology of the Mare. Basic and Applied Aspects.* Published by the author, Cross Plaines, WI, 1979. pp 83-168, 306-311.

49. Smith JA : The development and descent of the testes in the horse.*Vet Annual* 15:156-161, 1975.

50. Allen TD, in Negro-Vilar A: *Male Reproduction and Fertility.* Raven Press, New York, 1983. pp 351-361.

51. Engle ET: Experimentally induced descent of the testis in the macacus monkey by hormones from the anterior pituitary and pregnancy urine. *Endocrinology* 16:513-520, 1932.

52. Wolf FR *et al:* Prepuberal behavior and puberal characteristics of beef bulls on high nutrient allowances. *J Anim Sci* 24:761-765, 1985.

53. Naden J *et al:* Testicular growth, hormone concentrations, seminal characteristics and sexual behavior in stallions. *J Reprod Fertil* 88:167-176, 1990.

54. Nishikawa Y: *Studies on Reproduction in Horses.* Japan Racing Association, Tokyo, 1959. pp 2-27.

55. Skinner JD and Bowen J: Puberty in the Welsh stallion. *J Reprod Fertil* 16:133-135, 1968.

56. Cornwell JC: Seasonal variation in stallion semen and puberty in the Quarter Horse colt. MS thesis, Louisiana State University, 1972.

57. D'Occhio MJ: Brain-pituitary-testicular function. *Proc Intl Cong Anim Reprod Artif Insem,* 1988. pp 330-337.

58. Thompson DL Jr and Honey PG: Active immunization of prepubertal colts against estrogens: hormonal and testicular responses after puberty. *J Anim Sci* 59:189-196, 1984.

59. Amann RP and Walker OA: Changes in the pituitary gonadal axis associated with puberty in Holstein bulls. *J Anim Sci* 57:433-332, 1983.

60. Foster DL *et al:* Ontogeny of pulsatile luteinizing hormone and testosterone secretion in male lambs. *Endocrinology* 102:1137-1142, 1978.

61. Regaud C: Etude sur la structure des tubes seminiferes et sur la spermatogenese chez les mammiferes. *Arch Anat Microscop Morphol Expt* 4:101-156, 231, 1901.

62. Von Ebner H: *Kolliker's Handbuch der Gewebelehre des Menschen Leipzig.* Vol III. Engelmann, Leipzig, 1902.

63. Johnson L: Seasonal differences in equine spermatocytogenesis. *Biol Reprod* (in press 1991).

64. Leblond CP and Clermont Y: Spermiogenesis of rat, mouse, hamster, and guinea pig as revealed by the periodic acid-fuchsin sulfurous acid technique. *Am J Anat* 90: 167-206, 1952.

65. Swierstra EE *et al:* Reproductive physiology of the stallion. 1. Spermatogenesis and testis composition. *J Reprod Fertil* 40:113-123, 1974.

66. Johnson L: Spermatogenesis (animal species and humans). *Proc 1988 Serono Intl Symp Gamete Physiol,* 1989.

67. Johnson L: Increased daily sperm production in the breeding season of stallions is explained by an elevated population of spermatogonia. *Biol Reprod* 32:1181-1190, 1985.

68. Johnson L *et al:* Staging equine seminiferous tubules by Nomarski optics in unstained histologic sections and in tubules mounted "in toto" to reveal the spermatogenic wave. *Anat Record* 227:167-174, 1990.

69. Roosen-Runge EC and Giesel LO: Quantitative studies on spermatogenesis in the albino rat. *Am J Anat* 87:1-30, 1950.

70. Ortavant R *et al,* in Cole HH and Cupps PT: *Reproduction in Domestic Animals.* 3rd ed. Academic Press, New York, 1977. p 203.

71. Johnson L *et al:* Scanning electron and light microscopy of the equine seminiferous tubule. *Fertil Steril* 29:208-215, 1978.

72. Johnson L, in Cupps PT: *Reproduction in Domestic Animals.* 3rd ed. Academic Press, New York, 1991.

73. Parvinen M: Regulation of the seminiferous epithelium. *Endocrin Rev* 3:404-417, 1982.

74. Parvinen M and Vanha-Perttula T: Identification and enzyme quantification of the stages of the seminiferous epithelial wave in the rat. *Anat Record* 174:435-450, 1972.

75. Johnson L *et al:* Isolation and staging of horse seminiferous tubules by transillumination. *J Reprod Fertil* (in press 1990).

76. Huckins C: The morphology and kinetics of spermatogonial degeneration in normal adult rats: an analysis using a simplified classification of the germinal epithelium. *Anat Record* 190:905-926, 1978.

77. Johnson L: A new approach to quantification of Sertoli cells that avoids problems associated with the irregular nuclear surface. *J Anat Rec* 214:231-237, 1986.

78. Jones LS and Berndtson WE: A quantitative study of Sertoli cell and germ cell populations as related to sexual development and aging in the stallion. *Biol Reprod* 35:138-148, 1986.

79. Berndtson WE and Jones LS: Relationship of intratesticular testosterone content of stallions to age, spermatogenesis, Sertoli cell distribution and germ cell-Sertoli cell ratios. *J Reprod Fertil* 85:511-518, 1989.

80. Matsumoto AM, in Burger H and de Kretser DM: *The Testis.* 2nd ed. Raven Press, New York, 1989. pp 181-196.

81. Risbridger GP and de Kretser DM, in Burger H and de Kretser DM: *The Testis.* 2nd ed. Raven Press, New York, 1989. pp 181-196.

82. Sharpe RM *et al:* Re-evaluation of the intratesticular level of testosterone required for quantitative maintenance of spermatogenesis in the rat. *J Endocr* 177:19-26, 1988.

83. Nankin HR *et al,* in Moore WT and Eastman RC: *Diagnostic Endocrinology.* Decker, Philadelphia, 1990. pp 247-281.

84. Thompson DL *et al:* Patterns of secretion of luteinizing hormone, follicle stimulating hormone and testosterone in stallions during the summer and winter. *J Anim Sci* 60:741-748, 1985.

85. Clay CM *et al:* Influences of season and artificial photoperiod on stallions: Luteinizing hormone, follicle-stimulating hormone and testosterone. *J Anim Sci* 66:1246-1255, 1988.

86. Rabb MH *et al:* Effects of sexual stimulation, with and without ejaculation, on serum concentrations of LH, FSH, testosterone, cortisol and prolactin in stallions. *J Anim Sci* 67:2724-2729, 1989.

87. Clay CM *et al:* Influences of season and artificial photoperiod on stallions: pituitary and testicular responses to exogenous GnRH. *J Anim Sci* 67:763-770, 1989.

88. Thompson DL *et al:* Concentrations of prolactin, luteinizing hormone and follicle stimulating hormone in pituitary and serum of horses: Effect of sex, season and reproductive state. *J Anim Sci* 63:854-860, 1986.

89. Garza F *et al:* Active immunization of intact mares against gonadotropin releasing hormone: differential effects on secretion of luteinizing hormone and follicle-stimulating hormone. *Biol Reprod* 35:347-352, 1986.

90. Garza F *et al:* Effects of active immunization against gonadotropin releasing hormone on gonadotropin secretion after ovariectomy and testosterone propionate administration to mares. *J Anim Sci* 66:479-486, 1988.

91. Burns PJ and Douglas RH: Effects of a single injection of GnRH or equine pituitary extract on plasma LH and FSH concentrations in stallions. *J Equine Vet Sci* 4:281-283, 1984.

92. Rommerts FFG: How much androgen is required for maintenance of spermatogenesis? *J Endocr* 116:7-9, 1988.

93. Sharpe RM *et al:* Cell-cell interactions in the control of spermatogenesis an studied using Leydig cell destruction and testosterone replacement. *Am J Anat* 188:3-20, 1990.

94. Martin-Ritzen E *et al,* in Burger H and de Kretser DM: *The Testis.* 2nd ed. Raven Press, New York, 1989. pp 269-302.

95. Courot M: The regulation of testicular function by pituitary gonadotrophins. *Proc Intl Cong Anim Reprod Artif Insem,* 1980. pp 155-162.

96. Jakubowiak A *et al:* The effect of varying FSH pulses on transferrin secretion in superperfused Sertoli cell cultures. *J Androl* 8:30-P, 1987.

97. Robertson DM *et al,* in Burger H and de Kretser DM: *The Testis.* 2nd ed. Raven Press, New York, 1989. pp 231-254.

98. Pickett BW *et al:* Effect of month and stallion on seminal characteristics and sexual behavior. *J Anim Sci* 31:713-728, 1970.

99. Thompson DL *et al:* Reproductive physiology of the stallion. VIII. Artificial photoperiod, collection interval and seminal characteristics, sexual behavior and concentrations of LH and testosterone in serum. *J Anim Sci* 44:656-664, 1977.

100. Berndtson WE *et al:* Spermatogenesis, testicular composition and the concentration of testosterone in the equine testis as influenced by season. *Theriogenology* 20:449-457, 1983.

101. Clay CM *et al:* Influences of season and artificial photoperiod on stallions: Testicular size, seminal characteristics and sexual behavior. *J Anim Sci* 64:517-525, 1987.

102. Harris JM: Seasonal changes in serum levels of FSH, LH and testosterone and in semen parameters in stallions. *Theriogenology* 19:311-322, 1983.

103. Silvia PJ *et al:* Pituitary responsiveness of mares challenged with GnRH at various stages of the transition into the breeding season. *J Anim Sci* 64:790-796, 1987.

104. Hart PJ *et al:* Seasonal variations in hypothalamic content of gonadotropin-releasing hormone (GnRH), pituitary receptors for GnRH, and pituitary content of luteinizing hormone and follicle stimulating hormone in the mare. *Biol Reprod* 30:1055-1066, 1984.

105. Fitzgerald BP and Millbye LB: Effect of administration of an alpha-2 agonist, xylazine, on pulsatile gonadotrophin secretion in anoestrous horse mares. *J Reprod Fertil* 84:693-700, 1988.

106. Grubaugh W *et al:* Effects of pinealectomy in pony mares. *J Reprod Fertil* Suppl 32:293-295, 1982.

107. Bartels JE *et al:* Angiography of the corpus cavernosum penis in the pony stallion during erection and quiescence. *Am J Vet Res* 45:1464-1468, 1984.

108. Beckett SD*et al:* Corpus spongiosum penis pressure and penile muscle activity in the stallion during coitus. *Am J Vet Res* 36:431-433, 1975.

109. Tischner M *et al:* Analysis of the pattern of ejaculation in stallions. *J Reprod Fertil* 41:329-335, 1974.

2

Breeding Soundness Examination

The objective of a breeding soundness examination is to determine whether a stallion has the mental and physical faculties necessary to deliver semen, containing viable spermatozoa and no infectious disease, to the mare's reproductive tract at the proper time. The examination not only evaluates quality and quantity of ejaculated spermatozoa but also tests the libido and mating ability of a stallion, attempts to recognize congenital defects that may be transmissible to offspring and/or decrease a stallion's fertility, seeks infectious diseases that may be transmitted venereally, and searches for lesions that may reduce breeding longevity. Abbreviated examinations also can be performed to assess specific lesions of the stallion's genital tract with only the well-being of the horse in mind and no immediate concern for the stallion's potential as a breeding candidate. Thus, the breadth of the examination varies with individual horses and should be designed to answer specific client queries.

History and Identification

Pertinent historical information regarding a patient is an indispensable part of a diagnostic plan. Historical data should be gathered in a well-devised unassuming manner to ensure completeness and avoid inaccuracies. Possible environmental and heritable causes for the admitting problem should be addressed, and previous modes of therapy for an existing problem investigated when applicable. A historical review of stallions to be examined for breeding soundness should include their present use, lineage, previous breeding performance, results of prior fertility evaluations, illnesses, injuries, medications and vaccinations, with explicit information regarding previous and current reproductive management and medical programs.

Positive identification of the stallion, often considered a mundane procedure, is an integral part of the examination process, especially when sale of the horse is involved. Identification of a stallion must be accurate to avoid any ambiguity in identity at a subsequent date. Name, age, breed and registration number of the stallion are recorded, in addition to identifying marks, such as a lip tattoo, hide brands, color markings and hair whorls. When possible, photographs of the stallion should be taken for permanent identification.

General Physical Examination

Though this chapter focuses on the genital health of stallions, general physical condition cannot be ignored. Assessment of general body condition is first in order, followed by an appraisal of conformation. Particular attention should be given to defective traits that will affect mating ability (*eg,* lamenesses or back problems) or that are potentially heritable (*eg,* cryptorchidism, brachygnathia, wobbler syndrome; Figs 1, 2).[1] All abnormalities are recorded. Methodic examination of the various body systems (respiratory, cardiovascular, digestive, nervous, urinary, neuromuscular, skeletal) also is recommended, followed by a careful

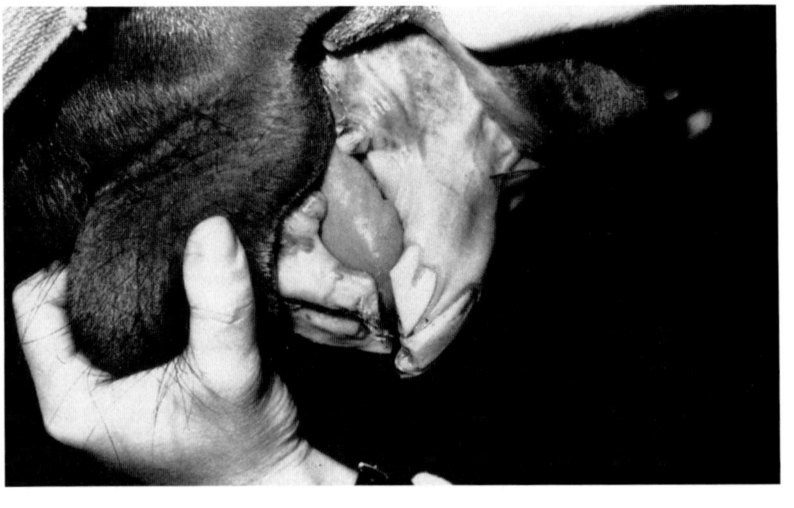

Figure 1. Oral deformity (parrot mouth) in a stallion.

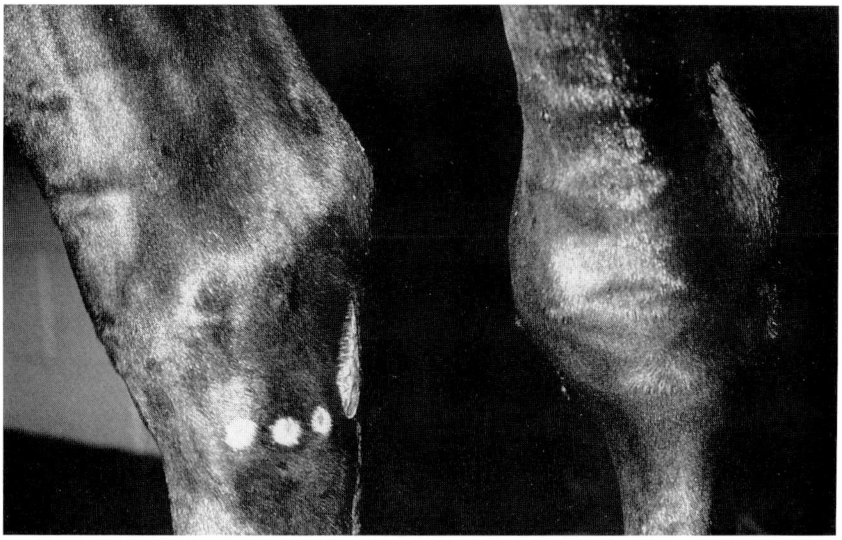

Figure 2. Hock lameness in a stallion hindered its mating ability.

ophthalmic examination. Common laboratory tests (Coggins test, hematologic examination, serum chemistry assays, urinalysis, fecal egg counts) can support physical examination findings in determining the general health of a stallion.

Physical Examination of the Reproductive Tract

An appreciation of normal genital anatomy is essential to competent physical examination of the stallion's reproductive tract (see Chapter 1). The extent of the examination is dependent on the type of medical problem presented. A thorough physical examination of both external and internal genital organs always should be incorporated into procedures for predicting stallion fertility.

External Genitalia

Close inspection of the penis is aided by first stimulating penile tumescence through exposure of the stallion to a mare in estrus (Fig 3). This procedure also permits assessment of sexual behavior, including erection capability. Manual extraction of the penis from the prepuce for examination is difficult and usually met with resistance from the stallion. The penis can be examined while the horse urinates. Urination can sometimes be stimulated by placing the horse in a freshly bedded stall; shaking the bedding may increase the horse's urge to urinate. Intrave-

Figure 3. Exposure of a stallion to a mare in estrus to stimulate penile erection.

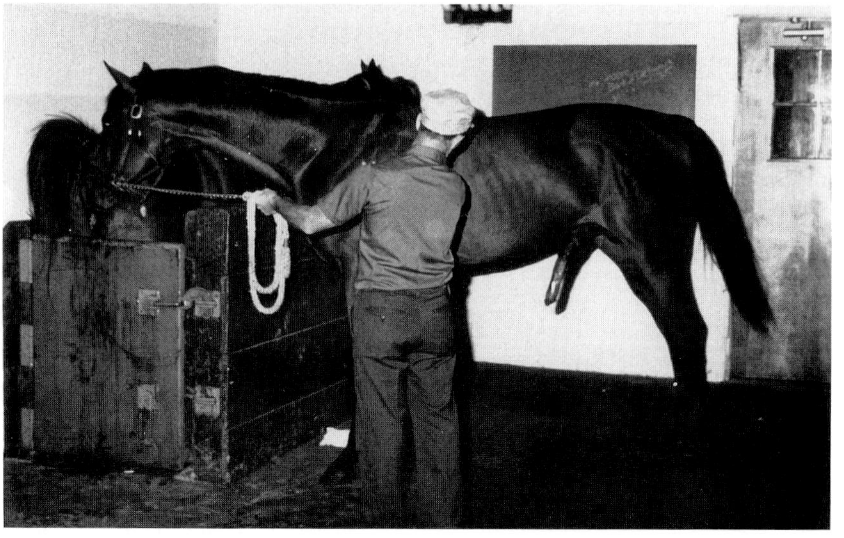

nous administration of a diuretic should result in urination within 10-15 minutes. Tranquilization (acepromazine, xylazine) elicits penile prolapse, making the penis accessible; however, tranquilizers, especially phenothiazines (*eg,* acepromazine), can result in penile paralysis or priapism and, therefore, should not be used indiscriminately (see Chapter 14).

The penis may require cleansing before inspection, as epithelial debris mixed with secretions from the preputial glands tends to accumulate in the preputial cavity and on the exterior of the penis. The root and proximal body of the penis are buried in tissue, thereby limiting the examination to the exposed body and glans. The penis should be examined thoroughly, and any palpable or visual lesions recorded. Because the fossa glandis and urethral process are partially concealed, particular attention should be given to these areas (Fig 4). Common penile lesions include those of traumatic origin as well as vesicles/pustules of coital exanthema, habronema granulomas, squamous-cell carcinomas and papillomas (see Chapter 14).

During penile tumescence, the prepuce also is readily available for examination. The skin of the prepuce should be thin and pliable, with no evidence of inflammatory or proliferative lesions. Developmental abnormalities of the penis and prepuce are rare.

Figure 4. Examination of the glans penis, including the urethral process and fossa glandis, for lesions during fertility evaluation of a stallion.

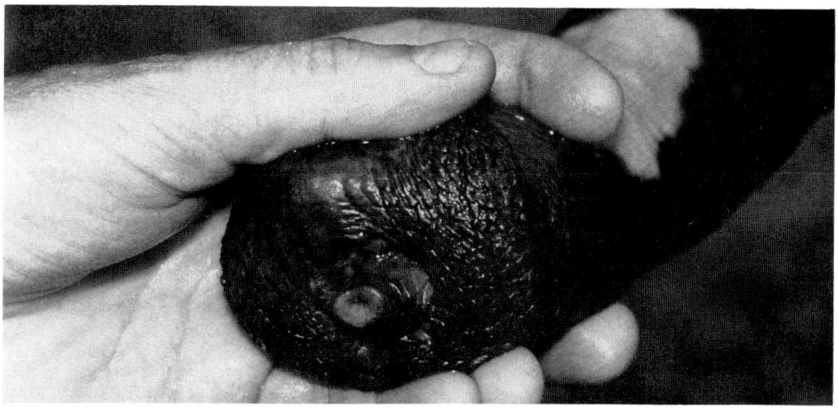

The scrotum of the stallion should be thin and elastic, with a distinct neck (Fig 5). The scrotum and its contents are normally pendulous (except during cold weather due to contractions of the tunica dartos) but may be drawn toward the body during palpation because of voluntary contractions of the cremaster muscles. Both testes and attached epididymides should be freely movable within their respective scrotal pouches. Size, texture and position of each testis always should be determined as part of a breeding soundness examination (Fig 6). Testicular size correlates highly with daily sperm production, so this measurement helps predict a stallion's breeding potential (Figs 7,8). Measurement of total scrotal width can be used to estimate daily

Figure 5. Scrotum of a stallion containing 2 testes and their attached epididymides. The scrotum is slightly pendulous with a distinct longitudinal indentation on its ventral surface, the scrotal raphe.

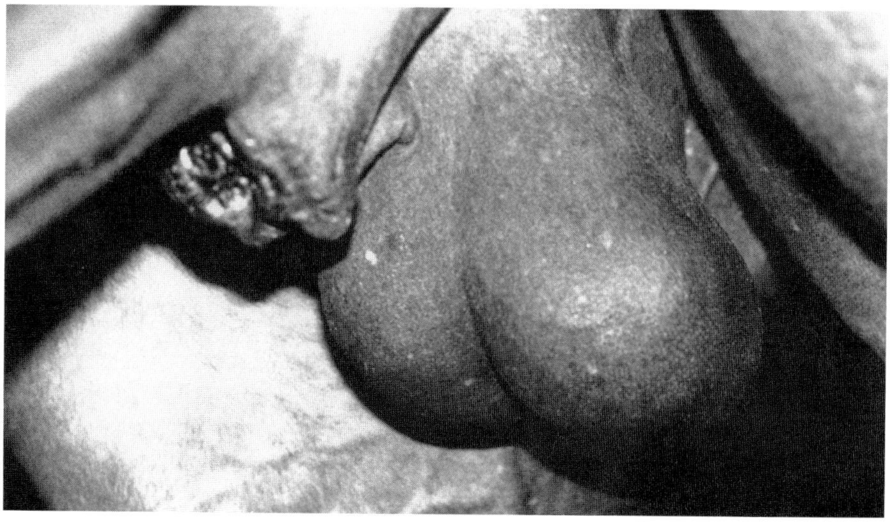

sperm production or daily sperm output in stallions.[2] One study, however, suggests that testicular volume may provide a more accurate estimate of daily sperm output.[3] Testicular volume can be calculated from linear measurements (testicular width, length and height), obtained using calipers or real-time ultrasonography, or from cross-sectional area through the widest part of the testis using ultrasonography (see Chapter 3). If daily sperm output in a stallion is significantly lower than that estimated by combined testicular volume, then testicular hypoplasia or degeneration is the likely cause.

Both testes should be oval, with a smooth regular outline and a slightly turgid resilient texture. The position of each testis within the scrotum can be determined accurately by palpation of the attached epididymis. The caudal ligament of the epididymis, a remnant of the gubernaculum, remains palpable during adult life as a small (1-2 cm) fibrous nodule adjacent to the epididymal tail, which itself is attached to the caudal pole of the testis. Therefore, this remnant serves as a landmark for determining testicular orientation within the scrotum. The epididymis normally is palpable in its entirety as it courses over the surface of the testis; however, its borders sometimes are difficult to identify.

Exploration of the spermatic cord is possible via palpation through the neck of the scrotum, though its specific contents often are not definable. Spermatic cords should be of equal size

Figure 6. Palpation of the external genitalia of a stallion for identification of abnormalities.

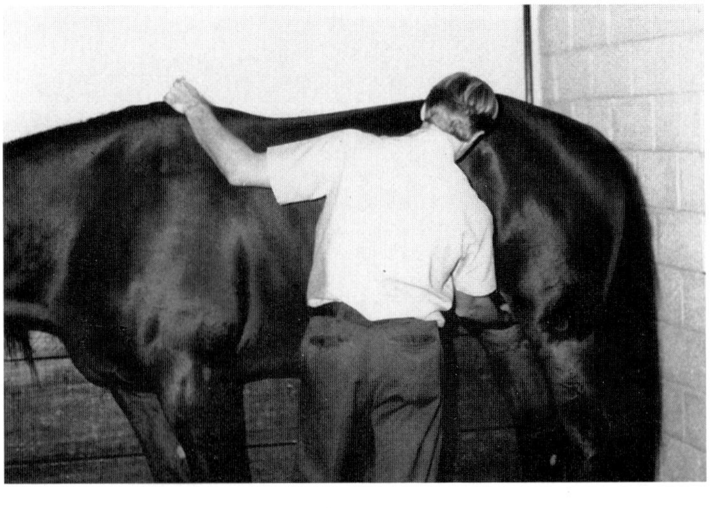

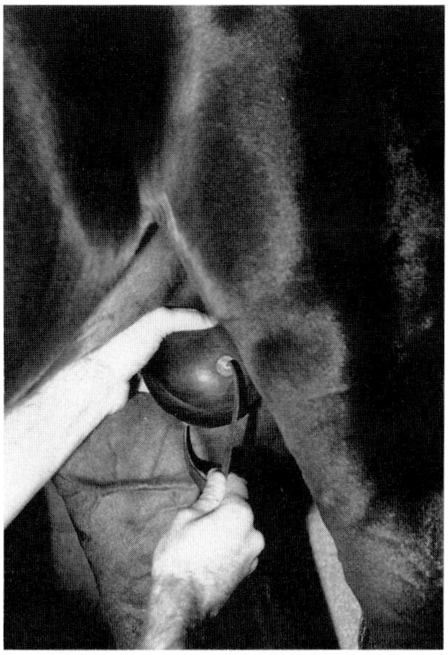

Figure 7. Measurement of total scrotal width in a stallion, using specially designed calipers.

and uniform diameter (2-3 cm). Acute pain in this area usually is associated with inguinal herniation or torsion of the spermatic cord.

Internal Genitalia

The internal genital organs can be examined by palpation per rectum (Fig 9). Adequate restraint is of paramount importance to this procedure. Minimal but effective restraint is the key to a

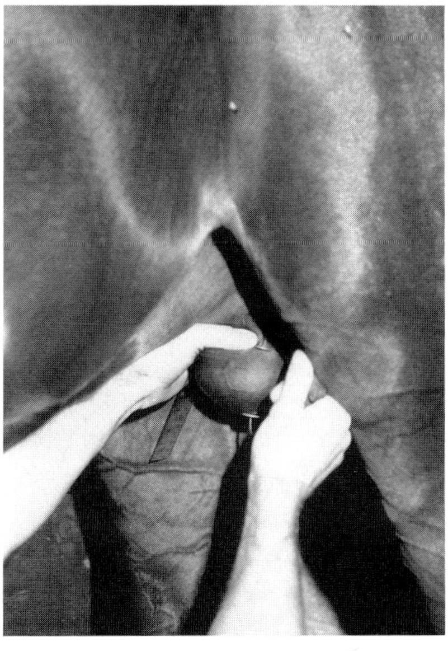

Figure 8. Measurement of left testicular height in a stallion, using calipers. Testicular dimensions (height, width, length) can also be measured accurately using real-time ultrasonography.

Figure 9. Examination of the internal genital organs and vaginal rings of a stallion by rectal palpation, after first restraining the animal in stocks.

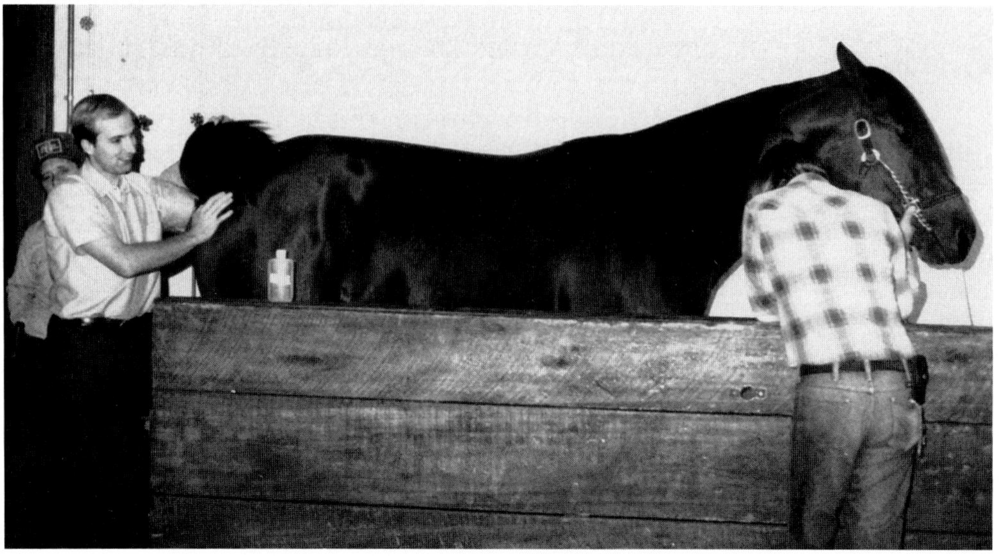

safe examination and varies from stallion to stallion. The disposition of the stallion should be determined at the onset and the examination canceled if the risk factor is high. Such precautions can protect both the stallion and operator from severe injury.

Before the examination, stallions should be placed in stocks, if available. Ideally, the stocks should be equipped with a solid rear door to help prevent leg extension if the stallion decides to kick. The height of the door should be level with the midgaskin region of the stallion's hindquarters. Higher doors can damage the operator's arm if a stallion squats abruptly while the operator's arm is in the rectum. Lower doors permit the stallion to easily kick over this barrier. Poorly designed doors do not afford protection to the examiner and increase the likelihood of unnecessary injury to the stallion.

If stocks are not available for the examination, the stallion should be placed in a doorway of a stall, with the hindquarters remaining 2 feet beyond the doorway. Thus, the operator is protected by the door frame. If a stallion must be examined in an open area, breeding hobbles should be properly secured to the stallion's hind legs to reduce the range of limb motion, should it decide to kick. If necessary, a twitch also can be placed on the stallion's muzzle for additional restraint. Tranquilization may be required to adequately restrain an anxious stallion, but usually this is discouraged because of the possible complicating effects on the penis (priapism or penile paralysis). Remember, overrestraint can be as dangerous to the stallion and operator as underrestraint.

The hand should be well lubricated and all manure in the rectum and distal colon removed before evaluation of pelvic and abdominal structures is attempted. The 2 vaginal rings (abdominal orifices of the inguinal canals) are palpable as slit-like openings ventrolateral to the pelvic brim. The deferent duct and pulse of the testicular artery often can be detected at the opening. The site is evaluated for size as well as for evidence of adhesions or herniation of viscera. The diameter of the opening is normally 2-3 cm. A larger opening may predispose the stallion to inguinal herniation. Some of the accessory genital organs also can be detected by palpation per rectum. The anatomic features of these structures are discussed in Chapter 1. Lesions of the accessory genital glands are uncommon and generally not evident by palpation.

Observation of Libido and Mating Ability

Excellent semen quality in a breeding prospect is inconsequential unless that stallion also has the desire and ability to deliver the semen to the mare's reproductive tract or an artificial vagina. Sexual behavior can be analyzed by bringing the stallion in contact with a mare in estrus. Typically, a stallion with good libido shows immediate and intense desire for the mare, manifested by restlessness, pawing, vocalization, intimate precopulatory activity, such as sniffing, licking and nipping the mare, exhibition of the "Flehmen" reaction (curling of the upper lip; primarily a response to sniffing of the mare's genitalia or urine) and development of an erection (Fig 10). The onset, intensity and duration of this courtship phase are affected by the stallion's genetic makeup, learned behavior (through both positive and negative experiences), limited seasonal variation and disease. A common cause for reduced or arrested libido in stallions is mismanagement, especially overuse or repetitive abusive punishment for expression of sexual interest. Length of the courtship phase and number of mounts required for ejaculation tend to increase in winter as compared to summer.[4,5] The physiologic mechanisms of stallion sexual behavior are not well understood but involve an intricate relationship between endocrine and neural systems.

Figure 10. "Flehmen" reaction (curling of the upper lip) in a stallion exposed to a mare in estrus.

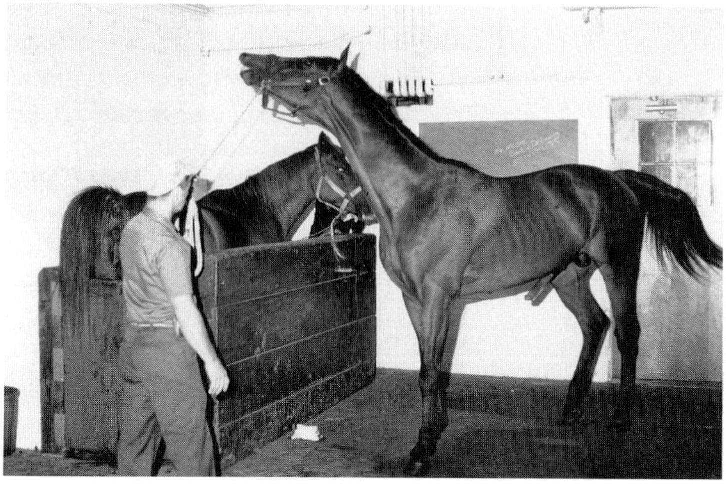

The ability of a stallion to copulate normally (develop an erection, mount without hesitation, insert the penis, perform intravaginal thrusts and ejaculate) should be assessed properly before the stallion is considered a satisfactory breeding prospect. The most common physical abnormalities associated with inability to mount are hindlimb lamenesses, such as hock problems or laminitis (Fig 11). The cause of erection and/or ejacu-

Figure 11. Mating disability resulting from hind limb lameness. The hocks of this stallion are pictured in Figure 2.

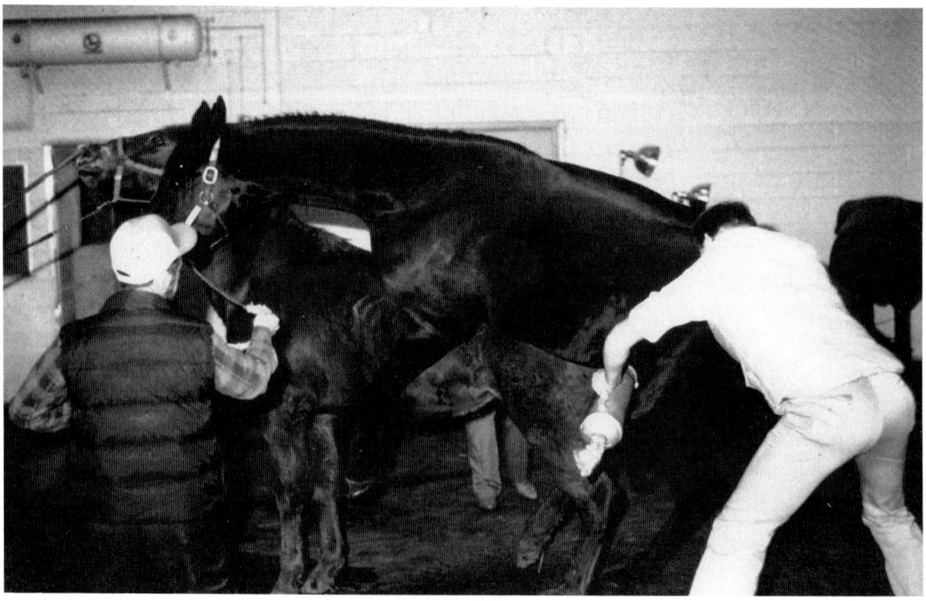

latory failure, unrelated to psychologic malfunction, can be difficult to determine. Penile injuries, spinal cord lesions and idiopathic organic dysfunctions can lead to impotence.

Examination for Venereal Disease

Various pathogenic microorganisms are transmitted by sexual contact, including bacteria, viruses and protozoa. The role of fungi, chlamydiae, mycoplasmata and ureaplasmata in venereal disease is unknown but is not considered significant. Depending on the etiologic agent involved, venereal disease may manifest itself through overt clinical signs in the stallion or, more commonly, "infected" stallions may be asymptomatic carriers.

Bacterial Genital Infections

Constant superficial bacterial colonization of the equine prepuce, penis and distal urethra results in unavoidable contamination of the mare's reproductive tract during coitus. A variety of environmental bacteria can be isolated from these sites, many contributing to the normal nonpathogenic bacterial flora of healthy stallions. These commensal bacteria tend to prevent overpopulation of the external genitalia with potentially harmful organisms (*Klebsiella pneumoniae*, *Pseudomonas aeruginosa*). Mismanagement of breeding stallions (through frequent penile washings, or poor selection and upkeep of bedding) may convert the bacterial population on the surface of the penis from a mixed group of harmless bacteria to a population teeming with potential pathogens.[6] The external genitalia of some stallions harbor large numbers of these opportunistic bacteria despite the lack of evidence for precipitating factors. The organism that causes contagious equine metritis, *Taylorella equigenitalis*, represents the only known bacterium capable of consistently producing venereal disease in horses. The stallion serves as a lesionless carrier of this disease, harboring the bacteria on its external genitalia, with subsequent horizontal transmission to the mare's reproductive tract at breeding (see Chapter 14).[7-9]

Internal genital infections in the stallion are rare. Such infections usually are associated with hemospermia in addition to accumulations of leukocytes and the inciting bacteria in ejaculates.

Documentation of a bacterial infection depends on serial isolation of a pathogen, preferably in large numbers and in relatively pure culture. The exception is culture of *Taylorella equigenitalis*, for which a single isolation is considered diagnostic. To identify organisms on the exterior of the penis or prepuce, swabs of these areas should be obtained for bacteriologic culture before scrubbing the penis to obtain urethral swabs. Ideally, specimens should be retrieved from the fossa glandis, free portion of the penile body, and folds of the external prepuce to provide an overall perspective of the microbial population. The stallion should be placed near a mare in estrus to achieve an erection and facilitate procurement of samples.

If one is to gain insight into a possible infection of the internal genital tract, the penis and prepuce of the stallion should be washed meticulously with a surgical scrub before collection of appropriate samples for culture. Particular attention is given to removal of debris and organisms from the glans penis and fossa glandis. A thorough rinse should follow the scrub, and the procedure should be repeated twice (Fig 12). After the final rinse, the penis is dried thoroughly (Fig 13), allowing no contamination of the urethral orifice. Briskly rubbing the glans penis during the washing process usually stimulates volumi-

Figure 12. Washing the stallion's penis with surgical scrub, in preparation for collection of urethral cultures, should be followed by thorough rinsing with water. Particular attention should be given to removing soap from the fossa glandis. Note the stimulating effect of washing the penis, as evidenced by "belling" of the glans penis.

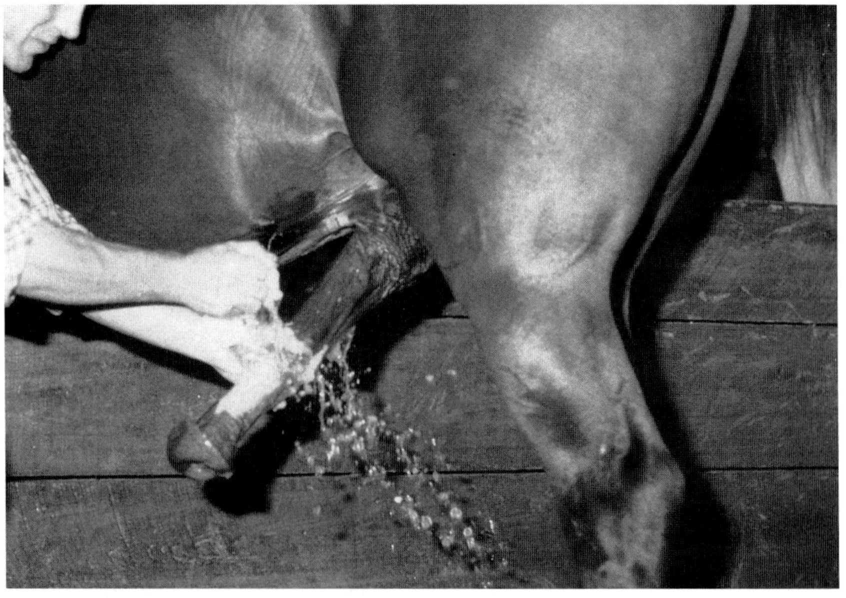

Figure 13. After the penis of the stallion is washed and rinsed, it should be thoroughly dried with clean disposable towels before attempting collection of urethral cultures. Care should be taken to avoid contamination of the urethral orifice during the drying process.

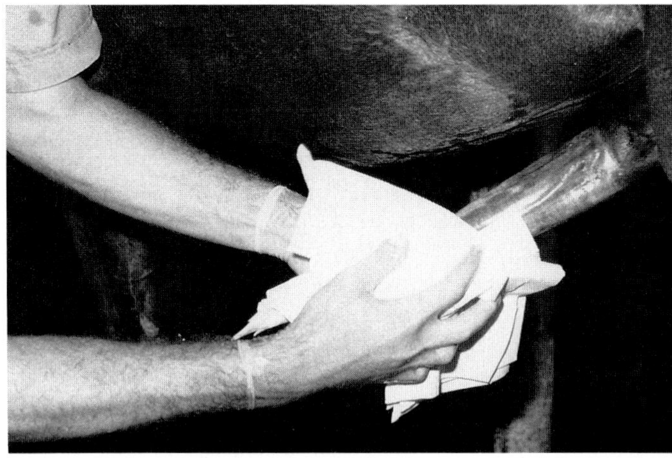

nous secretion of clear fluid (presperm fraction of ejaculate), originating from the urethral and/or bulbourethral glands, into the urethral lumen. This procedure helps remove any bacterial contaminants from the urethral lumen that may have gained access via the external urethral orifice. Some of this fluid may be collected for culture and cytologic examination if an infection of the urethra or bulbourethral glands is suspected. A cotton swab is inserted 3-5 cm into the urethra to procure a sample for bacterial culture before semen collection (preejaculation swab, Fig 14).

Semen then can be collected in an artificial vagina and a postejaculation urethral swab taken immediately upon removal of the penis from the artificial vagina; the urethral opening should not be contaminated before or during the swabbing process. Semen also can be sampled for bacteriologic culture. Collection of semen using an open-ended artificial vagina minimizes contamination of the penis with organisms still residing on the exterior of the penis during the semen collection process and, therefore, allows more meaningful interpretation of semen cultures (Fig 15). Vesicular gland fluid can be collected selectively for culture by first teasing the stallion vigorously during the penile washing process to distend the lumen of these bladder-like glands with secretions.

A 1 x 100-cm sterile catheter with an inflatable cuff then is passed into the urethra to the level of the seminal colliculus (origin of the excretory ducts of the vesicular glands), the cuff

Figure 14. To obtain a urethral culture, the distal tip of the glans penis is first deflected dorsally with a thumb to allow better exposure of the urethral orifice for swab insertion.

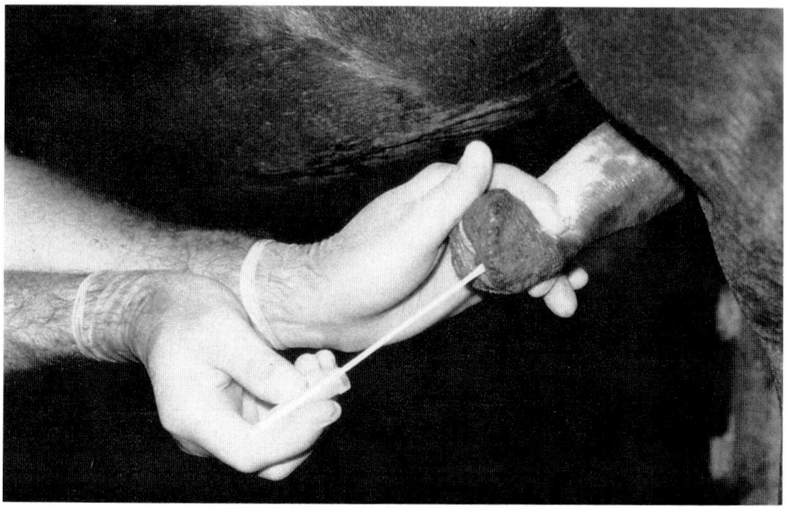

inflated, and the fluid in each vesicular gland expressed manually by palpation per rectum for collection and study.[8] Secretions from the prostate gland, ampullae and ductus deferens may be collected in the first jet of an ejaculate using an open-ended artificial vagina, as this fraction contains secretions primarily from these sites. Infections originating from the epidid-

Figure 15. Collection of semen with an open-ended artificial vagina effectively reduces contamination of semen with microorganisms on the surface of the penis. Semen can be collected using a funnel or urethral prosthetic device. (See Chapter 4 for more information regarding this semen-collection method.)

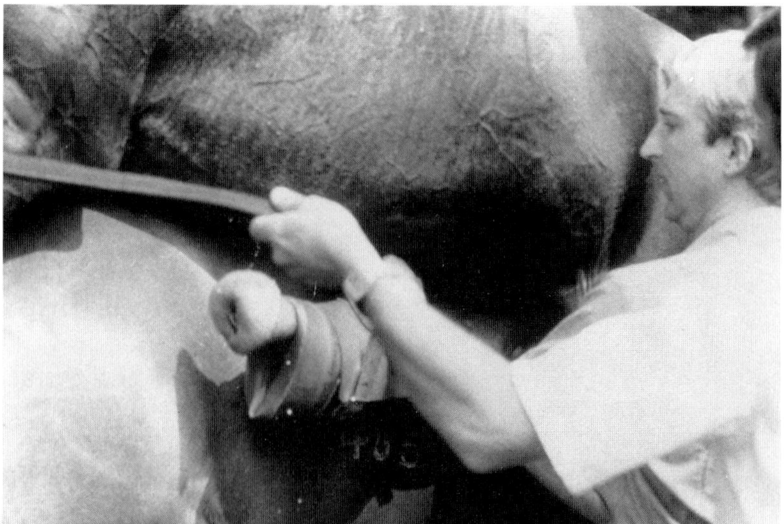

ymides or testes usually induce changes that are palpable through the scrotum. Additionally, the incriminating organism may be recoverable from the semen.

Viral Genital Infections

The 2 known venereal diseases attributed to viruses are coital exanthema, caused by equine herpesvirus-3, and togavirus-induced equine viral arteritis. Coital exanthema, diagnosed by physical examination, produces characteristic blisters on the penile body and prepuce that subsequently form pustules and ulcerations that resolve within 2-4 weeks (Fig 16). Clinical disease is self-limiting in the stallion, and fertility is not affected unless lesions are so painful as to interfere with breeding. Venereal transmission to mares is possible during the active stage of infection and results in similar lesions on the external genitalia of the mare.[11-14] Stallions can venereally transmit the disease before development of penile lesions. Chapter 14 contains more information on this disease.

The venereal mode of transmission is considered a major pathway for dissemination of equine viral arteritis, a disease associated with systemic illness and abortion. Once the acute phase of the disease has subsided, infected stallions can remain

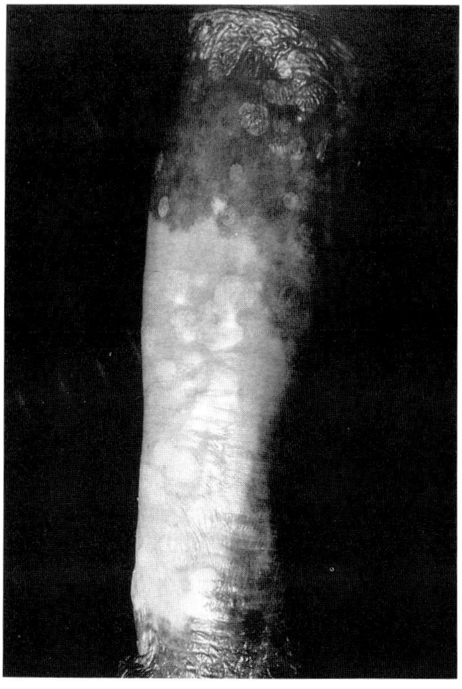

Figure 16. Lesions of coital exanthema on the penile body of a breeding stallion.

long-term asymptomatic carriers, with viral sequestration in the genital tract and shedding in the semen.[15] The venereal route appears to be the sole means of virus transmission from chronically infected stallions. Diagnosis of the disease in a stallion presumed to be a carrier is based on isolation of the causative virus from ejaculated semen or, alternatively, development of serum neutralization antibodies in seronegative mares that are bred to the suspect stallion.

Protozoal Genital Infections

Trypanosoma equiperdum, the causative organism of dourine, is the only protozoan known to produce venereal disease in horses. The disease, presently eliminated from the United States, is characterized initially by edematous swelling of the external genitalia, attendant mucopurulent discharge from the urethra, formation of 2- to 10-cm-diameter urticarial cutaneous plaques, and progressive emaciation, sometimes in conjunction with penile paralysis. Diagnosis is based on a complement-fixation test and isolation of trypanosomes from the urethral exudate, blood or urticarial plaques. Treatment is possible but generally impractical, and euthanasia is recommended.

Semen Collection

Accurate assessment of semen quality relies heavily on proper semen collection techniques. Ejaculated semen is very susceptible to environmental influences, so mishandling semen samples before evaluation negates their value for representing a stallion's innate fertility. Specific semen collection procedures, including artificial vagina selection and preparation, and use of a live mare or phantom mare as a mount, are outlined in Chapter 4. Once semen is collected, it should be taken promptly to a laboratory, avoiding injury to spermatozoa induced by sunlight, temperature shock, physical agitation or contact with various chemicals. Upon arrival at the laboratory, the semen should be placed in a 37 C incubator while awaiting examination (Fig 17).

Semen Evaluation

Workers involved with male fertility evaluation have long tried to develop laboratory methods of semen analysis that will deliver a precise estimate of spermatozoal fertilizing capacity in a given animal. Despite exhaustive attempts to find these elusive probes, no single semen characteristic evaluated has an absolute correlation to fertility. Nonetheless, a battery of semen quality tests of assumed scientific merit currently are incorporated into laboratory-based semen evaluations in an effort to predict stallion fertility. The aim of these tests is to bypass field fertility trials with their attendant drawbacks of expense and time consumption. A laboratory-based semen evaluation provides insight into the possible underlying cause of infertility in suspect stallions and, as such, may produce meaningful information on how to manage such a stallion to maximize fertility. Additionally, the examination can help management personnel determine the optimal number of mares that a stallion can breed effectively during a given breeding season.

To enhance the reliability of the examination, semen evaluation should be performed in a thorough, methodic manner by an experienced person in an adequately equipped laboratory. Both routine and in-depth diagnostic tests are available, so test selection must fit within the time and economic constraints of the stallion owner. Routine tests include gross evaluation of the sample, determination of semen volume and sperm concentration (to calculate total sperm number), pH determination, and assessment of spermatozoal motility and morphology. More involved tests include chemical analysis of semen plasma and

Figure 17. A semen laboratory should be equipped with an incubator, a heated stage for temporary holding of microscope slides, and a heated microscope stage so that spermatozoa can be consistently evaluated under optimal temperature conditions (37-38 C).

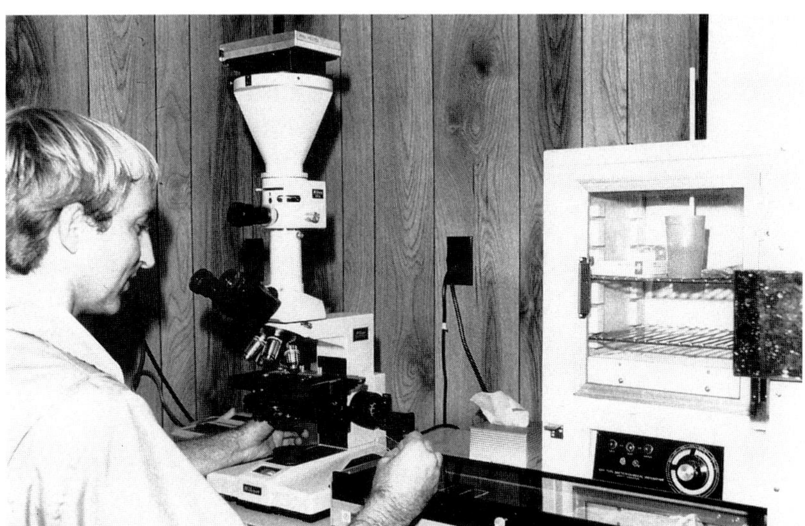

electron microscopic study of spermatozoal ultrastructure. The prohibitive costs associated with electron microscopic techniques limit their use to selected stallions.

Gross Evaluation

The gel is separated from the gel-free fraction of the ejaculate in the laboratory by aspiration if a filter was not placed in the artificial vagina to perform this function during semen collection. Filtration also is required to help remove extraneous debris, such as smegma, hair and dirt, from the gel-free semen. Volumes of gel and gel-free semen are then measured, and the color and consistency of the sample noted. Though volume itself is not important to fertility, it is used in calculation of total sperm number in an ejaculate. Consequently, accurate measurement of volume is essential. Semen volume can be increased by excessive precopulatory teasing, but the total sperm number in such ejaculates remains unchanged.[16] Semen volume also is affected by season, with smaller volumes produced in the winter months as compared to summer months.[17] The gel-free portion of an ejaculate contains the majority of spermatozoa, so the gel fraction usually is discarded after its volume is recorded without measurement of its sperm content. Gross evaluation of a semen sample provides a rough estimate of its sperm concentration and permits detection of color changes that may be associated with blood, urine or purulent material in the ejaculate.

Spermatozoal Concentration

Accurate measurement of sperm concentration is critical because total sperm number in an ejaculate is derived by multiplying sperm concentration and semen volume. An imprecise estimate of sperm concentration produces a corresponding inaccurate calculation of sperm number in an ejaculate. Such errors can produce misleading judgments and should be avoided. Sperm concentration of the gel-free semen can be determined using a hemacytometer (Fig 18). This method of measurement is time-consuming and can be replaced with a spectrophotometer (Fig 19) or densimeter (Fig 20) that is properly calibrated using hemacytometer measurements to establish a standard curve.[1,18] These instruments allow faster measurement of sperm concentration, and their accuracy is good if sperm concentration is not exceedingly high or low, and the ejaculate is free of debris, blood, purulent material or premature germ cells (*eg,* spermato-

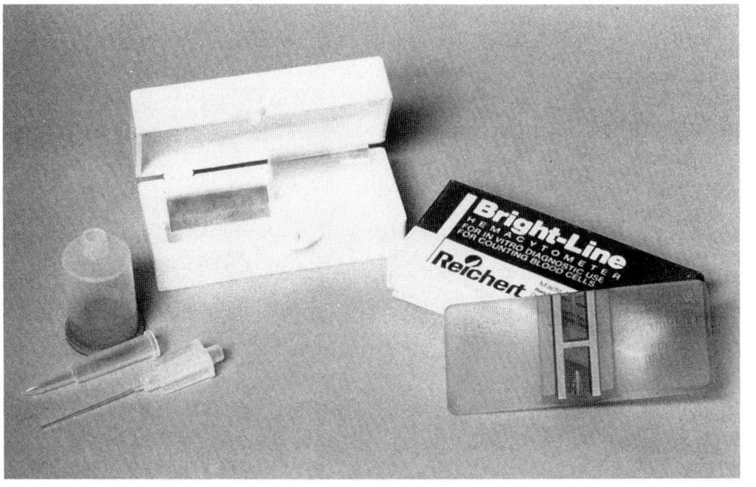

Figure 18. Hemacytometer (American Optical, South Bridge, MA) and dilution reservoir (WBC Unopette: Becton-Dickinson, Rutherford, NJ) with capillary pipettes (20 μl) for estimation of spermatozoal concentration in semen.

cytes). Mixing semen with an extender before measuring spermatozoal concentration also produces erroneous measurements with a spectrophotometer or densimeter if the extender is not optically clear. Dilution factors must be taken into account when estimating sperm concentration, as semen always is diluted before spermatozoal concentration is measured.

Total sperm number, calculated from sperm concentration and semen volume, is probably one of the more important measurements used in estimating a stallion's fertility. Total sperm number per ejaculate is subject to seasonal variation but also is affected by numerous other factors, including frequency of ejaculation, age, testicular size, size of extragonadal sperm reserves and various forms of reproductive disease.[17]

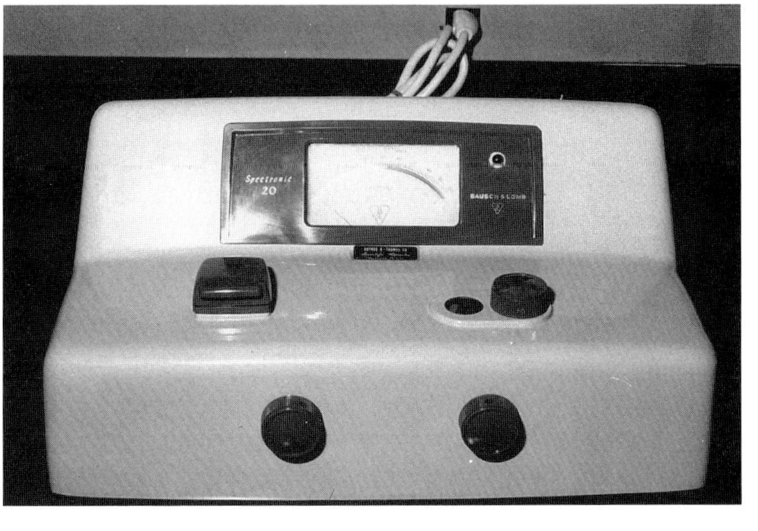

Figure 19. A spectrophotometer can often be used to accurately measure spermatozoal concentration in stallion semen, provided the instrument is properly calibrated using hemacytometer counts. Transmission is read after setting light wavelength at 550 nm.

Figure 20. A densimeter (with accessories) is commercially available (Animal Reproduction Systems, Chino, CA) for estimation of spermatozoal concentration in stallion semen.

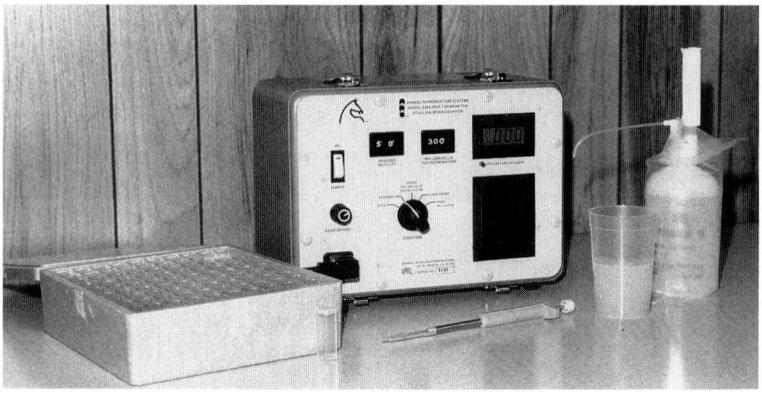

pH Determination

The pH of gel-free semen should be determined using a properly calibrated pH meter, preferably within an hour after semen collection. Measurements obtained using pH paper are much less precise than those derived with a meter, so this method of pH determination should be used only as a last resort. The pH of normal semen is slightly basic, with a reported range of 7.2-7.7.[1,17] Season of the year, frequency of ejaculation, and spermatozoal concentration can affect the pH of normal stallion semen. Abnormally high semen pH can be associated with contamination of the ejaculate by urine or soap, or with inflammatory lesions of the internal genital tract.

Spermatozoal Motility

Spermatozoal motility reflects the viability of a sperm population. A positive relationship between spermatozoal motility and fertilizing capacity has been demonstrated in many species, though this correlation cannot be considered absolute. Several different instruments and methods have been developed for objective assessment of equine spermatozoal motility, including time-lapse photomicrography (Fig 21), frame-by-frame playback videomicrography, spectophotometry, and computerized analysis (Fig 22), but these methods are usually too tedious or expensive to be incorporated into routine procedures for semen evaluation.[19-25] Subjective analysis of spermatozoal motility by visual estimation, using a microscope equipped with phase-contrast optics and a heated stage, is acceptable when personnel are experienced in analysis of spermatozoal motility.

Figure 21. One-second time-lapse photomicrograph of stallion semen, demonstrating immotile spermatozoa (solid arrows) and "tracks" of motile spermatozoa (open arrows).

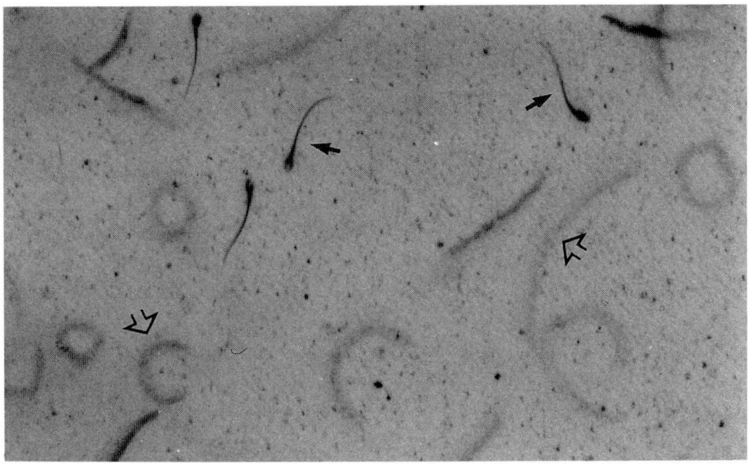

Visual assessment of spermatozoal motility should include gross or total motility (percentage of spermatozoa exhibiting motility of any form), progressive motility (percentage of spermatozoa which are progressively motile), and spermatozoal velocity (on an arbitrary scale of 0 to 4 or 5). Progressive spermatozoal motility generally is considered the most credible gauge of spermatozoal motion for predicting the fertilizing capacity of a semen sample.

Both initial spermatozoal motility and longevity of spermatozoal motility should be assessed and recorded. It is best to estimate initial spermatozoal motility of raw (undiluted) semen

Figure 22. Commercially available computerized system for objective analysis of spermatozoal motility.

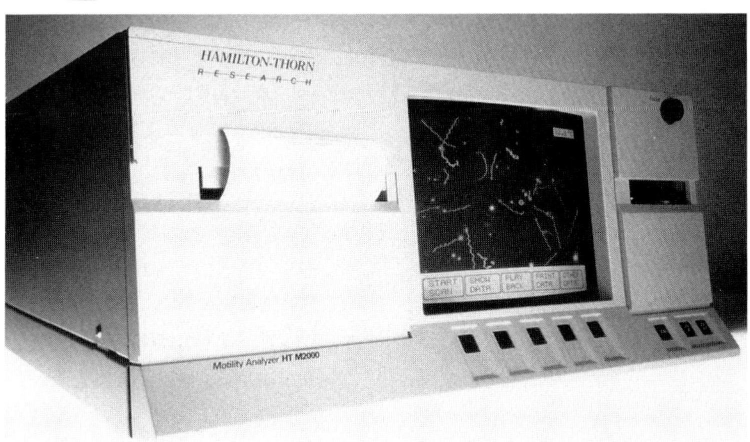

samples as a control for testing possible detrimental effects of seminal extenders on spermatozoal motility. However, the accuracy and repeatability of the spermatozoal motility evaluation can be improved markedly by diluting the semen in an appropriate extender before analysis. Warmed (37 C) nonfat dry milk-glucose extender (Table 1) serves this purpose well, as it supports spermatozoal motility and does not interfere with microscopic visualization of the spermatozoa. To standardize the spermatozoal motility testing protocol, all semen samples should be diluted to a specific concentration (*ie,* 25 x 10^6 sperm/ml) with extender before analysis.

Longevity of spermatozoal motility can be determined on raw semen samples stored at room temperature (20-25 C) and on samples diluted in extender (preferably to a final sperm concentration of 25 x 10^6 sperm/ml) and stored at room temperature or refrigerated (4-5 C). Longevity of spermatozoal motility is enhanced by semen dilution with extender and refrigerated storage.[26,27]

The relationship between spermatozoal motility characteristics and male fertility has been a controversial issue. The biologic relevance of spermatozoal motility to fertilizing capacity can probably be more adequately and objectively addressed now

Table 1. Semen extender formulations.

Non-Fat Dry Skin Milk (NFDSM)-Glucose Extender I

NFDSM	2.4 g
Glucose	4.9 g
Penicillin, crystalline	150,000 units
Streptomycin, crystalline	150,000 μg
Deionized H_2O	qs 100 ml

Non-Fat Dry Skim Milk (NFDSM)-Glucose Extender II

NFDSM	2.4 g
Glucose	4.9 g
Gentamicin sulfate (reagent grade)	100 mg
8.4% $NaHCO_3$	2 ml
Deionized H_2O	92 ml

(Mix liquids before adding NFDSM or the acidity of the antibiotic will curdle the milk)

Cream Gel Extender

1. Dissolve 1.3 g unflavored Knox gelatin in 10 ml sterile distilled water. Sterilize.
2. Heat hal & half cream in a double boiler to 92-95 C for 2-4 minutes. Remove film from surface.
3. Mix gelatin solution with 90 ml heated half & half cream (100 ml total volume). Cool.
4. Add penicillin (100,000 units), streptomycin (100,000 μg) and polymixin B sulfate (20,000 units).

Heated Skim Milk Extender

1. Heat 100 ml nonfortified skim milk to 92-95 C for 10 minutes in a double boiler. Cool.
2. Add polymixin B sulfate (100,000 units).

because of the advent of computerized sperm-motility analyzers. Studies in bulls suggest that objective measures of spermatozoal motility are more reliable than visual estimates for predicting fertility.[28,29] However, conflicting results have been obtained using stallion spermatozoa.[30] In the latter study, visual determination of percent spermatozoal motility was more highly correlated with fertility than other semen characteristics, such as percent of morphologically normal sperm, spermatozoal concentration, mean spermatozoal velocity or mean angular head displacement.[30]

Spermatozoal Morphology

The morphology or structure of spermatozoa is typically examined with a light microscope at 1000X magnification. Standard bright-field microscope optics can be used to examine air-dried semen smears, provided appropriate stains are used in slide preparation. Specific sperm stains include those developed by Williams and Casarett. General-purpose cellular stains (*eg,* Wright's, Giemsa, hematoxylin-eosin) also have been used to accent both germinal and somatic cells in semen smears. Background stains (*eg,* eosin-nigrosin, India ink) probably are the most widely used stains because of their ease of use. Visualization of sperm structural detail can be enhanced by fixing the cells in buffered formol-saline or buffered glutaraldehyde solution, then viewing the unstained cells as a wet mount with either phase-contrast or differential interference-contrast microscopy. Sperm fixation also is simplified by this method and the incidence of artifactual changes is reduced in comparison with stained smears.

At least 200 spermatozoa should be evaluated for evidence of morphologic defects. The type and incidence of each defect should be recorded (Figs 23-29). Abnormalities in spermatozoal morphology traditionally have been classified as primary, secondary or tertiary. Primary abnormalities are considered to be associated with a defect in spermatogenesis and, therefore, are of testicular origin. Secondary abnormalities are created in the excurrent duct system. Tertiary abnormalities, as opposed to the previous 2 types, develop *in vitro* as a result of improper semen collection or handling procedures.

The current trend is to record the numbers of specific morphologic defects, such as knobbed acrosomes, proximal protoplasmic droplets, swollen midpieces and coiled tails. This method of

Figure 23. Phase-contrast micrograph of a stallion spermatozoan with normal morphology. Refer to Chapter 1 for anatomy of spermatozoa.

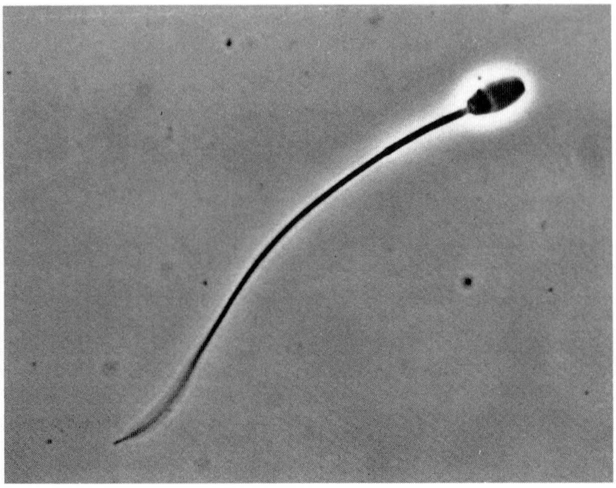

Figure 24. Phase-contrast micrograph of a stallion spermatozoan with an acrosomal defect (arrow).

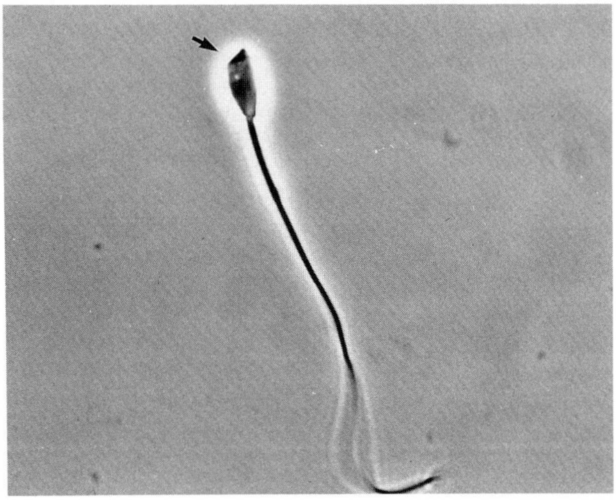

Figure 25. Phase-contrast micrograph of stallion spermatozoa with separated heads and flagella. Note the abnormal flagellar morphology.

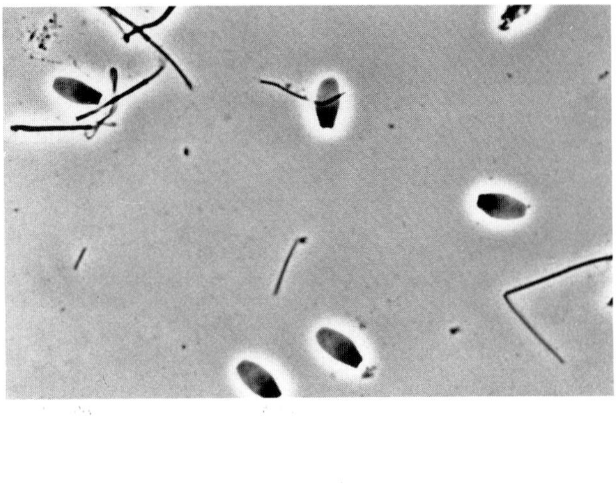

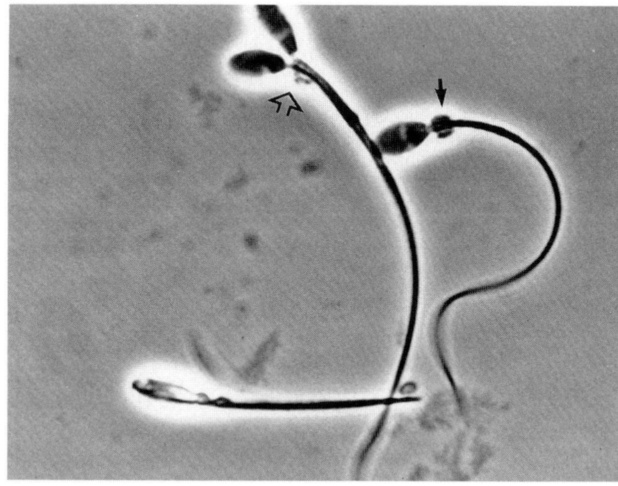

Figure 26. Phase-contrast micrograph of a stallion spermatozoan with a proximal cytoplasmic droplet (solid arrow), and another spermatozoan with 2 heads, a proximal cytoplasmic droplet, and a malformed midpiece (open arrow). Note the degenerative spermatozoan at the bottom of the field.

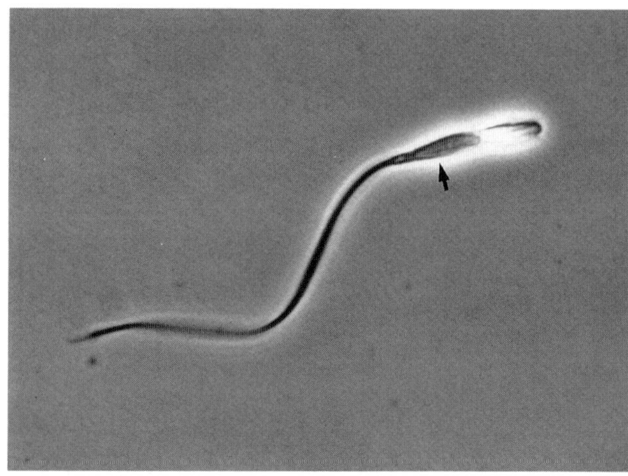

Figure 27. Phase-contrast micrograph of a stallion spermatozoan with a malformed midpiece (arrow).

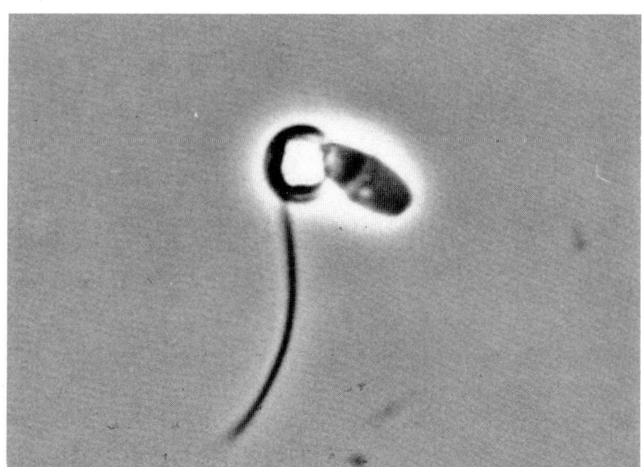

Figure 28. Phase-contrast micrograph of a stallion spermatozoan with a coiled flagellum.

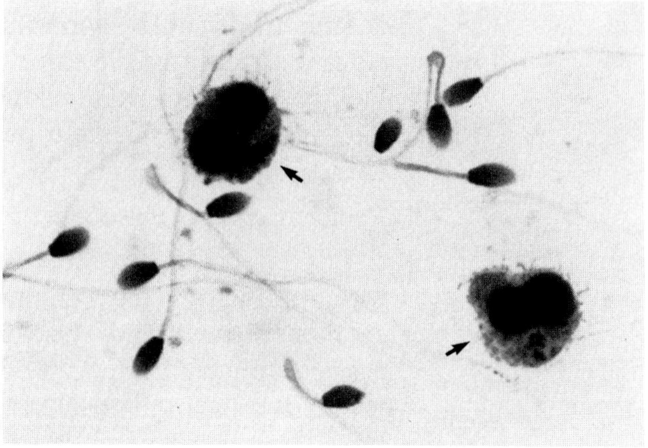

Figure 29. Photomicrograph of stallion semen containing premature (round) germ cells (arrows) (hematoxylin & eosin stain).

classification is considered superior to the traditional system because it reveals more specific information regarding a population of sperm while avoiding erroneous assumptions about the origin of these defects. The origin of some spermatozoal morphologic defects is unknown. Additionally, some morphologic abnormalities like detached heads can be primary, secondary or tertiary in nature, thereby introducing the possibility of error when using this classification system exclusively.

The value of spermatozoal morphology studies in predicting the fertility of a stallion is met with a degree of skepticism, as some stallions can have many sperm abnormalities yet display normal fertility. Conversely, some stallions exhibit decreased fertility even though the percentage of morphologically normal sperm in their ejaculates is high (based on light microscopic studies). It is assumed that morphologically abnormal sperm do not exert a negative influence on normal sperm. Therefore, the total number of morphologically normal sperm in ejaculates may provide more information regarding the fertility of a stallion than the percentage or absolute number of morphologically abnormal sperm.[1]

Chemical Analysis of Seminal Plasma

The chemical composition of equine seminal plasma has been reported, but the relationship of its various components to sperm fertilizing capacity has not been established. One study revealed that electrolyte concentration, protein concentration and specific protein composition of seminal plasma do not provide good predictive information regarding postthaw motility of cryopreserved spermatozoa.[31] Our understanding of the biochemistry of equine seminal plasma is too rudimentary to consider it a meaningful part of a breeding soundness examination. Isolation of chemical markers in seminal plasma is an important diagnostic aid for some types in infertility in men.[32]

Transmission Electron Microscopy

Light microscopy affords limited magnification and, therefore, limited appraisal of spermatozoal morphology. This obstacle can be overcome by scanning and/or transmission electron microscopic techniques. Though expensive, these 2 microscopic methods offer high-resolution detail and permit closer examination of spermatozoal morphology. Subtle morphologic alterations, inapparent through light microscopy, often can be identified easily by electron microscopic analysis. Scanning electron microscopy offers 3-dimensional visualization of entire spermatozoa (Fig 30). Transmission electron microscopy permits cross-sectional viewing of spermatozoa and reveals their ultrastructure in detail (Fig 31). Both electron microscopic techniques may be economically justifiable diagnostic aids in selected circumstances.

Urethral Endoscopy

Urethral endoscopy generally is reserved for use in patients with hemospermia or those with suspected specific urethral, bladder or vesicular-gland lesions. Use of a flexible fibroscope or

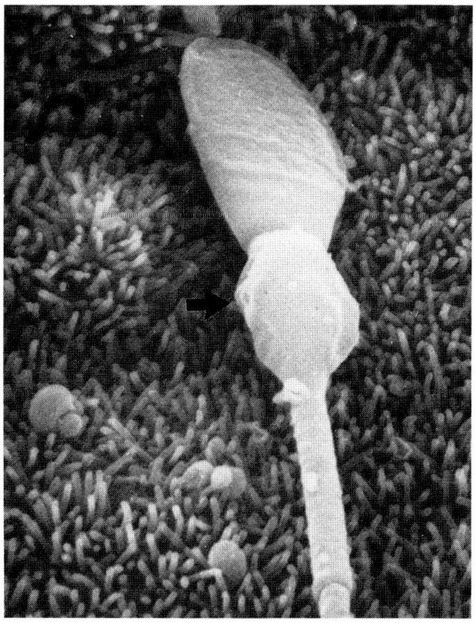

Figure 30. Scanning electron micrograph of a spermatozoan from an efferent ductule.[31] Note the proximal cytoplasmic droplet (arrow) components.

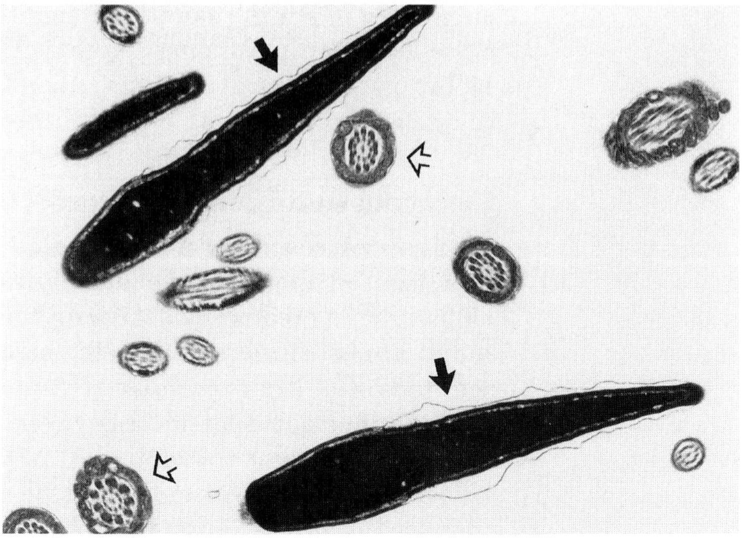

Figure 31. Transmission electron micrograph of a stallion spermatozoan, demonstrating both head (solid arrow) and flagellar (open arrow) components.

video endoscope is recommended because it easily negotiates the ischial arch when passed via the urethral orifice, avoiding the need for subischial urethrotomy (Fig 32). To permit easy passage through the urethral lumen, the insertion tube should have a maximum outside diameter of 10 mm. A working length of 100 cm permits access to the bladder lumen if the penis is not fully erect. Proper preoperative disinfection of equipment is critical. Endoscopic examination of the urethra and bladder may reveal mural and luminal abnormalities undetectable by other means. Urethral pathologic entities detectable by endoscopic examination include inflammation, ulcerations, lacerations, fistulae,

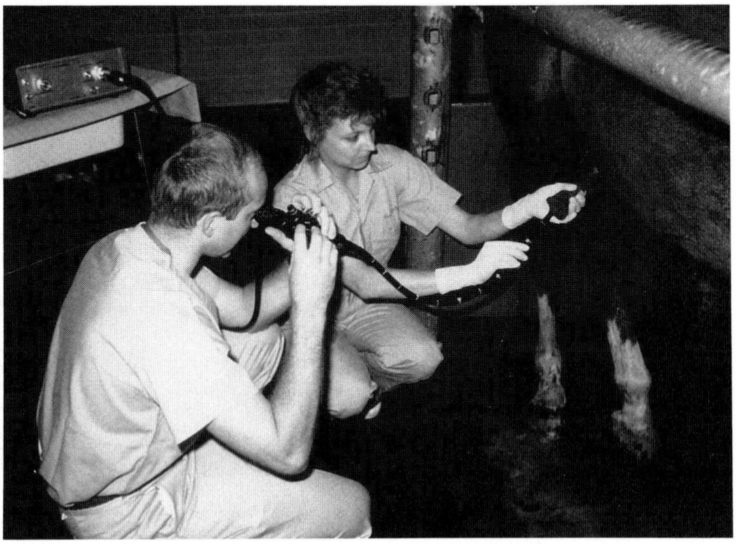

Figure 32. A flexible endoscope being passed into the urethra of a stallion sedated with xylazine.

strictures, growths, calculi and foreign bodies.[33] Cystitis, bladder calculi, and bladder tumors also may be revealed, as may lesions of vesicular adenitis.[34,35]

Ultrasonography

Though ultrasonography has been used to evaluate various abnormalities of the stallion genital tract, reports of this technique are scarce. Ultrasonography adds a new dimension to diagnostics because it permits noninvasive evaluation of otherwise inaccessible tissues. Its applications are numerous and include obtaining accurate testicular measurements (Fig 33), detection/assessment of intratesticular masses, evaluation of intrascrotal fluid accumulations (Fig 34) and examination of the cavernous spaces of the penis (Fig 35).[3,36] Ultrasonography is a useful adjunct to examinations made per rectum (*eg,* for evaluation of the accessory genital glands, Figs 36-39) or abdominal/inguinal exploration for an undescended testis in a suspected cryptorchid.[37,38]

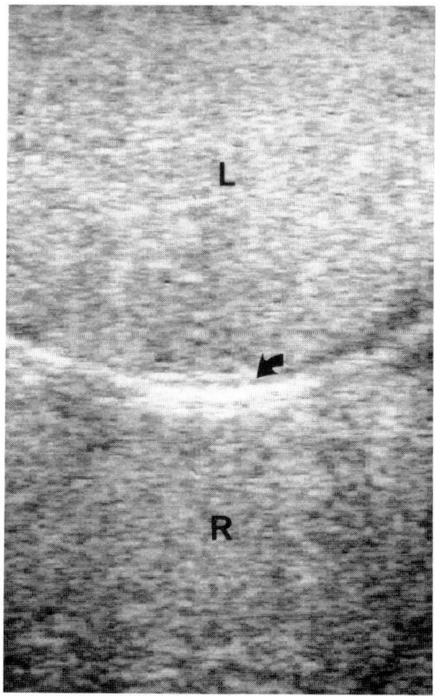

Figure 33. Ultrasonic image of the scrotal contents of a stallion in a left-to-right direction using a linear-array 5-mHz transducer held vertically. The left testis (L) width can be measured. The right testis (R) is only partially within the ultrasound field. A distinct scrotal septum (arrow) can be visualized.

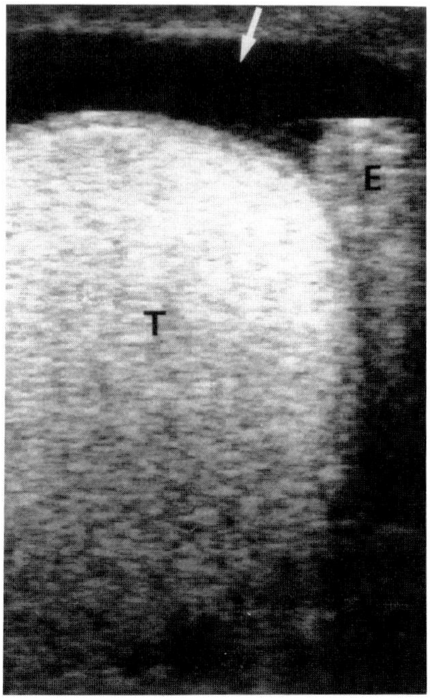

Figure 34. Ultrasonic image of the scrotal contents of a stallion with a hydrocele. Note the testicular parenchyma (T), cauda epididymidis (E) and anechoic fluid accumulation within the vaginal space (arrow).

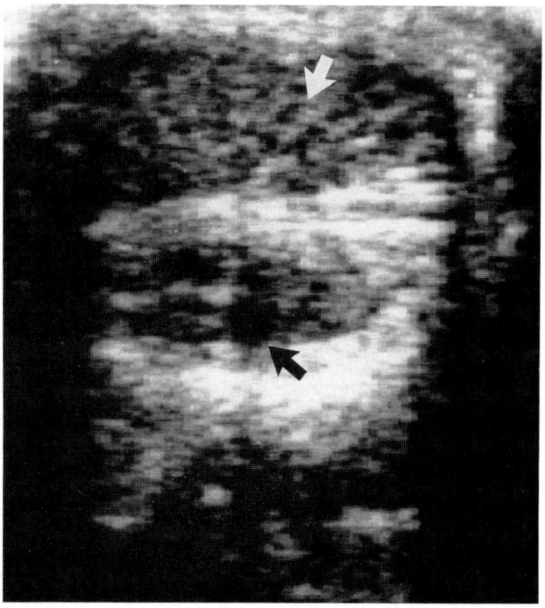

Figure 35. Ultrasonic image of the penile body of a stallion, revealing the corpus cavernosum penis (white arrow) and the urethral lumen, surrounded by the corpus spongiosum penis (black arrow).

Radiography

Radiographic techniques have been used effectively in stallions to evaluate patency of the urethra and ductus deferens. Contrast or double-contrast methods of radiography also may be useful for evaluation of the corpus cavernosum penis. Urethrograms (contrast and double-contrast radiography of the urethral lumen) have been used to diagnose urethral strictures and ulcerations, space-occupying lesions and urethral fistulae.[33,39] Contrast radiography has been used to detect bilateral luminal obstructions of the ductus deferens causing azoospermia.[40] Under general anesthesia, each ductus deferens was catheterized near its origin at the epididymal tail, contrast medium was injected toward the urethral opening, and radiographs made to locate the obstruction. Saline was injected after the contrast medium to relieve accumulations of spermatozoa obstructing the lumina. Contrast radiographic study of the corpus cavernosum penis also may be useful to evaluate patency of this cavernous space following chronic penile paralysis or priapism.

Chromosomal Analysis

Cytogenetics has become a popular area of clinical reproduction in stallions. Cause of infertility and reduced fertility often is not disclosed by conventional diagnostic methods; therefore, investigators are relying more heavily on chromosomal studies

Figure 36. Ultrasonic image of the pelvic urethra (open arrow) and surrounding stratum cavernosum (solid arrows) of a stallion, as viewed transrectally using a 5-mHz transverse linear-array transducer.

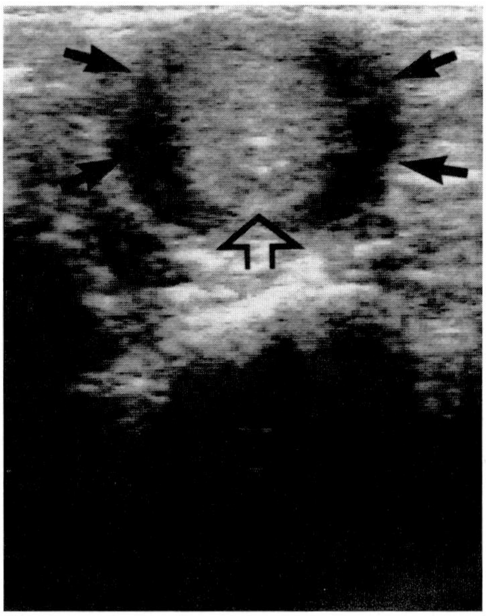

Figure 37. Ultrasonic image of the bulbourethral glands (B) and urethra (arrows) of a stallion, as viewed transrectally using a 5-mHz tranverse linear-array transducer.

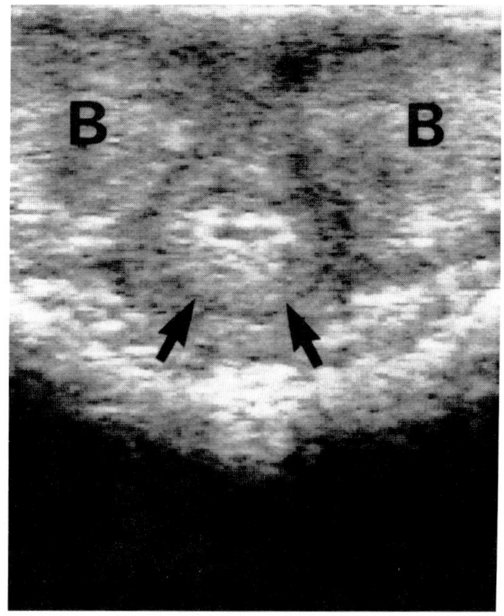

Figure 38. Ultrasonic image of the right prostatic lobe (arrows) of a stallion, as viewed transrectally using a 5-mHz transverse linear-array transducer.

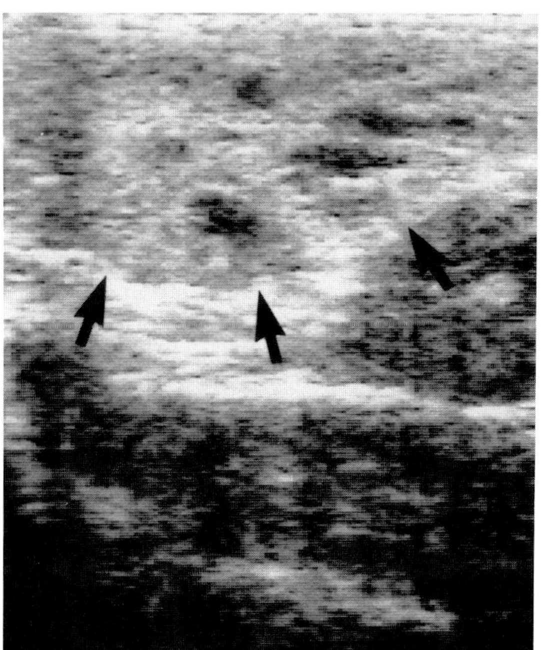

Figure 39. Ultrasonic image of the left vesicular gland (white arrow) and ampulla (black arrow) of a stallion, as viewed transrectally using a 5-mHz transverse linear-array transducer. The stallion was sexually stimulated before examination to facilitate partial dilation of the vesicular-gland lumen with anechoic secretions.

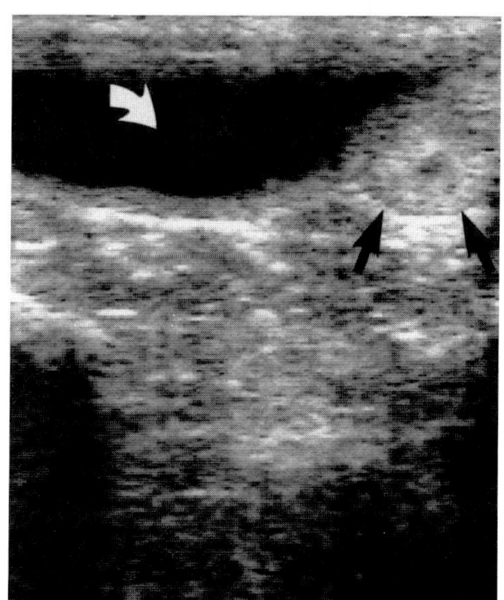

to isolate genetically derived causes for such problems. Karyotyping permits scrutiny for numeric and/ or structural changes in chromosome composition that could affect reproductive performance. This diagnostic technique shows great promise and soon may become an established tool for determining origin and pathogenesis of some types of infertility presently unresolved.[41-43] These procedures may become a required part of reproductive soundness exams for prospective breeding stallions.

A flow cytometric procedure has been developed to evaluate the structural integrity of sperm chromatin. The potential of the sperm-chromatin structure assay for predicting fertility has been evaluated in bulls, with encouraging results.[44]

Hormonal Analysis

An endocrine basis for reproductive malfunction in stallions has not been firmly established. An exception is administration of exogenous testosterone or anabolic steroids, both of which adversely affect spermatogenesis. It has been postulated that an abnormally high plasma concentration of follicle-stimulating hormone, sometimes with by a high plasma concentration of luteinizing hormone, indicates testicular degeneration in older stallions. Conversely, a low plasma luteinizing hormone concentration has been associated with poor fertility in young stallions.[45] Some investigators contend that low libido or impotence in stallions may be related to low plasma concentrations of luteinizing hormone and estradiol-17β, in the presence of normal testosterone levels.[46] Contradictory reports indicate that stallions with low plasma concentrations of luteinizing hormone and estradiol-17β can have excellent libido and semen quality.[47]

Obviously, the relationship of hormonal levels to specific reproductive abnormalities of the stallion is not completely understood, so hormonal assays cannot usually be considered diagnostically dependable. One unrefuted application of a hormonal assay is diagnosis of cryptorchidism in horses without scrotal testes, by measuring concentrations of blood testosterone and/or estrogens (see Chapter 8).

Intraepididymal Aspiration of Spermatozoa

Percutaneous aspiration of sperm from the epididymal tail has been used to differentiate azoospermia due to aspermatogenesis from azoospermia associated with an ejaculatory disturbance.[16] The effect of this procedure on reproductive performance has not been critically tested, so it should only be used diagnostically as a last resort. Local adhesions or sperm granulomas could develop secondary to epididymal aspiration and lead to interference with sperm passage through the epididymal tail. Formation of antisperm antibodies is another possible sequela.

Testicular Biopsy

Though testicular biopsy has been recommended by some investigators as an innocuous diagnostic procedure for stallion infertility, it cannot be endorsed on a routine basis.[48] More critical study of the potential adverse effects of this diagnostic method is required before it can be recommended. Postoperative complications, such as sperm granuloma formation or intratesticular hemorrhage and attendant increase in intratesticular pressure, could cause irreparable interference with spermatogenesis.

Aspiration biopsy is potentially less damaging than a punch biopsy but does not offer information regarding spermatogenesis. Aspiration biopsy may help differentiate causes of testicular enlargement, such as neoplasia, trauma or septic orchitis. The technique can be performed with the horse standing; local anesthesia of the scrotum is unnecessary. A 23- or 25-ga needle is inserted into the testicular parenchyma, and a 12-ml syringe is attached to the needle and its plunger withdrawn. The needle is redirected at several different angles without exiting the parenchyma. The plunger is then gently released, and the needle is pulled from the testicle. Aspirated material is expelled onto a slide, gently smeared, dried and stained. An experienced cytologist should examine the slide because normally developing spermatocytes are easily mistaken for neoplastic cells.

Other Diagnostic Tests

Glass wool-Sephadex filters have been used to help predict the fertilizing capacity of fresh or frozen/thawed stallion semen.[49] To perform this test, a small aliquot of semen is placed over a short column of glass wool and Sephadex, and then is flushed with a standard volume of buffer. The percentage of spermatozoa passing through the filter is then calculated using a hemacytometer counting chamber. The filter is thought to trap immotile, acrosome-damaged and capacitated spermatozoa.

Recovery of stallion spermatozoa from this filter system was more highly correlated with fertility than was objective assessment of spermatozoal motility.[49]

Evaluation of serum, semen plasma and spermatozoa for antisperm antibodies may evolve as a useful diagnostic test in stallions with idiopathic infertility.[50] The methodology and utility of this assay are under investigation.

Interpreting Examination Findings

An inherent drawback of a stallion fertility (or breeding soundness) examination is imprecision due to the biologic nature of the specimen under consideration. Though the examination process has scientific merit, precision is impossible. In addition, factors other than innate stallion fertility, including mare fertility and management procedures, markedly influence pregnancy and foaling rates for a given stallion, and often are difficult to control or assess.

The purpose of a fertility examination is to *estimate* a stallion's capability as a sire. Ideally, the testing process should produce sufficient information about a stallion to permit approximation of the number of mares to which that stallion can safely be booked during a breeding season. An indispensable ingredient in this formulation is the stallion's estimated daily sperm output. Numerous other factors also must be considered before a reasonable judgment can be made about a "stallion book" (see Chapter 3).

Stallions typically are classified as satisfactory, questionable or unsatisfactory breeding prospects. The categorizations are usually based on a stallion's ability to achieve a seemingly low seasonal pregnancy rate of 60%, but this percentage coincides with conditions for payment of fertility insurance the first year that insured stallions stand at stud. This pregnancy rate assumes that the stallion breeds a standard number of mares (*eg,* 40-45 mares by natural service or 120-140 mares by artificial insemination) during a typical breeding season of 135-150 days. An additional stipulation is that the stallion is bred to mares of normal fertility under good management conditions. Specific criteria that must be met before a prospective breeding stallion can be appropriately classified are discussed in depth in the Society for Theriogenology's *Manual for Clinical Fertility Evaluation of the Stallion.*[1] The reader should refer to this official manual for a thorough discussion of the subject.

In general, to be classified as a satisfactory breeding prospect, a stallion must be free of undesirable potentially heritable defects, behavioral disorders or transmissible diseases (venereal or otherwise); possess no physical traits that would interfere with mating ability, semen quality or spermatozoal output; and ejaculate $\geq 1 \times 10^9$ progressively motile, morphologically normal spermatozoa in the second of 2 ejaculates collected 1 hour apart following 1 week of sexual rest.

References

1. Kenney RM *et al: Manual for Clinical Fertility Evaluation of the Stallion.* Soc for Theriogenol, Hastings, NE, 1983.

2. Thompson DL *et al:* Testicular measurements and reproductive characteristics in stallions. *J Reprod Fertil* (Suppl) 27:13-17, 1979.

3. Love CC *et al:* Evaluation of measures taken by ultrasonography and calipers to estimate testicular volume and predict daily sperm output in the stallion. *Proc Intl Symp Equine Reprod,* 1990. pp 50-51.

4. Pickett BW *et al:* Reproductive physiology of the stallion. VI. Seminal and behavioral characteristics. *J Anim Sci* 43:617-624, 1976.

5. Clay CM *et al:* Influences of season and artificial photoperiod on stallions: testicular size, seminal characteristics and sexual behavior. *J Anim Sci* 64:517-525, 1987.

6. Bowen JM *et al:* Effects of washing on the bacterial flora of the stallion's penis. *J Reprod Fertil* 32:41-45, 1982.

7. Powell DG, in Morrow DA: *Current Therapy in Theriogenology 2.* Saunders, Philadelphia, 1986. pp 786-792.

8. Powell DG and Whitwell K: The epidemiology of contagious equine metritis (CEM) in England 1977-1978. *J Reprod Fertil* 27:331-335, 1979.

9. Timoney PJ: Isolation of the contagious equine metritis organism from colts and fillies in the United Kingdom and Ireland. *Vet Record* 111:478-482, 1982.

10. Cooper WC: Methods of determining the site of bacterial infections in the stallion reproductive tract. *Proc Ann Mtg Soc Theriogenol,* 1979. pp 1-4.

11. Krogsrud J and Onstad O: Equine coital exanthema: isolation of a virus and transmission experiments. *Acta Vet Scand* 12:1-14, 1971.

12. Pascoe RR: The effect of equine coital exanthema on the fertility of mares covered by stallions exhibiting the clinical disease. *Aust Vet J* 57:111-114, 1981.

13. Bitsch V: Cases of equine coital exanthema in Denmark. *Acta Vet Scand* 13:281-283, 1972.

14. Pascoe RR and Bagust TJ: Coital exanthema in stallions. *J Reprod Fertil* 23:147-150, 1975.

15. Timoney PJ *et al:* The carrier state in equine arteritis virus infection in the stallion with specific emphasis on the venereal mode of virus transmission. *J Reprod Fertil* 35:95-102, 1987.

16. Pickett BW *et al: Normal and Abnormal Sexual Behavior of the Equine Male.* Colorado State University Exp Sta Anim Reprod Lab Gen Series Bull 1004, 1981. pp 3-25.

17. Pickett BW *et al: Management of the Stallion for Maximum Reproductive Efficiency* - II. Colorado State University Exp Sta Anim Reprod Lab Gen Series Bull 05, 1989. pp 39-120.

18. Pickett BW *et al: Procedures for Collection, Evaluation and Utilization of Stallion Semen for Artificial Insemination.* Colorado State University Exp Sta Anim Reprod Lab Gen Series Bull 04, 1987. pp 11-26.

19. Van Huffel XM *et al:* Photomicrographic evaluation of stallion spermatozoal motility characteristics. *Am J Vet Res* 46:1272-1275.

20. Palmer E: Personal communication, 1984.

21. Jasko DJ *et al:* A spectrophotometric procedure for the determination of objective measurements of equine spermatozoan motility. *Theriogenology* 31:945-954, 1989.

22. Amann RP: Computerized evaluation of stallion spermatozoa. *Proc Ann Mtg AAEP,* 1987. pp 453-473.

23. Jasko DJ *et al:* Objective analysis of stallion sperm motility. *Theriogenology* 30:1159-1167, 1988.

24. Blach EL *et al:* Changes in quality of stallion spermatozoa during cryopreservation: Plasma membrane integrity and motion characteristics. *Theriogenology* 31:283-298.

25. Varner DD *et al:* Use of a computerized system for evaluation of equine spermatozoal motility. *Am J Vet Res,* accepted for publication, 1990.

26. Varner DD *et al:* Effects of semen fractionation and dilution ratio on equine spermatozoal motility parameters. *Theriogenology* 28:709-723, 1987.

27. Varner, DD *et al:* Effects of cooling rate and storage temperature on equine spermatozoal motility parameters. *Theriogenology* 29:1043-1054, 1989.

28. Budsworth PR *et al:* Relationships between computerized measurements of motion of frozen-thawed bull spermatozoa and fertility. *J Androl* 9:41-54, 1988.

29. Budsworth PR *et al:* A microcomputer-photographic method for evaluation of motility and velocity of bull sperm. *J Dairy Sci* 70:1927-1936, 1987.

30: Jasko DJ *et al:* Determinations of stallion semen quality and their relationship with fertility. *Proc Intl Symp Equine Reprod,* 1990. pp 206-207.

31. Amann RP *et al:* Proteins in stallion seminal plasma. *J Reprod Fertil* (Suppl) 35:113-120, 1987.

32. Wetterauer U: Recommended biochemical markers for routine semen analysis. *Urol Res* 14:241-246, 1986.

33. Voss JL and Pickett BW: Diagnosis and treatment of haemospermia in the stallion. *J Reprod Fertil* 23:151-154, 1975.

34. Sullins KE and Traub-Dargatz JL: Endoscopic anatomy of the equine urinary tract. *Compend Cont Ed Pract Vet* 6:S663-S668, 1984

35. Varner DD, unpublished observations, 1990.

36. Blanchard TL *et al:* Priapism in a stallion with generalized melanosarcoma. *JAVMA,* in press, 1990.

37. Little TV and Woods GL: Ultrasonography of accessory genital glands in the stallion. *J Reprod Fertil* 35:87-94, 1987.

38. Jann HW and Rains JR: Diagnostic ultrasonography of evaluation of cryptorchidism in horses. *JAVMA* 195:297-300, 1990.

39. Walker DF and Vaughan JT: *Bovine and Equine Urogenital Surgery.* Lea & Febiger, Philadelphia, 1980. pp 105- 182.

40. Hughes JP: Significance of fertility evaluation of the stallion. *Proc Ann Mtg Soc Theriogenol,* 1983. pp 167- 175.

41. Halnan CRE: Equine cytogenetics; role in equine veterinary practice. *Eq Vet J* 17:173-177, 1985.

42. Hare WCD and Singh EL: Equine cytogenetics. *Compend Cont Ed Pract Vet* 2:S111-S118, 1980.

43. Ballachey BE *et al:* Heterogeneity of sperm nuclear chromatin structure and its relationship to bull fertility. *Biol Reprod* 36:915-925, 1987.

44. Burns PJ and Douglas RH: Reproductive hormone concentrations in stallions with breeding problems: case studies. *J Eq Vet Sci* 5:40-42, 1985.

45. Wallach SJR *et al:* Sexual behavior and serum concentration of reproductive hormones in impotent stallions. *Theriogenology* 19:833-840, 1983.

46. Irvine CHG *et al:* Sexual behavior and serum concentration of reproductive hormones in normal stallions. *Theriogenology* 23:607-617, 1985.

47. Threlfall WR and Lopate C: Testicular biopsy. *Proc Ann Mtg Soc Theriogenol,* 1987. pp 65-73.

48. Samper JC *et al:* Relation between the fertility of fresh and frozen stallion semen and semen quality measured as sperm motility and with glass wool/Sephadex filters. *Proc Intl Symp Equine Reprod,* 1990. pp 52-53.

49. Kenney RM: Personal Communication, 1990.

50. Blanchard TL *et al:* Priapism in a stallion with generalized melanosarcoma. *JAVMA* (accepted for publication, 1991).

3

Management of the Breeding Stallion

General Considerations

Feeding Program

In most instances, the nutritional requirements of a mature breeding stallion are fulfilled by a maintenance ration. A maintenance ration consists of a balanced amount of dietary nutrients required for support of basic bodily functions, such as respiration, digestion, maintenance of body temperature, and repair or replacement of damaged body tissues. These conditions usually can be met with adequate pasture or good-quality hay (1.5-2% body weight/day), free access to a trace-mineralized salt, and unrestricted fresh water.[1] Stallions exposed to cold environmental temperatures may require grain as an energy supplement. Though stallions should be maintained in good body condition, overfeeding is discouraged. This subject has not been critically investigated in the stallion, but a high-energy diet in beef bulls has been associated with reduced epididymal sperm reserves and semen quality.[2] Obesity also may adversely affect libido and mating ability or predispose to various conditions, such as laminitis.

Contrary to popular belief, supplementation with vitamins A or E beyond NRC requirements does not improve reproductive function of stallions.[3,4] Immature stallions and those that are worked regularly in addition to usual breeding activities require a ration that has been adjusted for these additional needs.

Proper dental care complements the success of good nutritional management. All stallions should be checked at 6-month intervals for dental problems.

Exercise Program

Moderate daily exercise is conducive to good mental and physical health. Vices attributed to boredom, such as stall weaving, cribbing and self-mutilation, may be averted by offering stallions adequate daily exercise. The inactivity of total stall confinement has long been considered by many stallion managers as a possible cause of lethargy and reduced sexual desire of some stallions, and hyperexcitability and viciousness in others. The semen quality of stallions receiving controlled daily exercise and stall-confined stallions is similar.[5] Interestingly, one study revealed the mean libido score of nonexercised stallions to be higher than that of stallions receiving forced but light daily exercise.[6] Thus, stallions with decreased libido may benefit from reduction or elimination of daily exercise, whereas highly aggressive stallions may be more manageable when kept on a controlled exercise program. This area certainly warrants further study.

Immunization Program

Vaccine selection for breeding stallions generally follows that adopted for other horses on the same premises. A vaccination program cannot be uniformly devised to fit all management systems; rather, each farm should implement its own program tailored to its particular needs. Though the effect of various vaccines on the stallion's genital system has not been investigated thoroughly, in general, vaccines are not considered to have a deleterious effect on reproductive functions of stallions. Always read package inserts that accompany vaccines for possible contraindications in breeding stallions.

Tetanus toxoid is essential and should be given annually. Bivalent (A1 and A2) influenza and rhinopneumonitis vaccines should be given to breeding stallions exposed to horses not normally stabled on the premises. The frequency of administration of these 2 vaccines has not been firmly established and varies from 2-month intervals to annual boosters. Annual vaccination against encephalitis (Eastern, Western, Venezuelan) and rabies also may be indicated if the diseases are enzootic in the locale. Strangles (*Streptococcus equi*) bacterins have questionable efficacy and generally are not included in vaccination programs for stallions.

Interest in viral arteritis has revived because of the recent outbreak in Kentucky horses.[7] Breeding of infected stallions is considered the primary mode of viral transmission, as the virus is sequestered in the semen after the acute phase of the infection has subsided.[8] The duration of the carrier state in stallions is quite variable. A modified-live vaccine against viral arteritis (Arvac: Fort Dodge) has been developed in an attempt to curb outbreaks of disease. Vaccination of susceptible mares appears to provide good protection against the disease. One study showed that vaccinated mares did not develop clinical disease when bred to a chronically infected carrier stallion that shed virus in his semen.[9] Vaccination of stallions does not appear to affect their reproductive function and does not result in viral transmission to seronegative mares bred 10-25 days after stallion vaccination.[10] The vaccine is regulated by state governments and is not approved for use in some states.

Parasite Control

As with an immunization program, a deworming program must be suited to the requirements of each farm. Few critical studies have been performed to evaluate the effect of various antiparasitic drugs on reproductive function in stallions. However, such drugs are considered safe unless otherwise indicated on their package inserts. Any deworming program must be combined with good paddock/pasture management, including use of individual paddocks for each stallion, pasture rotation and regular harrowing. The effectiveness of the program can be evaluated by periodic fecal examinations for parasitic egg levels.

Initial use of ivermectin may result in transient edematous swelling of the scrotal wall and edema along the ventral midline of the abdomen. The tissue reaction is thought to be associated with death of *Onchocerca* microfilariae (see Chapter 2).[11]

Breeding Soundness Examination

All stallions introduced into a stud should receive a breeding soundness examination well in advance of their first breeding season at the stud. The examination tests libido and mating ability, may uncover transmissible congenital defects, permits detection of infectious venereal diseases, and allows close scrutiny of semen quality and quantity.[12] The examination also helps management personnel determine the number of mares that can be contracted to the stallion for the coming breeding season without jeopardizing the stallion's fertility.

Experienced stallions should receive a breeding soundness examination before each breeding season as a precautionary measure. The examination may reveal otherwise undetected changes in reproductive function from the previous season. Specific guidelines for performing a breeding soundness examination are discussed in Chapter 2 and in the *Official Manual for Clinical Fertility Evaluation of the Stallion,* published by the Society for Theriogenology.[12]

Artificial Lighting Program

The effect of season on equine reproduction is well documented. Horses seem to have an endogenously established annual reproductive cycle that is influenced greatly by photoperiod. Reproductive function is not arrested in stallions during the winter months as it is in most mares; however, reproductive functions in stallions still follow a circannual rhythm. Testicular size and weight, daily sperm production, semen volume, hormonal concentrations and libido are increased during the natural breeding season (summer), as compared to the nonbreeding season (winter).[13-16] Chapter 1 contains a discussion of seasonal (photoperiodic) effects on reproductive characteristics of stallions.

The breeding season of horses can be accelerated by providing broodmares with an artificial lighting program.[18] Photoperiod manipulation accelerates ovulatory receptivity in mares earlier in the calendar year, at a time when mares under natural lighting would exhibit erratic anovulatory reproductive behavior. Providing stallions with an artificial lighting schedule similar to that used for mares (ie, equivalent of 16 hours of daylight, beginning December 15) results in increased testicular size and, possibly, increased spermatozoal output earlier in the following year (January or February) as compared to stallions exposed to only natural daylight.[16,19] Age of stallions and individual stallion variation are likely to influence the effect of artificial photoperiod on these reproductive characteristics.[16,19] Young (4-7 years) and middle-aged (8-14 years) stallions seem to be most responsive to the artificial increase in photoperiod.[16]

The increase in these reproductive traits seems to be short lived, as light-supplemented stallions appear to become refractory to increased photostimulation. As the breeding season progresses, testicular size regresses to near that of stallions exposed to natural day length only. Because the percentage of mares presented to a stallion is relatively low in February as compared to April-June, providing stallions with artificial lighting to increase testicular size and spermatozoal output early in the breeding season may not be warranted. It has not been determined conclusively whether an artificially increased photoperiod for stallions will result in regression of testicular size and spermatozoal output below that of stallions receiving only natural light late in the breeding season. To encourage stallions to respond maximally to an artificial lighting program, it may be beneficial to expose them to only 8 hours of daylight between October 1 and December 15, rather than the natural decrease in day length that occurs during this period of the year.[17,19]

Estimating a Stallion's Book

Predicting the maximum number of mares to which a stallion can be contracted for a given breeding season, without reducing fertility, poses a continual and perplexing management problem. Numerous factors must be taken into account when devising strategies to determine this figure; no simple equation can calculate this number accurately.

Stallion Factors

Stallion Selection: Stallion candidacy to a breeding career is generally based on pedigree, athletic ability and conformation. Little emphasis is placed on reproductive potential. The longevity of breeding sires depends largely on performance of their progeny. Propagation of subfertile stock is intrinsic in this selection process, and the percentage of subfertile stallions in the domestic-horse population will likely escalate unless evaluation of reproductive potential is included in the selection criteria for stallion breeding prospects.

Method of Breeding: Breeding stallions can be mated naturally (by pasture breeding or controlled hand-mating) or used in artificial insemination programs. The number of mares that can be booked to a stallion for a breeding season usually is much greater when the stallion is used in an artificial insemination program, as each ejaculate can be divided into several insemina-

Semen Quality: Daily sperm output, percentage of progressively motile sperm, mean velocity of progressively motile sperm, and percentage of morphologically normal sperm in ejaculates should be estimated to determine the number of viable sperm available for insemination if a stallion is used daily. Daily sperm output is affected by photoperiod, but the other values appear to be independent of changes in day length. While not studied extensively, longevity of ejaculated spermatozoal motility may be another factor that affects the fertility of stallions. Daily sperm output (DSO) can be calculated in the horse by 1 of 4 methods:

The *10-ejaculate collection series* involves collecting semen once daily from a stallion for 10 consecutive days.[33] If possible, the stallion should have at least 1 week of sexual rest before initiating this semen collection sequence. Semen collection for the first 7 days serves to stabilize extragonadal sperm reserves. Mean sperm output from semen collected on days 8-10 represents the DSO of the stallion. In some stallions, especially young stallions, extragonadal reserves of sperm are small. In these cases, 10 days may not be required to attain DSO. Semen from the stallions is simply collected once daily until 3 consecutive ejaculates are obtained in which spermatozoal number does not vary by more than 10%. The average sperm number of these 3 ejaculates would represent DSO for that stallion. Occasionally stallions require more than 10 days to stabilize extragonadal sperm reserves, especially stallions that tend to accumulate abnormally high numbers of spermatozoa in the cauda epididymides and deferent ducts if not ejaculated frequently (see Chapters 9 and 16).

With *extrapolation from extragonadal reserves,* 2 ejaculates are obtained from a stallion, 1 hour apart, after allowing the stallion to have at least 2 weeks of sexual rest.[34] If the total sperm number in the second ejaculate is between 20% and 70% of the total sperm number in the first ejaculate, DSO is computed as 27.5% of the total sperm number in the first ejaculate.

Extrapolation from scrotal width uses the regression equation for predicting daily sperm output from scrotal width:[35]

$$\text{DSO} = -3.36 \times 10^9 + 0.066 \times 10^9 X$$

where X = scrotal width (mm).

Alternatively, daily sperm production (DSP) can be calculated from a regression equation, then DSO is considered 87% of DSP:

$$DSP = -4.88 \times 10^9 + 0.093 \times 10^9 X$$

where X = scrotal width (mm).

$$DSO = DSP \times 0.87$$

Using extrapolation from testicular volume, testicular volume (TV) is computed from 1 of 2 equations:[36]

$$TV = 4/3\pi\, abc$$

where a = testicular height/2,
b = testicular width/2, and
c = testicular length/2,

or

$$TV = 4/3\, Ac$$

where A = cross-sectional area through the widest part of the testis, and
c = testicular length/2.

Testicular measurements can be determined using a real-time ultrasound unit with a 5-mHz linear-array transducer. Alternatively, testicular height, width and length for the first equation can be measured using calipers.

Extrapolation of DSO from TV uses the following regression equation:

$$DSO = 0.024X - 0.76$$

where X = TV

Prediction of daily sperm output is probably most reliable when 10 ejaculates are collected (Method 1), followed by extrapolation from testicular volume. Extrapolation from extragonadal reserves or scrotal width is likely to produce more variable results. Remember also that a stallion's DSO is subject to seasonal variation; therefore, DSO computations reflect sperm output from a stallion only for that particular time of the year.

Mare Factors

Prediction of a "stallion book" must take into account the fertility of mares that will be presented to the stallion. Ignoring this critical factor can result in stallion overuse and/or a reduced season conception rate for a stallion. Age, condition and estimated fertility of mares should be ascertained.

The percentages of maiden, barren and lactating (foaling) mares that will be presented to a stallion for the forthcoming breeding season also should be estimated. These percentages are important in formulation of a stallion book because a stallion can breed more mares if they are spaced evenly throughout the breeding season. Parturition occurs between March and May for most pregnant mares, while the typical breeding season for horses begins in mid-February and continues through early to mid-July.

If an overly large proportion of lactating mares is booked to a stallion for a breeding season, the stallion's book will not be spread evenly over the entire breeding season. Instead, a large number of mares will be ready for breeding later in the breeding season, putting extra breeding demand on the stallion. Breeding most barren and maiden mares early in the breeding season reduces the number of mares that a stallion must breed later in the season, when most lactating mares are presented. However, excessive demand on the stallion early in the breeding season should be avoided because overuse may depress libido and breeding performance.

Management Factors

Management Motives: Mares should be managed in such a manner to optimize their fertility so that determination of a stallion book is not further complicated by management deficiencies. Good nutritional and deworming programs are crucial to good reproductive performance. Intensive reproductive management of mares through proper artificial lighting programs, conscientious estrus detection and ovulation synchronization/prediction techniques ensures that mares are bred in a most efficient manner for the stallion.

Artificial Lighting Program: The operational breeding season for most breeds begins in mid-February, which does not coincide with the natural breeding season. Mares are reproductively responsive to day length; providing them with supplemental light to artificially increase day length accelerates the onset of reproductive cyclicity in nonpregnant mares so they can be bred earlier in the calendar year. Hormonal therapy can be used in conjunction with artificial lighting programs. Supplemental lighting programs also encourage reproductive cyclicity in mares that give birth early in the year. The effect of artificial light on stallion reproductive performance has been discussed previously. Because, under an artificial lighting program, reproductive functions of the stallion peak in February, this practice may be especially beneficial on stud farms expecting to breed large numbers of mares early in the breeding season.

Length of Breeding Season: The breeding season lasts 4.5-5 months (February 15 to July 1-15) for most breeding operations. This is especially true for breeds that strive to maximize foal growth in preparation for competitive events at 2-3 years. If the breeding season is unrestricted or extended, the number of mares a stallion can breed during a season increases accordingly.

Insemination Dose: One distinct advantage of artificial insemination programs over natural mating is that ejaculates from fertile stallions can be divided into several insemination units, each containing a prescribed number of viable spermatozoa. An insemination dose containing 500 million progressively motile sperm is the industry standard. In some fertile stallions, however, the sperm number per insemination can be reduced to 100 million progressively motile cells without reducing the pregnancy rate.[37] Obviously the sperm number chosen per insemination has a dramatic effect on the number of mares that can be booked to a stallion in a breeding season.

Natural Service Programs

Some breed registries do not register foals produced by artificial insemination; only those conceived by a natural mating. This conservative program restricts the number of mares a stallion can impregnate during a breeding season, as compared to stallions in artificial insemination programs. A major advantage of this breeding system is that it effectively limits the number of marketable get from a sire, thereby preventing overproduction. Unfortunately, the many positive features of artificial insemination cannot be realized in natural service programs (see Artificial Insemination Programs below).

The major difference between natural service and artificial programs is the number of times a stallion ejaculates daily. Because an ejaculate of a stallion in a natural service program cannot be subdivided into several insemination units, it is not uncommon for a popular stallion to breed 2-3 different mares per day, 7 days per week, during the peak of the breeding season. Thus, management of mares becomes a critical feature of the breeding program. Accurate ovulation prediction should be stressed so that mares are bred as close to ovulation as possible.

This helps prevent stallion overuse. Mares must also be receptive to the stallion at the time of breeding to reduce the risk of stallion injury during mating. Proper mare restraint during the act of breeding is of paramount importance. Methods of restraint are described in Chapter 4.

If a stallion is scheduled to breed >1 mare/day, breeding sessions should be distributed evenly to help ensure uniformity in sperm output per ejaculate (*eg,* 8-12 hours apart if 2 mares are to be bred per day). Increasing the frequency of ejaculations per day does not increase daily sperm output.[38] Factors that limit the number of mares a stallion can breed per day include sperm output and libido.

Stallion preparation for breeding is similar in both natural service and artificial insemination programs. Specific methods are described below.

Artificial Insemination Programs

Artificial insemination has become a key feature of many equine breeding programs in recent years, as nearly all breed organizations now permit its use. Only 3 United States breed registries currently do not allow artificial insemination: the Jockey Club (Thoroughbred breed), the American Miniature Horse Association and the Standard Jack and Jennet Registry of America.[39] Some associations have allowed artificial insemination for decades. For instance, the United States Trotting Association incorporated artificial insemination into its breeding procedures in the early 1950s.

Advantages of artificial insemination over natural mating are numerous:

- *Artificial insemination permits more efficient use of semen.* By dividing the ejaculate of a fertile stallion into several insemination units, the number of mares that can be bred per ejaculate is increased several fold. The number of mares that are booked to a stallion per breeding season can be increased accordingly.
- *Semen extender* that is mixed with ejaculated semen before artificial insemination *contains supportive and protective factors* that may improve pregnancy rates from subfertile stallions.
- *Addition of antibiotics* to seminal extenders *reduces the potential for venereal transmission of bacterial diseases* by stallions.

- *Semen collection for artificial insemination using a breeding phantom (dummy mare) greatly reduces the risk of injury due to breeding accidents.* The breeding phantom provides a non-variable breeding stimulus, and usually minimizes the number of personnel and time required for semen collection.
- *Semen collection in an artificial vagina permits close scrutiny of semen quality* in the laboratory before insemination.
- *Extended semen can be preserved for prolonged periods* after ejaculation and transported from the site of collection, increasing availability of the stallion's semen to mare owners. Restrictions of various breed registries regarding these procedures must be observed.

Semen Collection

The semen collection process is a very vital part of artificial insemination programs, whether the ejaculates are to be inseminated immediately or preserved. Intercepting semen and exposing it to a hostile environment before insemination can have devastating effects on eventual fertilizing capacity of sperm. Sunlight, temperature shock, chemical shock, osmotic shock and physical agitation, singularly and in combination, can irreparably damage sperm. Therefore, it is extremely important that ejaculated semen be handled delicately. Recommended methods of semen collection and handling techniques are discussed in Chapter 4.

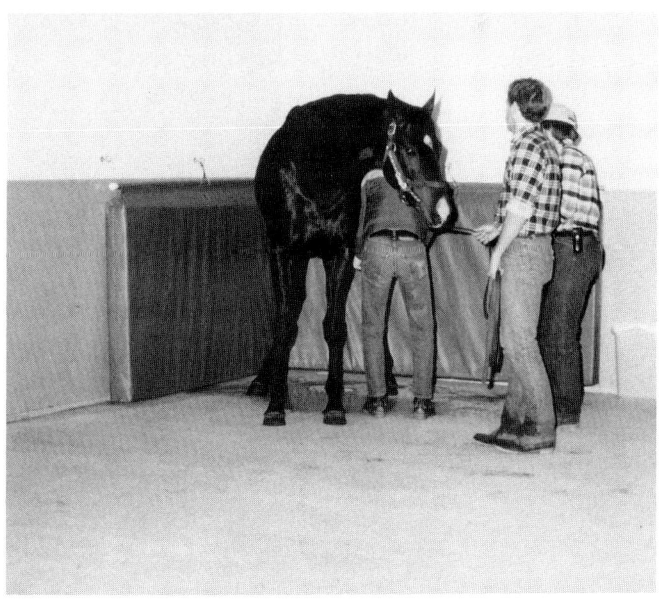

Figure 1. Penis being cleansed in preparation for breeding, with stallion in a padded corner.

Breeding Shed Specifications

Semen can be collected outdoors, provided the area is free of obstructions and has a dry, nonslippery surface and a perimeter fence. An outdoor paddock with a dry grass surface serves this purpose well. If one anticipates collecting semen on a regular basis, a lighted indoor breeding area is recommended. Such a facility reduces distractions to the stallion during breeding and permits work to continue during night hours and inclement weather.

Ideally, a breeding shed used in an artificial insemination program should have the following features: breeding area of adequate size; nonslippery floor; padded teasing rail; breeding phantom (dummy mare); and laboratory for semen evaluation and processing.

The breeding area should be sufficiently large (400-500 sq ft) to prevent interference with breeding activities and permit coordinated movement of a stallion and mount mare. The minimum height of ceiling and light fixtures is 10 ft. One corner of the breeding shed can be equipped with padded walls and washable floor with a drain. This area is designated for inspection and cleansing of external genitalia of stallions (Fig 1).

A padded teasing rail installed at the edge of the breeding arena accommodates an estrous mare to stimulate sexual behavior in stallions. A properly constructed breeding phantom situated adjacent to the teasing rail allows a stallion to remain near an estrous mare while mounting the apparatus for semen collection (Fig 2).

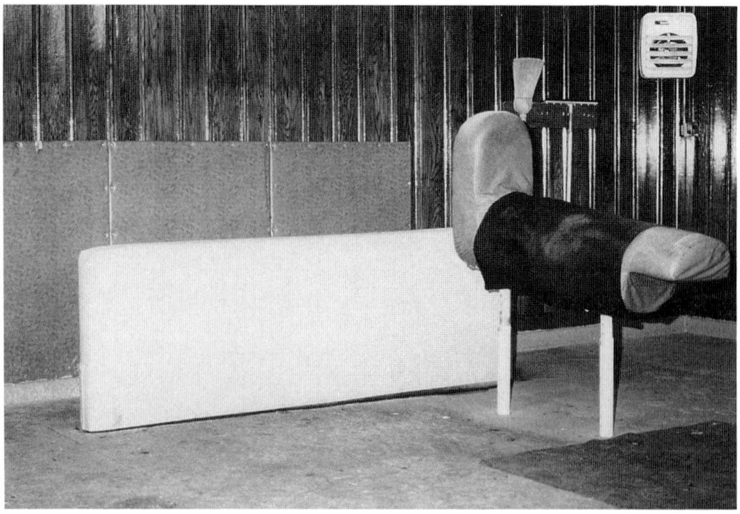

Figure 2. Breeding phantom adjacent to a padded teasing rail in a stallion breeding area.

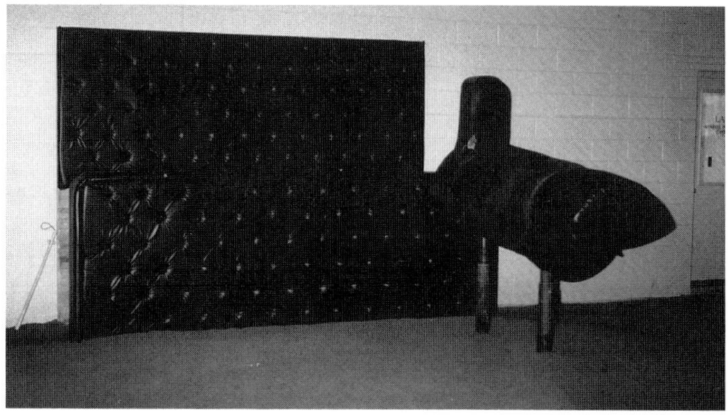

Figure 3. A well-packed surface of stone dust in a stallion breeding area.

The primary requirement of a breeding shed floor is good footing for stallions during breeding. Sand, stone dust, clay, dirt, pea gravel and tan bark are commonly used as floor surfaces (Figs 3-5). All furnish a nonslippery base but are difficult to clean. Artificial floors have been installed in some breeding sheds (Figs 6, 7). These floors are usually made of a durable and easy-to-clean rubberized material. The surfaces are expensive, however, and some types do not provide good footing, especially when wet.

Figure 4. A floor of pea gravel with a central mat for varied surfaces in a stallion breeding area.

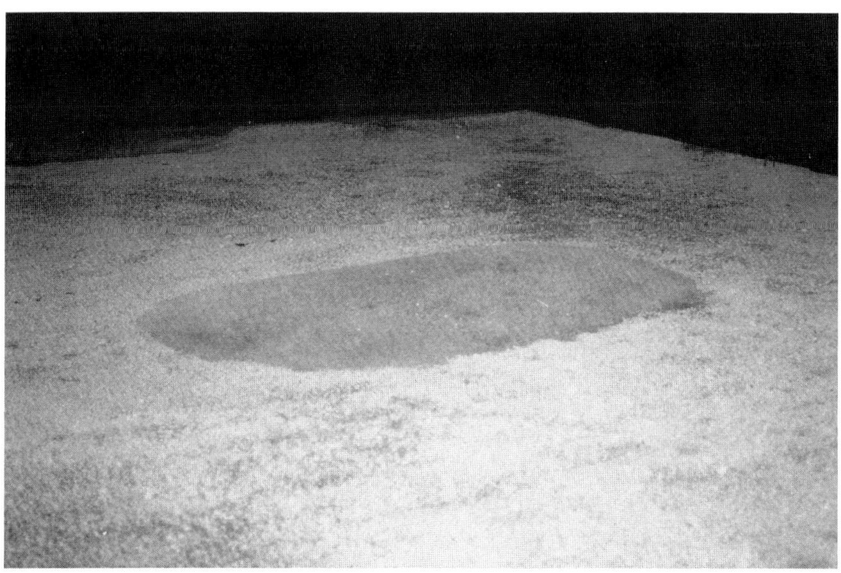

Figure 5. A stallion breeding area with tan bark on the periphery and an artificial surface with a raised removable mat in the center.

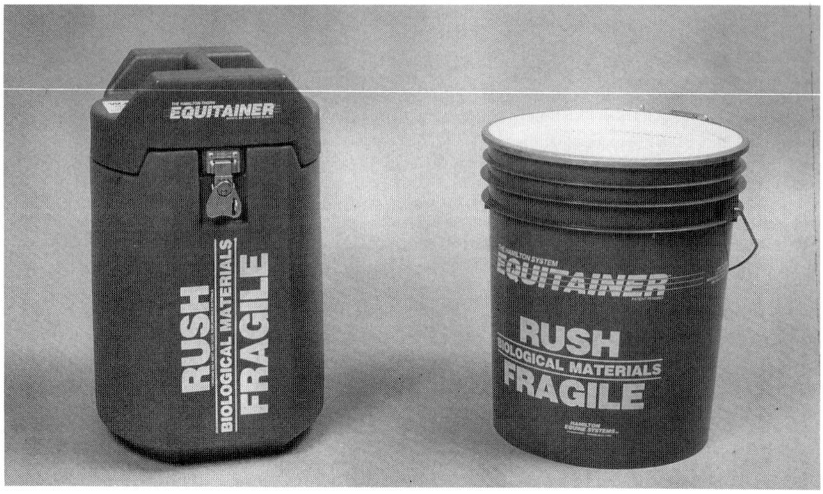

An environmentally controlled laboratory should adjoin the breeding area. The laboratory should be properly equipped for artificial-vagina preparation and maintenance, semen evaluation and *in-vitro* semen preservation.

Figure 6. Pavers of compressed rubber fibers used as a breeding surface for stallions.

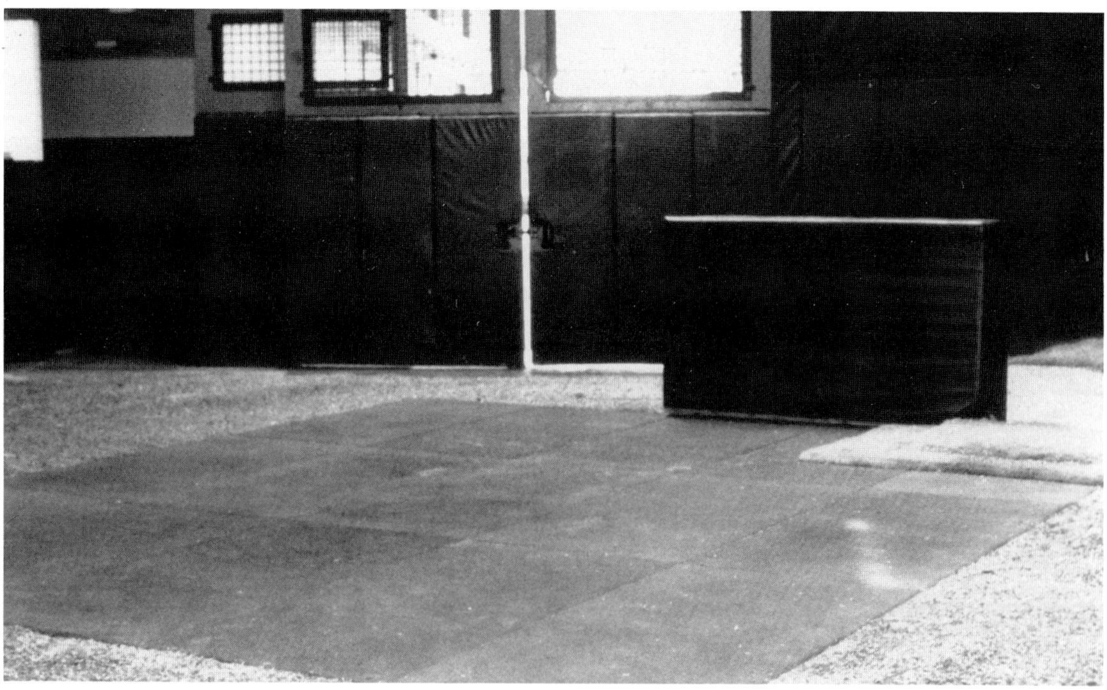

Figure 7. A poured waterproof surface containing rubberized material as a breeding surface for stallions.

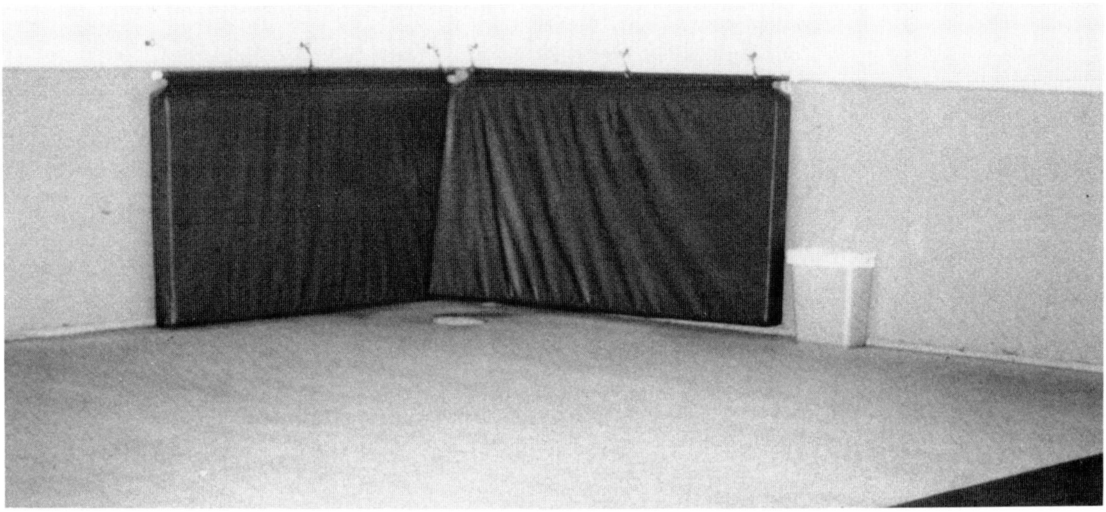

Artificial Insemination Techniques

Insemination Timing and Frequency: The pregnancy rate of fertile stallions usually is maintained when mares are inseminated 48-72 hours before ovulation.[40] Daily insemination, or even twice-daily insemination, until ovulation is detected may be required to enhance pregnancy rates of subfertile stallions. Though good fertility has been reported using postovulation breeding, this method of insemination requires further study before it can be endorsed for maximizing reproductive efficiency in stallions.[41] One obvious disadvantage to postovulation breeding in natural-service programs is that some mares go out of behavioral estrus within 12-24 hours after ovulation, making it very dangerous for the stallion to attempt mating at this time.

Insemination Dose (Sperm Number): The optimum number of sperm in a standard artificial insemination dose is 500 million progressively motile sperm. This sperm insemination number can be reduced to 100 million progressively motile cells from some stallions without reducing fertility.[37]

Insemination Volume: Insemination volume apparently is not as important to good fertility as sperm number. A typical insemination volume of extended equine semen is 10-25 ml, though larger or smaller volumes can be used successfully. Insemination volumes of <2 ml (raw semen) have produced acceptable pregnancy rates.[37] Conversely, mares bred by natural service generally receive 60-70 ml of semen (average volume of stallion ejaculate), and sometimes the uterus is infused with 100-125 ml of semen extender immediately before breeding to improve fertility of some stallions.[42]

References

1. Hintz HF, in Mansmann RA and McAllister ES: *Equine Medicine and Surgery.* 3rd ed. American Veterinary Publications, Goleta, CA, 1982. pp 87-116.

2. Coulter GH and Kozub GC: Testicular development, epididymal sperm reserves and seminal quality in two-year-old hereford and angus bulls: effects of two levels of dietary energy. *J Anim Sci* 59:432-440, 1984.

3. Ralston SL *et al:* The effect of vitamin A supplementation on seminal characteristics and vitamin A absorption in stallions. *J Equine Vet Sci* 6:203-207, 1986.

4. Rich GA *et al:* Effect of vitamin E supplementation on stallion seminal characteristics and sexual behavior. *Proc Intl Cong Anim Reprod Artif Insem,* 1984. pp 11-163.

5. Dinger JE *et al:* Effect of controlled exercise on semen characteristics in two-year-old stallions. *Theriogenology* 25:525-535, 1986.

6. Dinger JE and Noiles EE: Effect of controlled exercise on libido in two-year-old stallions. *J Anim Sci* 62:1220-1223, 1986.

7. Timoney PJ and McCollum EH: The epidemiology of equine viral arteritis. *Proc Ann Mtg AAEP,* 1985. pp 545-551.

8. Timoney PJ *et al:* The carrier state in equine arteritis virus infection in the stallion with specific emphasis on the venereal mode of virus transmission. *J Reprod Fertil* 35: 95-102, 1987.

9. McCollum WH *et al:* Response of vaccinated and non-vaccinated mares to cervical insemination with semen from a stallion persistently infected with equine viral arteritis virus. *Proc Ann Conf Res Workers Anim Dis,* 1986. p 12.

10. McKinnon AO *et al:* Vaccination of stallions with a modified live equine viral arteritis virus. *J Equine Vet Sci* 6:66-69, 1986.

11. Herd RP and Donham JC: Efficacy of ivermectin against *Onchocerca cervicalis* microfilarial dermatitis in horses. *Am J Vet Res* 44:1102-1105, 1983.

12. Kenney RM *et al: Manual for Clinical Fertility Evaluation of the Stallion.* Soc for Theriogenol, Hastings, NE, 1983. pp 3-100.

13. Pickett BW *et al:* Reproductive physiology of the stallion. VI. Seminal and behavioral characteristics. *J Anim Sci* 43:617-625, 1976.

14. Johnson L and Thompson DL: Age-related and seasonal variation in the Sertoli cell population, daily sperm production and serum concentrations of follicle-stimulating hormone, luteinizing hormone and testosterone is stallions. *Biol Reprod* 29:777-789, 1983.

15. Thompson DL *et al:* Patterns of secretion of luteinizing hormone, follicle-stimulating hormone and testosterone in stallions during the summer and winter. *J Anim Sci* 60:741-748, 1985.

16. Burns PJ *et al:* Effects of season, age and increased photoperiod on reproductive hormone concentrations and testicular diameters in Thoroughbred stallions. *J Equine Vet Sci* 4:202-208, 1984.

17. Clay CM *et al:* Influences of season and artificial photoperiod on stallions: testicular size, seminal characteristics and sexual behavior. *J Anim Sci* 64:517-525, 1987.

18. Ginther OJ: *Reproductive Biology of the Mare. Basic and Applied Aspects.* Published by the author, Cross Plaines, WI, 1979. pp 83-168.

19. Pickett BW *et al: Management of the Stallion for Maximum Reproductive Efficiency* - II. Colorado State University Exp Sta Anim Reprod Lab, Gen Series Bull 05, 1989. pp 39-58.

20. Johnson L and Thompson DL: Age-related and seasonal variation in the Sertoli cell population, daily sperm production and serum concentrations of follicle-stimulating hormone, luteinizing hormone and testosterone in stallions. *Biol Reprod* 29:777-789, 1983.

21. Johnson L *et al:* Establishment of adult levels of spermatogenesis in the horse. *J Reprod Fertil* (in press, 1990)

22. Johnson L *et al:* No effect of age on Sertoli Cell number or germ cell: Sertoli cell ratio in adult stallions. *Proc Am Soc Androl,* 1988. p 31.

23. Jones LS and Berndtson WE: A quantitative study of Sertoli cell and germ cell populations as related to sexual development and aging in the stallion. *Biol Reprod* 35: 138-148, 1986.

24. Berndtson WE *et al:* Spermatogenesis, testicular composition and the concentration of testosterone in the equine testis as influenced by season. *Theriogenology* 20: 449-457, 1983.

25. Thompson DL *et al:* Concentrations of prolactin, luteinizing hormone and follicle stimulating hormone in pituitary and serum of horses: Effect of sex, season and reproductive state. *J Anim Sci* 63:854-860, 1986.

26. Johnson L and Thompson DL: Effect of seasonal changes in Leydig cell number on the volume of smooth endoplasmic reticulum in Leydig cells and intratesticular testosterone content in stallions. *J Reprod Fertil* 81:227-232, 1987.

27. Harris JM: Seasonal changes in serum levels of FSH, LH and testosterone and in semen parameters in stallions. *Theriogenology* 19:311-322, 1983.

28. Clay CM *et al:* Influences of season and artificial photoperiod on stallions: Luteinizing hormone, follicle-stimulating hormone and testosterone. *J Anim Sci* 66: 1246-1255, 1988.

29. Clay CM *et al:* Influences of season and artificial photoperiod on stallions: pituitary and testicular responses to exogenous GnRH. *J Anim Sci* 67:763-770, 1989.

30. Squires EL *et al:* Restoration of reproductive capacity of stallions after suppression with exogenous testosterone. *J Anim Sci* 53:1351-1359, 1981.

31. Squires EL *et al:* Effect of anabolic steroids on reproductive function of young stallions. *J Anim Sci* 54:576-582, 1982.

32. Blanchard TL *et al:* The effects of stanozolol and boldenone undecylenate on scrotal width, testis weight, and sperm production in pony stallions. *Theriogenology* 20: 121-131, 1983.

33. Gebauer MR *et al:* Reproductive physiology of the stallion: daily sperm output and testicular measurements. *JAVMA* 165:711-713, 1974.

34. Dinger JE and Noiles EE: Prediction of daily sperm output in stallions. *Theriogenology* 26:61-67, 1986.

35. Thompson DL *et al:* Testicular measurements and reproductive characteristics in stallions. *J Reprod Fertil* 27:13-17, 1979.

36. Love CL *et al:* Evaluation of measures taken by ultrasonography and calipers to estimate testicular volume and predict daily sperm output in the stallion. *Proc Intl Symp Equine Reprod,* 1990. pp 50-51.

37. Pickett BW *et al:* Effect of seminal extenders on equine fertility. *J Anim Sci* 40: 1136-1143, 1975.

38. Voss JL *et al:* Effect of ejaculation frequency on sperm output. *J Reprod Fertil* 35:643, 1987.

39. Varner DD: Collection and preservation of stallion spermatozoa. *Proc Ann Mtg Soc Theriogenol,* 1986. pp 13-33.

40. Palmer E: Factors affecting stallion semen survival and fertility. *Proc Intl Cong Anim Reprod Artif Insem,* 1984. pp 111-163.

41. Belling TH Jr: Postovulation breeding and related reproductive phenomena in the mare. *Equine Pract* 6(2):12-19, 1984.

42. Blanchard TL *et al:* Use of a semen extender containing antibiotic to improve the fertility of a stallion with seminal vesiculitis due to *Pseudomonas aeruginosa*. *Theriogenology* 28:541-546, 1987.

4

Preservation of Spermatozoa

Collecting Semen

Artificial Vagina Selection

A properly constructed and prepared artificial vagina (AV) increases the efficiency of semen collection in artificial insemination programs and optimizes the quality of ejaculated semen. Several well-designed AVs are available. Each type has distinct attributes and peculiarities, so AV selection is based on specific requirements and personal preference. Homemade AVs also have been constructed to meet specific needs of the user. Initial cost, maintenance costs, types of accessories, durability, weight, temperature maintenance and spermatozoal losses incurred during semen collection should all be considered when contemplating purchase of an equine AV.

The *Missouri-model AV* (Nasco, Ft. Atkinson, WI) is probably the most widely used AV in the United States (Fig 1). It is composed of a double-walled rubber liner containing a permanently sealed water chamber and a leather carrying case. This AV is relatively inexpensive, lightweight, and easy to assemble and clean. It has fairly good heat retention and, because the glans penis should extend beyond the waterjacket at the time of ejaculation (Fig 2), internal temperature of the AV may exceed the 45-48 C spermatozoal-tolerance threshold without causing heat-related injury to ejaculated sperm.[1] This AV is equipped with an air valve so that it can be pressurized with water alone,

Figure 1. Missouri (Nasco)-model equine artificial vagina with accessories.

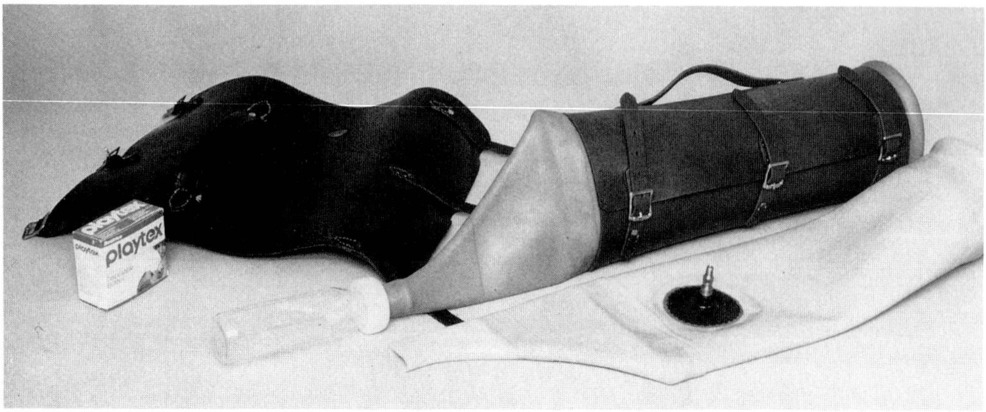

with an air valve so that it can be pressurized with water alone, or with air and water to reduce its weight. Because the liner is made of heavy rubber and the water chamber is permanently sealed, there is little chance of water leakage into the semen sample during collection.

The *Japanese (Nishikawa)-model AV* (Scott Medical Supply, Howard, CA) is composed of a small, rigid aluminium case and a single rubber liner, so it is lightweight and easy to maneuver

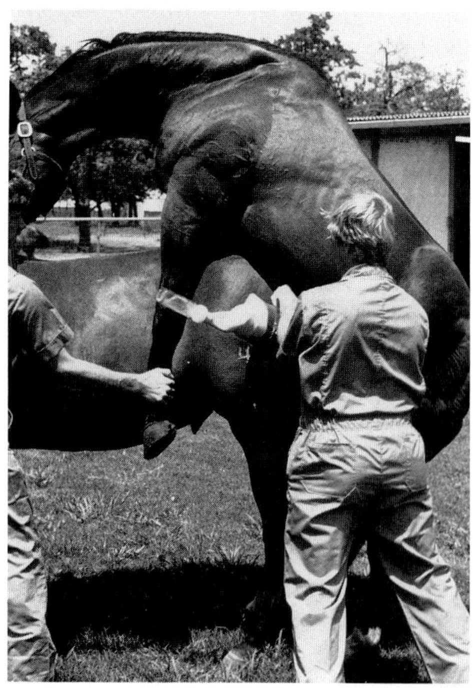

Figure 2. When the erect penis is inserted fully into a Missouri-model artificial vagina, the glans penis is usually beyond the water jacket. This method of semen collection prevents heat-related damage to ejaculated sperm.

Figure 3. Japanese (Nishikawa)-model equine artificial vagina with accessories.

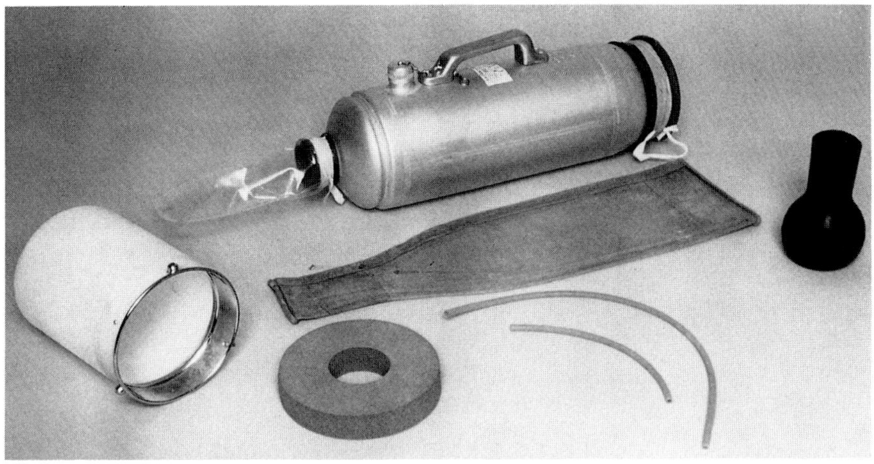

(Fig 3). This AV is easy to assemble and clean. Another attribute of this AV is direct attachment of a semen receptacle to the aluminum casing. This design permits the ejaculate to be discharged directly into the receptacle, allowing only minimal contact of semen with the rubber liner. The liner must be secured tightly to the aluminum case with rubber bands before adding water to the chamber between the liner and aluminum case. Water can leak out if this seal is not tight, reducing AV pressure and increasing the risk of water contamination of the ejaculate. The liner should be checked for defects before use because pinpoint holes in the rubber liner can develop, resulting in water leakage into the AV lumen.

The original *Colorado-model AV* is composed of 2 independent rubber liners and a heavy plastic case covered by a leather collar. It is more cumbersome than the above AVs but offers good heat retention. In addition, it has 2 rubber liners between the water chamber and AV lumen, thus greatly reducing the likelihood of water contamination of the semen sample. Because the water jacket of the AV is longer than the penis, the temperature must be critically regulated to prevent undue heat damage to ejaculated sperm.

The *CSU-model AV* (Animal Reproduction Systems, Chino, CA; Fig 4) and *Lane-model AV* (Lane Manufacturing, Denver, CO) are modified versions of the original Colorado model. Both models are lighter than the original and have a rigid handle to facilitate AV manipulation. These versions have the advantages described above for the Colorado model, and come with an

Figure 4. CSU-model equine artificial vagina with accessories.

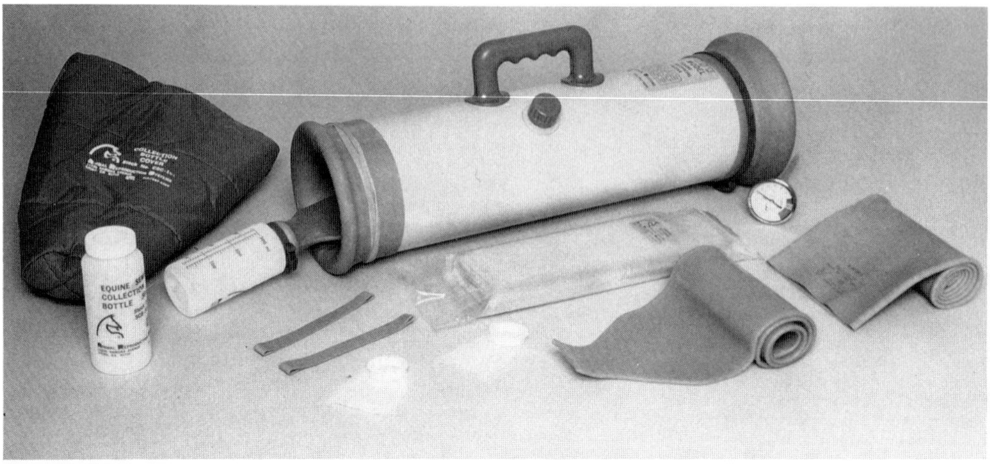

assortment of accessories, including several AV liners, semen filters and collection bottles, a thermometer to monitor internal temperature of the AV, and an insulated protector cone to cover the semen receptacle during the semen collection process.

The *Polish-model AV* can be used to collect sperm-rich ejaculates from breeding stallions. This method of semen collection increases spermatozoal concentration and likewise, reduces the volume contribution of semen plasma in ejaculates. The first 3 jets of an ejaculate contain 75-80% of the spermatozoa present in the total ejaculate, and comprise only about 50% of semen volume.[2-4] The result of this semen-fractionation step is a significant increase in spermatozoal concentration, sometimes exceeding 0.6 to 1 x 10^9 spermatozoa/ml. The technique is considered useful for *in-vitro* semen preservation programs because spermatozoal concentration can be increased without centrifugation, and toxic influences of semen plasma on spermatozoal viability may be diminished. Collection of semen by this method may also reduce contamination of ejaculates by bacteria from the exterior of the penis or reduce/eliminate urine contamination of ejaculates from stallions affected by urospermia (Chapter 16).[5] It may also prevent access of blood from a previous penile injury to semen collected in an AV.

The Polish-type AV is essentially an open-ended model (Fig 5).[2] The glans penis is allowed to protrude from the AV (Fig 6) and semen is collected using either a funnel system or urethral prosthetic device (Figs 7, 8).[6]

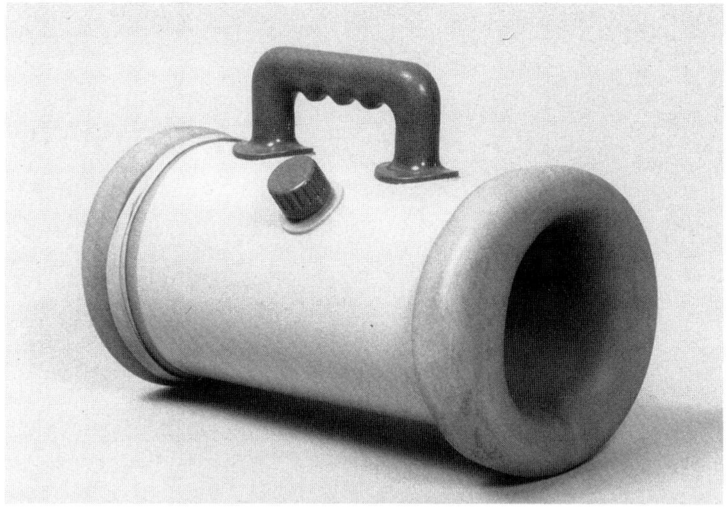

Figure 5. A CSU-model artificial vagina that was shortened to serve as an open-ended model (see Figures 6 and 8).

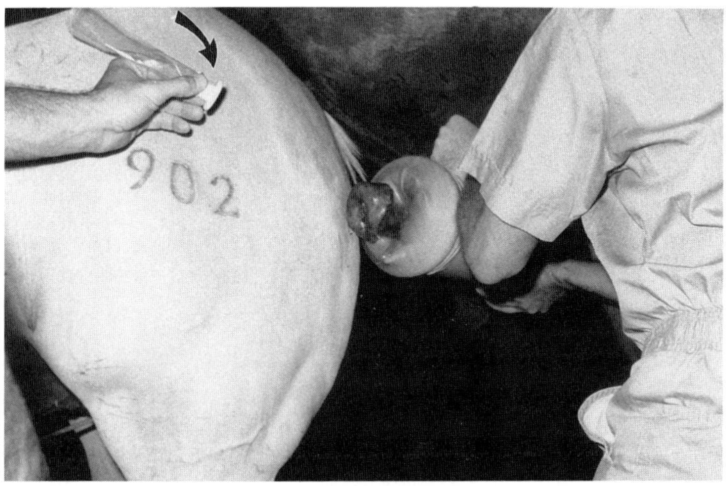

Figure 6. Collection of semen in an open-ended artificial vagina requires 2 individuals: one responsible for holding the artificial vagina and one responsible for collecting the ejaculated semen. In this instance, a urethral prosthetic device with an attached plastic bag (arrow) is ready for insertion into the fossa glandis of the penis, following its protrusion through the open-ended artificial vagina.

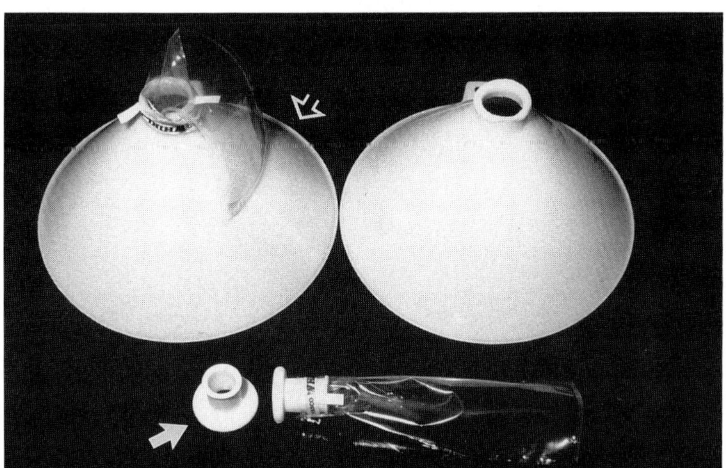

Figure 7. Using an open-ended artificial vagina, semen can be collected using either a funnel system (open arrow) or urethral prosthetic device (solid arrow).

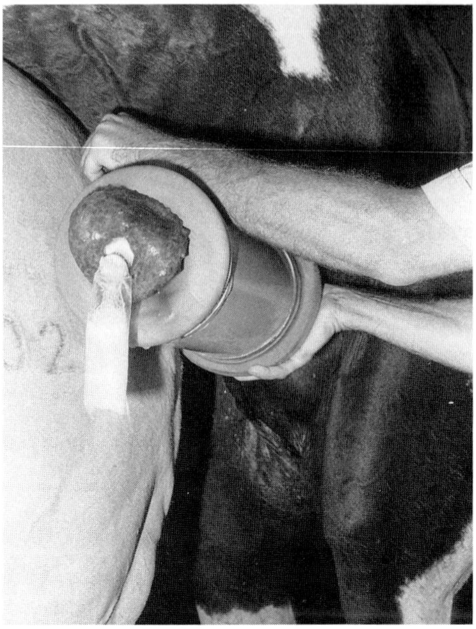

Figure 8. Collection of semen from a stallion using an open-ended artificial vagina and a urethral prosthetic device with attached plastic (Whirl-Pak) bag.

Artificial Vagina Maintenance

All AV components that come in contact with ejaculated spermatozoa must be nonspermicidal. Reusable items must be cleansed properly to render them chemically clean, then dried and, if possible, sterilized between uses. Soaps or disinfectants should not be used to clean AV liners, as the residue can be toxic to spermatozoa during subsequent semen collections. Used rubber AV liners hold be cleaned with hot running water soon after use. If smegma within a used AV is allowed to dry before cleaning, the chore becomes more difficult. Cleaned rubber liners can be submerged in ethyl or isopropyl alcohol for 2-24 hours for disinfection, followed by air drying in a dust-free cabinet. Missouri AVs can be gas sterilized with ethylene oxide, as long as an adequate "air-out" period is allowed (48-72 hours). Sterile, nontoxic disposable equipment should be used when possible to avoid chemical contamination of ejaculates or horizontal transmission of disease. Plastic disposable AV liners, with or without attached semen receptacles, are commercially available for the AVs described above (Fig 9). This equipment helps ensure a clean, nontoxic method of semen collection, as the reusable latex rubber liners may have spermicidal properties.[7] Unfortunately, some stallions do not readily accept AVs fitted with a disposable plastic liner rather than a reusable rubber liner.

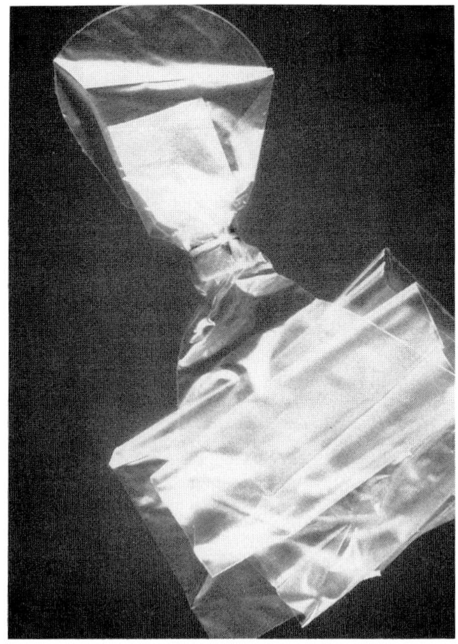

Figure 9. Plastic disposable liner for an equine artificial vagina, complete with a collection bag and filter.

Preparation of Artifical Vaginas for Semen Collection

Immediately before attempting semen collection, the water jacket of the AV is usually filled with warm (48-50 C) water to provide an internal AV temperature of 44-48 C (Fig 10). Providing an AV temperature above that of the body seems to aid penile stimulation during copulation. Spermatozoa can be damaged, however, by contact with surfaces above 45-48 C.[1] As mentioned above, the luminal temperatue of a Missouri-model AV can

Figure 10. Filling the water jacket of a Missouri-model artificial vagina can be facilitated by replacing thte spray nozzle of a sink hose with an air chuck, and securing this to the valve stem of the artificial vagina.

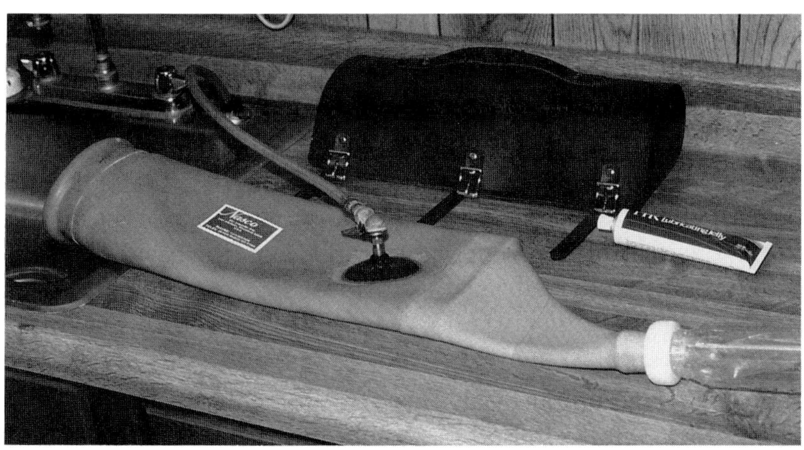

exceed 45-48 C without damaging spermatozoa, provided the glans penis is outside the water jacket when ejaculation occurs (Fig 2). Some stallions may respond more favorably to semen collection with an AV if its luminal temperature is 50-55 C.

Luminal pressure of the AV should be adjusted to provide uniformly good contact around the penis, without interfering with penile penetration. Proper AV pressure accommodates expansion of the penis to full erection. It is important to fully insert the penis into the AV during the first penile thrust, then maintain it in this fully inserted position; otherwise the glans penis will dilate near the opening of the AV and will be too large to permit full penile penetration into the AV. The result would be extended contact of ejaculated semen with the AV liner en route to the semen receptacle, or ejaculatory failure from inadequate penile stimulation. Both temperature and water pressure in the AV should be constant during collection to promote consistent performance and maximal spermatozoal harvest.

The inner surface of the AV should be lubricated with a sterile, nonspermicidal lubricant (*eg,* H-R Lubricating Jelly: Carter, New York) before penile insertion. The collection receptacle should be maintained near body temperature during semen collection and transport to the laboratory to prevent cold shock to the spermatozoa before they are placed in a protective extender. Semen should also be protected from light.

To maximize the number of spermatozoa available from each semen collection, an appropriate filter should be incorporated into the AV. The filter allows most of the gel-free (but sperm-rich) fractions to pass into the semen receptacle but traps the gel (which is presented in the final fractions of an ejaculate). Though some spermatozoa inevitably are trapped in the gel and filter, more would be lost if the semen were filtered *after* collection of the combined gel and gel-free portions, or if the gel were aspirated from the gel-free portion with a syringe. Nylon micromesh filters are superior to polyester matte for separating gel from gel-free fractions because they are nonabsorptive and do not trap as many sperm.[8] The filter with its contained gel should be removed immediately upon collection of the semen to prevent seepage of gel into the gel-free portion of the ejaculate.

Use of Condoms for Semen Collection

A condom is a poor alternative to an AV for semen collection, but it is the only viable option if the stallion will not breed an

AV, or if an AV is unavailable (Fig 11). Stallions most reluctant to breed an AV are those that have never bred before and those accustomed to breeding mares by natural service. The quality of semen collected in a condom is inferior to that obtained with an AV because of the marked contamination of the sample with bacteria and debris from the exterior of the penis.

Figure 11. An equine condom can be used for collection of semen, but the quality of the sample is generally inferior to that obtained using a properly prepared artificial vagina. The adjacent ruler is 6 inches long.

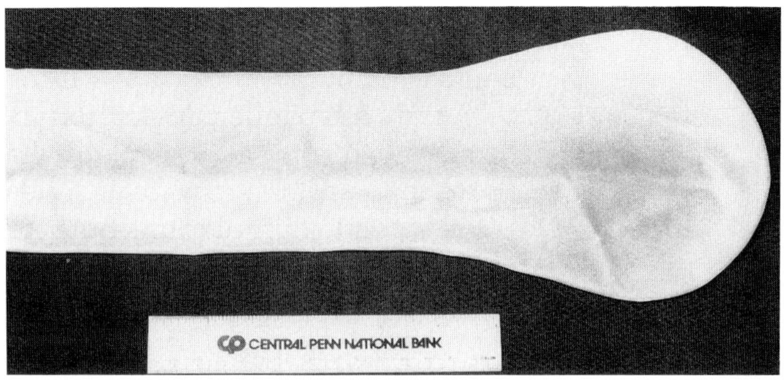

Stallion Preparation for Breeding

Before collecting semen from a stallion, the stallion should be teased with a mare in behavioral estrus to stimulate erection. The erect penis and associated external genitalia are then inspected for lesions and the penis cleansed to minimize contamination of the ejaculate with bacteria, dirt and epithelial debris. Particular attention should be given to the glans penis, fossa glandis and free body of the penis during the washing procedure (Fig 12). Repetitive cleansing of the penis with soap scrubs is contraindicated because it removes the normal bacterial flora of the penis, and may allow overgrowth of potentially pathogenic organisms that are transmissible to the mare.[9,10] Therefore, only water should be used in routine precollection washes in most instances. The penile washing procedure should be followed by thorough drying (Fig 13), as the water itself may be spermicidal. Ideally, the penis is washed with the stallion standing in an open area; if additional restraint is required, the stallion can be backed into a padded corner of a room before washing (Fig 14).

Some stallions harbor large populations of pathogenic bacteria on the exterior of the penis that are not precipitated by overzealous washing procedures. The penis of these stallions may be washed with an antibacterial scrub to reduce bacterial numbers on the penis immediately before breeding or semen

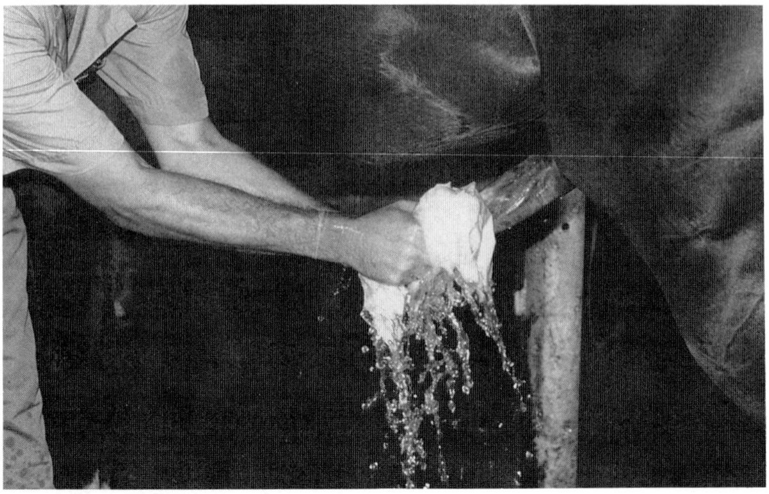

Figure 12. Washing the erect penis of a stallion with water before collection of semen. Particular attention is given to removal of debris from the distal penis, including the fossa glandis.

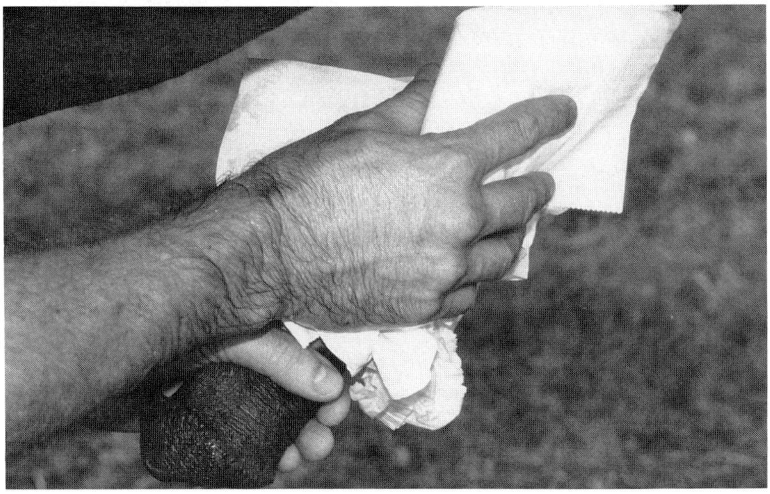

Figure 13. In preparation for semen collection, the penis shoud be dried after washing, as water itself may be spermicidal.

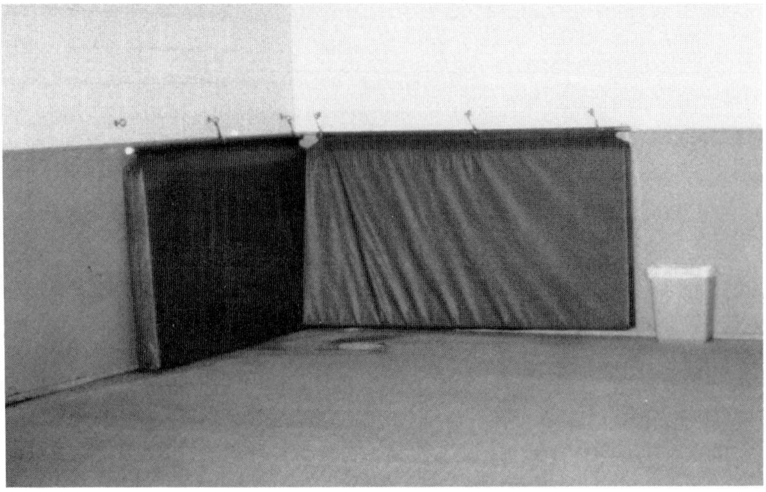

Figure 14. To aid in restraint when washing the penis before semen collection, the horse may first be backed into a padded corner of the breeding arena.

collection. Thorough rinsing is required if soap is used to cleanse the penis before breeding or semen collection because soap residue has spermicidal properties. Colony counts of bacteria may also be reduced or eliminated by rinsing the penis daily with a dilute solution of sodium hypochlorite (for *Klebsiella pneumoniae*) or hydrochloric acid (for *Pseudomonas aeruginosa*) until the organisms are no longer recoverable (Chapter 14).[11] In an artificial insemination program, bacteria-contaminated semen should be mixed with a semen extender containing appropriate antibiotics to kill any potentially pathogenic bacteria before insemination. Under natural-service conditions, the extender can be placed in the uterus of the mare immediately before breeding.[12]

The method and optimal duration of teasing (sexual preparation) required before semen collection has not been examined thoroughly in stallions. Studies in bulls indicate that extended teasing periods and false mounts (allowing the male to mount but deflecting the penis so that intromission and ejaculation do not occur) before semen collection increase spermatozoal output in ejaculates.[13] Sexually stimulating stallions for prolonged periods before semen collection does not apper to elevate the total spermatozoal number in ejaculates;[14] however, the effect of false mounting on spermatozoal output has not been addressed.

Preparation of the Stallion Mount

Semen collection using an AV ordinarily is performed by allowing the stallion to mount a mare or a breeding phantom. In certain situations, however, stallions have been trained to ejaculate using an AV or manual stimulation while standing on the ground.[15-17]

Either gonad-intact or ovariectomized mares can be used as mount mares. Intact mares should not be used unless they are exhibiting behavioral estrus. Ovariectomized mares generally are considered more appropriate than intact mares for daily semen collection activities because they are predictable and can be used at any time. Mares should be selected for ovariectomy based on their degree of receptivity to a stallion while in estrus as intact mares. Ovariectomized mares rarely require exogenous hormonal therapy to display behavioral signs of estrus. When needed, 1-2 mg of estradiol cypionate (ECP: Upjohn) can be given IM to intensify signs of estrus in ovarectomized mares.

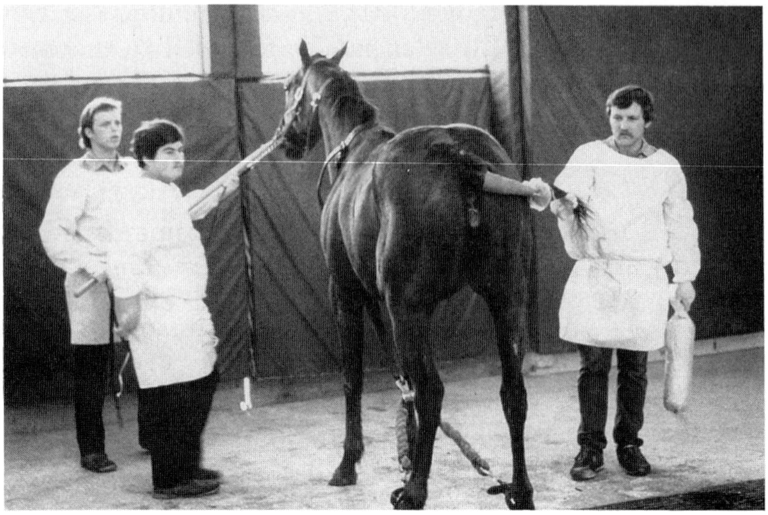

Figure 15. Restraint of a mare in preparation for natural breeding. Hobbles and a muzzle twitch are applied.

This regimen does not induce estrus in intact mares with a functional corpus luteum.

Mares should be physically restrained before the stallion is allowed to mount. Leg hobbles and a twitch on the muzzle can be applied to mares (Fig 15). Rarely is tranquilization needed. If a mare's reactions to an approaching stallion are unknown or unpredictable, it is wise to allow a relatively inexpensive stallion to mount the mare to test the mare's response before permitting a more valuable stallion to mount for semen collection (Fig 16). If the mare reacts unfavorably, another mount should be used. It is equally important that the stallion not be allowed to savage the mare during breeding. This behavior usually can be con-

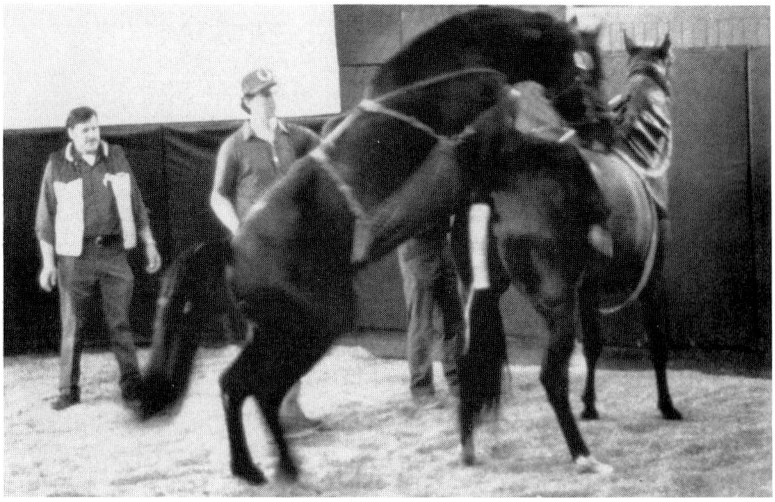

Figure 16. An inexpensive stallion, equipped with a shield to prevent penile insertion, is allowed to mount a mare without hobbles to evaluate her receptivity. This procedure may be performed to minimize undue breeding injuries to valuable stallions.

trolled with a chain shank passed through the stallion's mouth. Muzzles can be fastened to the halter of stallions if excessive biting cannot be controlled by other methods (Fig 17). If necessary, a leather breeding shield can be secured around the neck of the mount mare so that the stallion bites this apparatus rather than the mare during breeding (Fig 18).

For most stallions, semen collection is enhanced by use of a breeding phantom or dummy mare (Fig 19). These mounting devices provide several advantages over an estrous or mount mare for semen collection. They eliminate variability, allowing a more consistent semen collection protocol. Breeding phantoms also greatly reduce the likelihood of stallion injury during semen collection, and of mare injury resulting form the vicious biting of some stallions. Stallions with rear limb or back problems can

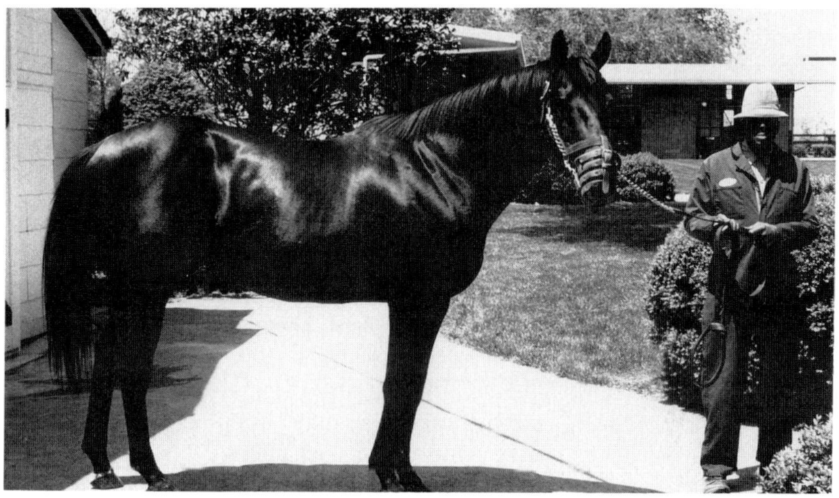

Figure 17. A muzzle applied over the mouth of a stallion to prevent biting of mares during mating.

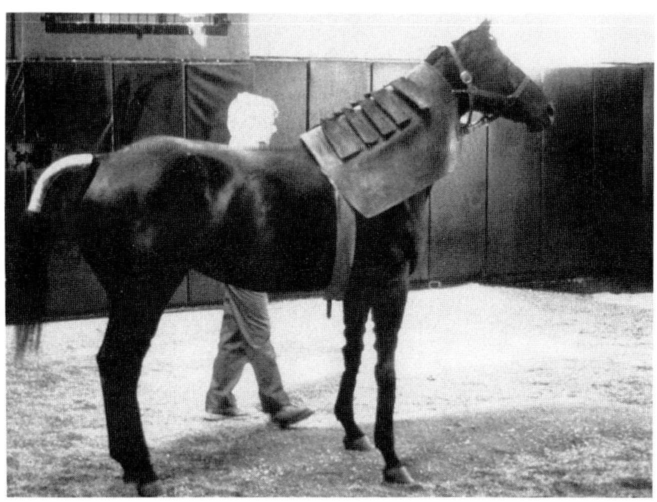

Figure 18. A breeding shield applied over the neck of a mare before breeding to prevent injury from bites of an aggressive stallion.

mount a stationary breeding phantom more easily than a live mare. The height of the phantom can be adjusted to accommodate the stallion. In addition, the phantom can be thoroughly cleaned between mounts, minimizing transmission of disease.

The size, shape and composition of breeding phantoms are quite diverse, ranging from padded hot-water tanks to sophisticated structures with mounted AVs and hydraulic controls for adjusting the height. Desirable elements of a dummy include:

- Adjustable height, with midheight slightly shorter than the average height of the breed involved.
- Width sufficient to permit the stallion to grasp the dummy firmly with the forelegs (total width, including padding, usually ≤ 22-24 inches).
- Adequate padding with an overlying cover that is durable, nonabrasive and easy to clean.
- A stand with a centrally placed upright support to prevent injury to the stallion's legs during collection.
- Installation in an area free of obstructions, with space for a live mare to stand adjacent to the dummy (Fig 20).

Most stallions readily accept the phantom as a mounting device. The novice stallion is trained by placing a mare alongside the phantom. This stimulates mounting behavior in the stallion, but the stallion is diverted so that it mounts the phantom rather than the live mare. Very little training is required in most instances. Sometimes a mare in estrus must be close to the phantom to stimulate the stallion to mount it. Once trained, some stallions do not even require the presence of an estrous

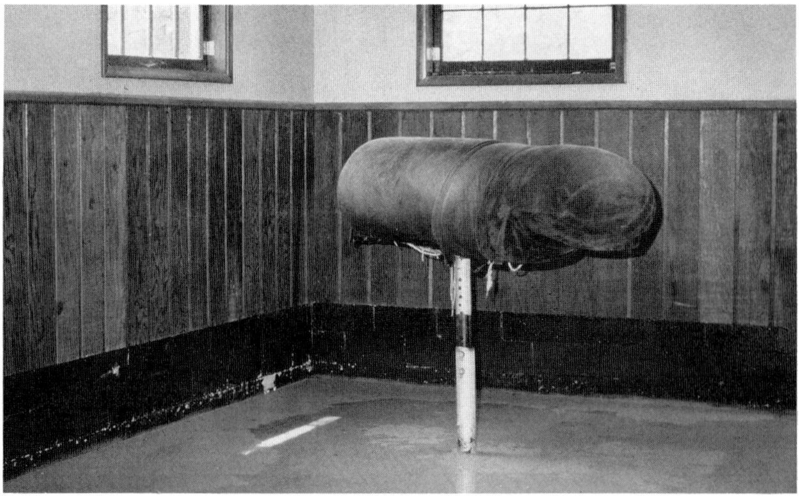

Figure 19. A model breeding phantom.

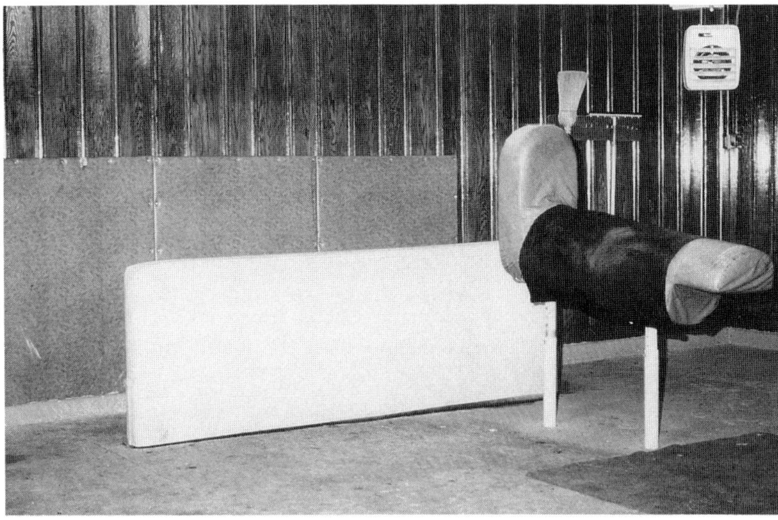

Figure 20. Breeding phantom adjacent to a padded teasing rail in a stallion breeding area.

mare to mount the phantom. When properly constructed, breeding phantoms greatly improve the efficiency and safety of semen collection.

General Semen-Handling Techniques

Semen should be transported to the lab immediately after collection while avoiding light, agitation and cold shock to the spermatozoa. All materials coming in contact with the semen sample before addition of semen extender should be prewarmed to body temperature, including the extender itself. If a filter was not placed in the AV during semen collection, upon arrival at the laboratory the ejaculate should be strained through a nontoxic filter to remove extraneous debris and the gel fraction. The volume, color and consistency of the gel-free semen are recorded, then the spermatozoal concentration and percentage of progressively motile spermatozoa in the gel-free ejaculate are estimated (Chapter 2). If possible, the semen should be combined with semen extender within 2 minutes after collection to optimize spermatozoal survival and longevity (Fig 21). In fact, it is customary on some farms to put warmed semen extender in the semen receptacle before collection so that the spermatozoa come in contact with this protective medium immediately after ejaculation. One disadvantage of this latter protocol is that the spermatozoal concentration cannot be measured accurately with a spectrophotometer or densimeter unless the extender used is optically clear (Chapter 2). Otherwise, only a hemacy-

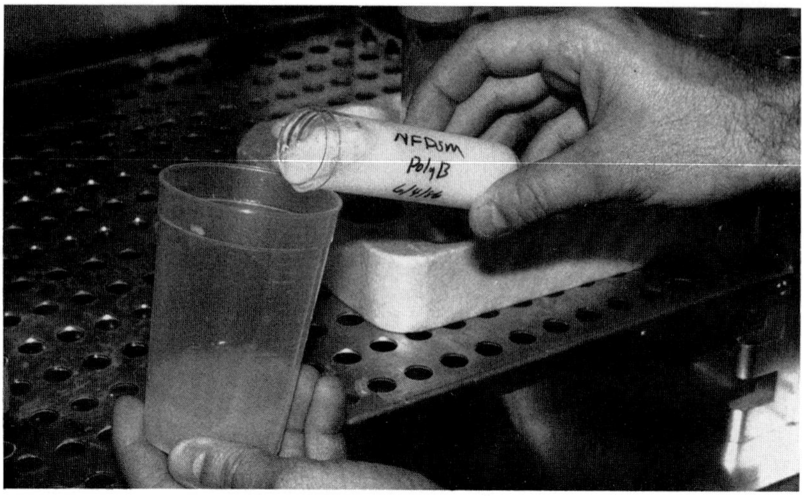

Figure 21. Semen extender, prewarmed to about 37 C, should be added to semen within 2 minutes after its collection.

tometer can be used to measure the spermatozoal concentration in the extended sample. A multiplication factor is used to estimate spermatozoal concentration in the raw semen sample.

Estimation of spermatozoal motility can be enhanced by first placing the semen in semen extender, provided the extender does not contain particles that obscure visualization of the spermatozoa (Chapter 2).

Semen collected for artificial insemination should first be mixed with an appropriate extender, whether the semen is to be inseminated immediately or preserved. Insemination of mares with raw, untreated semen is not recommended. Semen extender enhances spermatozoal survival outside the stallion's genital tract. Antibiotics in the extender reduce or eliminate bacterial contamination of the mare's reproductive tract at insemination. Conversely, artificial insemination of mares with raw semen collected using an AV provides no advantages over natural service other than division of the ejaculate for multiple inseminations. This may result in reduced conception rates if the semen is not handled properly and inseminated quickly, or if the semen contains potentially pathogenic organisms.

Satisfactory semen extenders are available commercially, or can be made readily in the laboratory (see Table 1).

Liquid Preservation of Semen

Semen collected from fertile stallions and not inseminated immediately can often be stored in the liquid state for 12-24 hours before insemination without affecting fertility. In fact, the fertilizing capacity of spermatozoa from some stallions has been maintained for up to 96 hours postejaculation through liquid preservation.[18] Successful semen preservation depends on initial semen quality. Semen that is inferior at the onset probably will have unsatisfactory spermatozoal longevity when stored *in vitro*. Therefore, it is very important to consider individual stallion variation when contemplating semen storage.

Gel-free semen should be mixed with warm (37 C) semen extender immediately after ejaculation, typically at a semen:extender ratio of 1:2 to 1:4. Generally speaking, the greater the ratio of semen dilution, the better the spermatozoal survival rate. Longevity of spermatozoal motility *in vitro* may be maximized by first diluting ejaculates with extender to a final concentration of 25×10^6 sperm/ml.[4]

The formulations for 3 commonly used and proven semen extenders are listed in Table 1. These extenders provide spermatozoa with metabolizable substrates, and accommodate spermatozoal pH and osmotic-pressure requirements. Milk protein in the extenders protects spermatozoa from cold shock, while antibiotics prevent or reduce bacterial proliferation. Bacteria in the semen sample must be susceptible to the antibiotics chosen in order to be eliminated. The antibiotics most commonly used in stallion semen extenders are penicillin G (1000-1500 units/

Table 1. Semen extender formulations.

Non-Fat Dry Skin Milk (NFDSM)-Glucose Extender I

NFDSM	2.4 g
Glucose	4.9 g
Penicillin, crystalline	150,000 units
Streptomycin, crystalline	150,000 μg
Deionized H_2O	qs 100 ml

Non-Fat Dry Skim Milk (NFDSM)-Glucose Extender II

NFDSM	2.4 g
Glucose	4.9 g
Gentamicin sulfate (reagent grade)	100 mg
8.4% $NaHCO_3$	2 ml
Deionized H_2O	92 ml

(Mix liquids before adding NFDSM or the acidity of the antibiotic will curdle the milk)

Cream Gel Extender

1. Dissolve 1.3 g unflavored Knox gelatin in 10 ml sterile distilled water. Sterilize.
2. Heat hal & half cream in a double boiler to 92-95 C for 2-4 minutes. Remove film from surface.
3. Mix gelatin solution with 90 ml heated half & half cream (100 ml total volume). Cool.
4. Add penicillin (100,000 units), streptomycin (100,000 μg) and polymixin B sulfate (20,000 units).

Heated Skim Milk Extender

1. Heat 100 ml nonfortified skim milk to 92-95 C for 10 minutes in a double boiler. Cool.
2. Add polymixin B sulfate (100,000 units).

ml), streptomycin sulfate (1000-1500 μg/ml), polymixin B sulfate (200-1000 units/ml), gentamicin sulfate (100-1000 μg/ml), amikacin sulfate (100-1000 μg/ml) or ticarcillin (100-1000 μg/ml). Any of these antibiotics can be incorporated into the extender formulations in Table 1. Use of gentamicin sulfate or amikacin sulfate generally requires adding a buffer, such as sodium bicarbonate, for adjustment to a pH that approximates neutrality.

All of the extenders described in Table 1 can be made immediately before use, or processed in bulk and stored frozen (-20 C) in packets for future use. Semen extenders are also available commercially. Milk-based extenders may be superior to those containing egg yolk as a protectant, based on both longevity of spermatozoal motility *in vitro* and fertilizing capacity following 24 hours of storage at 5 C.[19,20] Extenders prepared with nonfat dry milk solids and glucose may be superior to heated skim-milk extenders.[21]

A pH in the range of 6.5-7.5 for semen extenders appears to be compatible with maintenance of spermatozoal motility and fertilizing capacity. Slightly acidic conditions (pH 6.6-6.8) may be superior to slightly basic conditions (pH 7.2-7.4).[22] Likewise, some variation in osmolarity (300-400 mOsmol/L) of semen extenders is tolerated by spermatozoa, but an osmolarity of about 350 mOsmol/L seems to maximize longevity of stallion spermatozoal motility when semen is stored in a milk-based extender at refrigerated temperature.[23]

Once semen is extended, it should be promptly removed from the 37-C (incubator) environment to prevent rapid deterioration in viability.[24] Extended semen of many stallions retains it fertilizing capacity for 12-24 hours when stored near room temperature (about 20 C).[25,26] Spermatozoal survival can be enhanced by cooling the extended sample to refrigerated temperature (about 5 C).[19,24,26-28] Extended semen should be cooled slowly to refrigerated temperature because rapid cooling can reduce spermatozoal viability. The optimal cooling rate appears to be -0.3 C/min (initial cooling rate);[24,29] however, the phase of the cooling curve that is most critical to maintenance of spermatozoal integrity has not been adequately addressed.

Lowering the storage temperature for spermatozoa is thought to result in a corresponding reduction in metabolic acitvity, thereby delaying senescent changes in the spermatozoa. The underlying mechanism of this relationship is not well understood but is likely to stem from the effect of ambient temperature on enzyme kinetics. Extended semen that is cooled need not be warmed before insemination unless an extender is used that forms a gel when cooled (*eg,* cream-gel extender in Table 1).

A major factor that influences longevity of spermatozoal viability *in vitro* is the type of package in which the spermatozoa are stored. Extended semen can be maintained in plastic syringes; however, toxic materials in the rubber plunger seals of some syringes (*eg,* 2-[2-hydroxyethylmercapto]benzothiazole, used for curing rubber) may leach into the contents of the syringe.[30] The net effect on extended semen stored in these syringes is reduced spermatozoal motility and possibly reduced fertilizing capacity.[31-33] All-plastic syringes (*eg,* Air-Tite syringes: Air-Tite Products, Vineland, NJ) are recommended for storage of extended stallion semen.

Survival of stallion spermatozoa *in vitro* can be maximized by eliminating air space in the storage package.[34] This can be easily accomplished by storing the semen in capped plastic syringes, or by pouring extended semen into sterile disposable polyethylene bags (*eg,* Whirl-Pak bags: Nasco, Atkinson, WI) and closing the bags to eliminate air space. Semen can also be stored in capped glass or plastic vials, provided all air space is eliminated and the storage containers or cap liners are nontoxic to spermatozoa. For storage of stallion spermatozoa, the closed-package method seems even superior to storage in an atmosphere containing 5% CO_2 and 95% O_2.[34]

Cryopreservation of Semen

Semen cryopreservation involves maintaining semen samples at extremely low temperatures. Liquid nitrogen, the cryogen normally used, permits spermatozoal storage at -196 C. Provided spermatozoa can withstand the transition to and from the frozen state, they are essentially "suspended in time," as further damage and metabolism are negligible during storage. For cryopreserved spermatozoa to fulfill their sole biologic function (fertilization) upon emergence from a cryopreserved state, certain characteristics must have been retained: normal metabolism for production of energy, progressive motility, intact membranes, acrosomal enzymes, surface-associated proteins required for sperm-egg recognition and binding, and uninjured nucleoprotein/chromatin.[35,36] Many stresses encountered by spermatozoa during cryopreservation could disrupt these important characteristics, including alterations of metabolism, reorganization of membranes, and extreme fluctuations in cellular volume, any of which could lead to spermatozoal malfunction or death.[37] Given these extremely harsh conditions, it seems remarkable that any of the cells could survive.

A successful equine semen cryopreservation program could expand considerably the current artificial insemination applications in the equine industry. It could dramatically increase the availability of genetically superior stallions by permitting worldwide shipment of semen. The longevity of cryopreserved germ plasm would far exceed that of the donor stallion; therefore, frozen semen banks would serve as excellent economic protection against untimely stallion deaths. Incorporation of frozen semen in artificial insemination programs would greatly reduce expenses and stress associated with mare transport and boarding, as semen could be readily shipped to the mare for insemination. In addition, transmission of disease among farms could be minimized. The advent of semen freezing has revolutionized the dairy cattle industry, through massive exploitation of superior sires. Infinite longevity of cryopreserved bull spermatozoa now enables shipment of bull semen to virtually any herd in the world.

Unfortunately, the benefits of cryopreserved semen that have been realized with cattle have not been duplicated in the equine industry. Owing to biophysical and biochemical differences in the spermatozoa of these 2 species, the freezing techniques used for bull semen have not been extrapolated successfully to stallion semen.[37,38] Further, research funds are severely limited for perfection of semen cryopreservation techniques for stallions, as most equine breed registries in the U.S. are strongly opposed to commercial use of cryopreserved semen. Despite some progress in this area, there is no simple, reliable method for freezing semen from a large percentage of otherwise fertile stallions.

The per-cycle pregnancy rate achieved with frozen/thawed stallion semen is reported to range from 6% to 70%. Though some of this variation is likely due to differences in cryopreservation technique, insemination protocol or mare fertility, stallion-to-stallion variation also occurs.[35,36,38-41] Several semen-preservation protocols have been evaluated in an effort to maximize survival of frozen/thawed stallion spermatozoa.

The basic technique for cryopreservation of stallion spermatozoa involves several steps:

Increasing the Concentration of Spermatozoa: This step can be accomplished by either centrifuging the ejaculated semen or collecting only the sperm-rich portion of ejaculates. Either method helps remove the potentially detrimental contribution of semen plasma to the ejaculate, while increasing spermatozoal concentration. If centrifugation is performed, the semen must first be mixed with an appropriate centrifugation medium to minimize cellular injury.

Adding Cryopreservation Medium: The more popular extenders for cryopreservation of stallion semen were originally developed in China, Japan, Eastern Europe, France and Germany. These extenders consist of various mixtures of egg yolk, milk, sugars, buffers, electrolytes, antibiotics and glycerol.[36]

Packaging Semen: Though freezing stallion spermatozoa in pellets has been described, it is more commonly packaged in small-volume straws (0.5-ml, 4-ml or 5-ml capacity; usually polyvinylchloride or polypropylene; Fig 22) or flattened aluminum tubes (15- to 25-ml capacity).

Freezing Semen: The most common cryogen for semen cryopreservation today is liquid nitrogen. Packaged semen can be placed horizontally in the static nitrogen vapor at a recommended level above the liquid:gas interface (*eg,* 1-4 cm), using specially designed racks (Fig 23). Alternatively, packaged semen can be frozen in a programmable nitrogen freezer (Fig 24).

Storing Semen: Semen is submerged in liquid nitrogen (-196 C) using specially designed storage containers to maintain spermatozoa in a dormant state (Fig 25).

Figure 22. Polyvinylchloride straws (5 x 240 mm, 4-ml capacity) for packaging of equine semen before cryopreservation. Straw ends are sealed with stainless-steel balls.

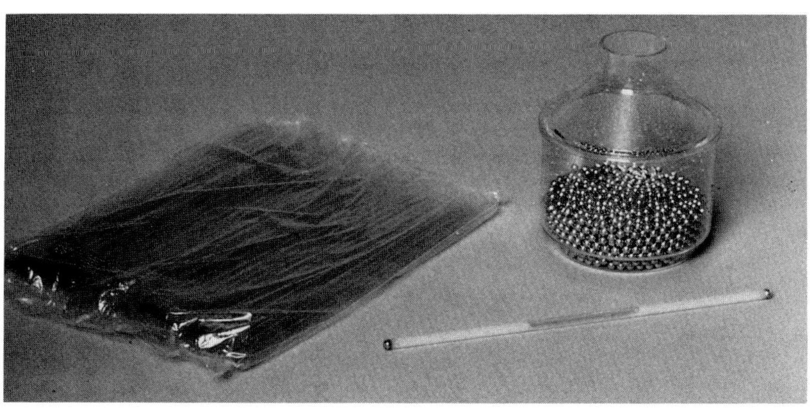

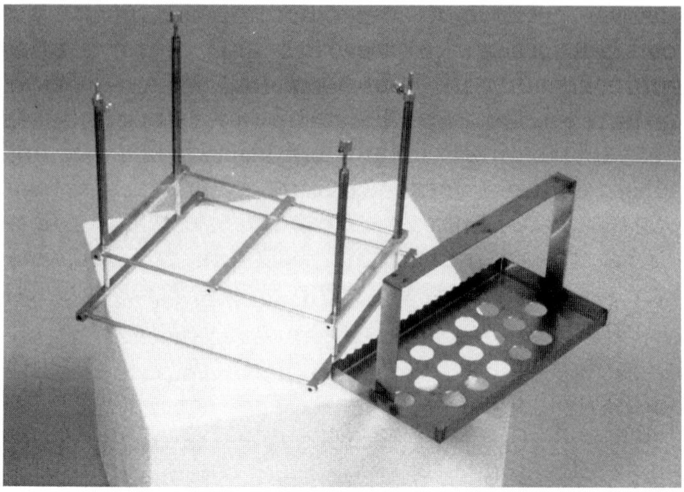

Figure 23. Specially designed rack and styrofoam container for freezing packaged equine semen in liquid-nitrogen vapor.

Thawing Semen: Packaged semen is thawed in a waterbath. Bath temperature and immersion time are designated by the company or individual responsible for freezing the semen.

Insemination: Immediately after thawing, packaged semen is inseminated, using the technique prescribed by the company or individual responsible for freezing the semen. The best pregnancy rates are probably achieved when mares are inseminated within 24 hours before or within 6-12 hours after ovulation.[40,42-44]

The principles of cryopreservation and its specific applications to stallion spermatozoa have been reviewed.[36] The reader is referred to this excellent source for specific information re-

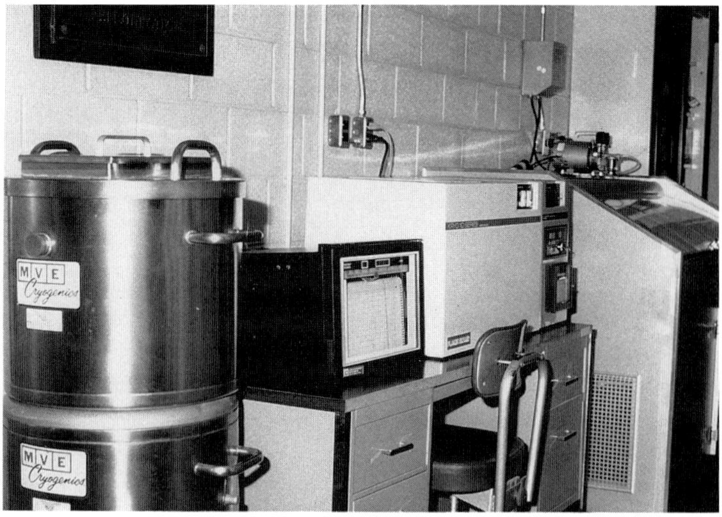

Figure 24. Well-equipped laboratory for cryopreservation of equine semen. Equipment includes a cold-handling cabinet containing an automatic device for filling and sealing straws, a programmable nitrogen freezer, a chart recorder with attached thermocouples for evaluating freeze rates, and 2 tanks designed for static-vapor freezing.

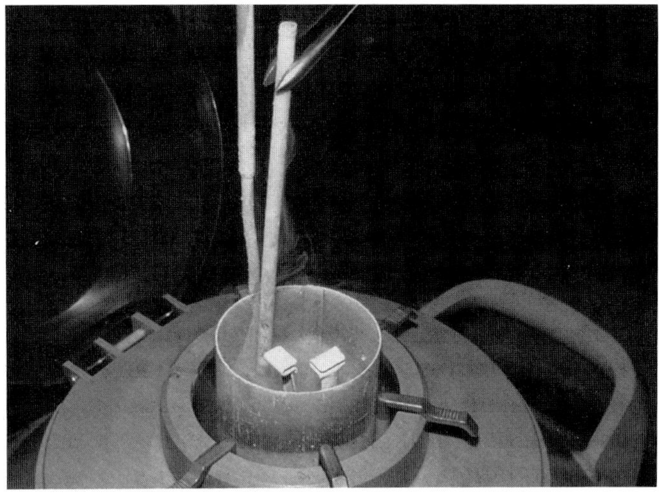

Figure 25. A canister in a liquid-nitrogen storage tank containing equine semen frozen in 4-ml straws.

garding methods of semen cryopreservation in stallions. Additional information is available from other sources.[35,37,48]

Semen Transport

Mare insemination with "mail order" semen is becoming commonplace in some breed organizations. Semen-handling techniques for transport of cooled liquid semen are similar to these for liquid preservation of semen maintained on the premises where it was collected. Special attention should be given to packaging to prevent undue damage from the concussive forces of shipment.

Transport of cooled semen has been simplified greatly by development of the Equitainer system (Hamilton-Thorn Research, Danvers, MA; Fig 26). This shipment container was designed to slowly cool extended semen (-0.3 C/min initial cooling rate) and maintain a final storage temperature of 4-8 C for 36-60 hours (depending on model). Semen can be transported in this lightweight, durable container to distant locations for insemination. Conception rates achieved using this semen transport system have been quite satisfactory.[28,29,34,46] If the semen is normal and handled according to manufacturer's directions, the fertility of the stored and transported semen is the same as with artificial breeding on the same farm. Cryopreserved semen can also be successfully transported in storage containers containing liquid nitrogen. Only semen storage tanks that cannot easily capsize should be used.

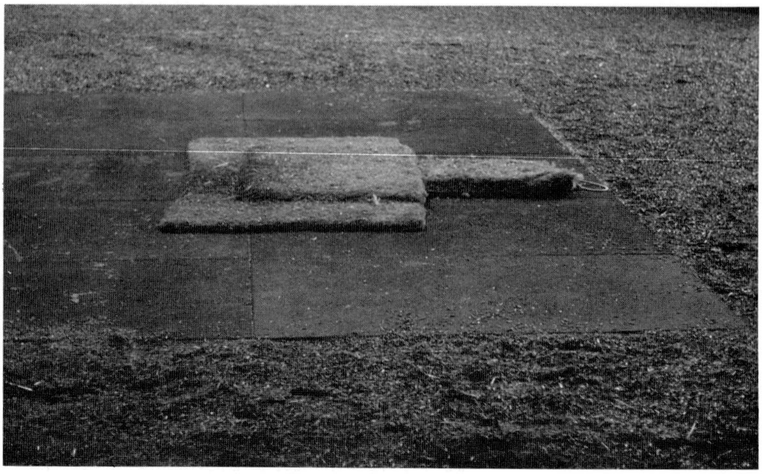

Figure 26. Commercially available containers for transport of equine semen. Recent model on left; early model on right.

References

1. Cooper WC: The effect of rapid temperature changes on oxygen uptake by and motility of stallion spermatozoa. *Proc Ann Mtg Soc Theriogenol,* 1979. pp 10-13.

2. Tischner M *et al:* Analysis of the pattern of ejaculation in stallions. *J Reprod Fertil* 41:329-335, 1974.

3. Kosiniak K: Characteristics of the successive jets of ejaculated semen in stallions. *J Reprod Fertil* (Suppl) 23:59-61, 1975.

4. Varner DD *et al:* Effects of semen fractionation and dilution ratio on equine spermatozoal motility parameters. *Theriogenology* 28:709-723, 1987.

5. Tischner M and Kosiniak K: Bacterial contamination of stallion semen and a collection technique. *Proc Equine Reprod Update Sem,* 1984.

6. McCarthy PF *et al:* A modified "open" artificial vagina and a urethral prosthetic device for the collection of gel-free semen. *Proc Ann Mtg Soc Theriogenol,* 1979. pp 5-9.

7. Merilan CP and Loch WE: The effect of artificial vagina liners on livability of stallion spermatozoa. *J Equine Vet Sci* 7:226-228, 1987.

8. Amann RP *et al:* Improved filter system for an equine artificial vagina. *J Equine Vet Sci* 3:120-125, 1983.

9. Bowen JM *et al:* Effects of washing on the bacterial flora of the stallion's penis. *J Reprod Fertil* 32:41-45, 1982.

10. Swerczek TW: Aggravation of strangles, equine clostridial typhlocolitis (colitis X) and bacterial venereal diseases in the horse by antibacterial drugs. *Proc Ann Mtg AAEP,* 1979. pp 305-311.

11. Kenney RM and Cummings MR: Potential control of stallion penile shedding of *Pseudomonas aeruginosa* and *Klebsiella pneumoniae. Proc Symp Voortplanting Paard,* 1990.

12. Blanchard TL *et al:* Use of a seminal extender containing antibiotic to improve the fertility of a stallion with seminal vasiculitis due to *Pseudomonas aeruginosa. Theriogenology* 28:541-546, 1987.

13. Hale EB and Almquist JO: Relation of sexual behavior to germ cell output in farm animals. *J Dairy Sci* 43:145, 1960.

14. Pickett BW *et al: Normal and Abnormal Sexual Behavior of the Equine Male.* General series 1004, Colorado State Uni, Fort Collins, 1981. pp 4-25.

15. Varner DD and Blanchard TL: Unpublished observations, 1986.

16. Crump J and Crump J: Stallion ejaculation by manual stimulation of the penis. *Theriogenology* 31:341-346, 1988.

17. McDonnell SM and Love CC: Manual stimulation collection of semen from stallions: training time, sexual behavior and semen. *Theriogenology* 33:1201-1210, 1990.

18. Hughes JP and Loy RG: Artificial insemination in the equine. A comparison of natural breeding and artificial insemination of mares using semen from six stallions. *Cornell Vet* 60:463-475, 1970.

19. Palmer E: Factors affecting stallion semen survival and fertility. *Proc 10th Intl Cong Anim Reprod Artif Insemin,* 1984. pp 377-379.

20. Province CA *et al:* Extenders for preservation of canine and equine spermatozoa at 5 C. *Theriogenology* 22:409-415, 1984.

21. Province CA *et al:* Cooling rates, storage temperatures and fertility of extended equine spermatozoa. *Theriogenology* 23:925-933, 1985.

22. Varner DD: Unpublished observations, 1989.

23. McIntosh A *et al:* Unpublished observations, 1990.

24. Varner DD *et al:* Effects of cooling rate and storage temperature on equine spermatozoal motility parameters. *Theriogenology* 29:1043-1054, 1989.

25. Franel AT *et al:* Motility and fertility of equine spermatozoa in a milk extender after 12 or 24 hours at 20 C. *Theriogenology* 27:517-525, 1987.

26. Varner DD *et al:* Fertilizing capacity of equine spermatozoa stored for 24 hours at 5 or 20 C. *Theriogenology* 32:515-525, 1989.

27. Squires EL *et al:* Fertility of equine spermatozoa cooled to 5 or 20 C. *Proc 11th Intl Cong Anim Reprod Artif Insemin,* 1988.

28. Zidane N *et al:* Fertility of fresh equine semen preserved for up to 48 hours. *Proc 5th Intl Symp Equine Reprod,* 1990. pp 200-201.

29. Douglas-Hamilton DH *et al:* A field study of the fertility of transported equine semen. *Theriogenology* 22:291-304, 1984.

30. Peterson MC *et al:* Leaching of 2-(2-Hydroxyethylmercapto)benzothiazole into contents of disposable syringes. *J Pharmaceutical Sci* 70:1139-1143, 1981.

31. Driscoll D and Douglas-Hamilton DH: Personal communication, 1984.

32. Shull JW *et al:* Spermatozoal motility parameters of equine semen stored in plastic syringes. *Proc Conf Res Workers Anim Dis,* 1986.

33. Broussard JR *et al:* The effects of Monoject and Air-Tite syringes on equine spermatozoa. *Theriogenology* 33:200, 1990.

34. Heiskanen M-L *et al:* Motility and ATP content of extended equine spermatozoa in different storage conditions. *J Reprod Fertil* (Suppl) 35:103-107, 1987.

35. Loomis PR: Techniques and applications of artificial insemination with frozen equine semen. *J Equine Vet Sci* 6:139-142, 1986.

36. Amann RP and Pickett BW: Principles of cryopreservation and a review of cryopreservation of stallion spermatozoa. *J Equine Vet Sci* 7:145-173, 1987.

37. Hammerstedt RH *et al:* Cryopreservation of mammalian sperm: What we ask them to survive. *J Androl* 11:73-88, 1990.

38. Amann RP: Preservation of the male gamete (bull, stallion, dog). *Proc 10th Intl Cong Anim Reprod Artif Insem,* 1984. pp 28-36.

39. Tischner M: Evaluation of deep-frozen semen in stallions. *J Reprod Fertil* (Suppl) 27:53-59, 1979.

40. Palmer E: Factors affecting stallion semen survival and fertility. *Proc 10th Intl Cong Anim Reprod Artif Insem,* 1984. pp 111-163.

41. Muller Z: Practicalities of insemination of mares with deep-frozen semen. *J Reprod Fertil* (Suppl) 35:121-125, 1987.

42. Aliev A and Ochkin D: The optimum time of insemination. *Anim Breed Abstr* 37:Abstr 5273, 1979.

43. Martin JC *et al:* Centrifugation of stallion semen and its storage in large-volume straws. *J Reprod Fertil* (Suppl) 27:47-51, 1975.

44. Kloppe LH *et al:* Effect of insemination timing on the fertilizing capacity of frozen/thawed equine spermatozoa. *Theriogenology* 29:429-439, 1988.

45. Varner DD: Collection and preservation of stallion spermatozoa. *Proc Soc Theriogenol,* 1986. pp 13-33.

46. Douglas-Hamilton DH *et al:* Fertility and characteristics of slow-cooled stallion semen. *J Reprod Fertil* (Suppl) 35:649-650, 1987.

47. Kenney RM *et al:* Minimal contamination techniques for breeding mares: technique and preliminary observations. *Proc Ann Mtg AAEP,* 1975. pp 327-336.

tized if it cannot be palpated safely. Absence of either testicle or detection of intestinal herniation into the inguinal canal may alter the method of anesthesia or technique of castration.

Castration in Lateral Recumbency

A variety of safe short-term IV anesthetics can be used, alone or in combination, for castrating a recumbent horse. The ultrashort-acting thiobarbiturates, alone or following administration of xylazine (Rompun: Haver) or acepromazine maleate (Prom-Ace: Fort Dodge), provide a short period of general anesthesia with moderate analgesia and muscle relaxation. Recovery usually is satisfactory if only a single dose of the thiobarbiturate is given.[1] Guaifenesin (Life Science Products), in combination with an ultrashort-acting barbiturate or ketamine HCl (with or without xylazine as a preanesthetic agent), gives good analgesia with smooth induction and recovery. Ketamine HCl (Ketaset: Bristol) produces general anesthesia with good analgesia for about 12-18 minutes if induction is preceded by sedation with xylazine.

After induction of general anesthesia, the horse is positioned in lateral recumbency with the upper (nondependent) hind limb drawn cranially toward the shoulder by a rope from the base of the neck to the pastern.[2] For the right-handed operator, the castration is performed most easily with the horse in left lateral recumbency. The following castration procedure is described for a right-handed surgeon:

The scrotum and sheath are prepared for aseptic surgery. The neck of the scrotum is grasped with the left hand and both testicles are identified and then immobilized by squeezing them toward the base of the scrotum. A long scrotal incision is made over each testicle, 1-2 cm lateral and parallel to the median raphe. The incisions are 8-16 cm long, depending on the size of the testicles. Alternatively, if the testicles are small or difficult to grasp, the median raphe is tensed by pulling the cranial end of the sheath cranially and upward while making a longitudinal incision on each side of the median raphe (Fig 1). The incision is carried through the skin, tunica dartos and underlying scrotal fascia. If an "open" castration technique is used, the common (parietal) vaginal tunic also is incised. The caudal ligament of the epididymis (a remnant of the gubernaculum), which affixes the common vaginal tunic to the epididymal tail and attached testicle, then is severed and the spermatic cord is transected

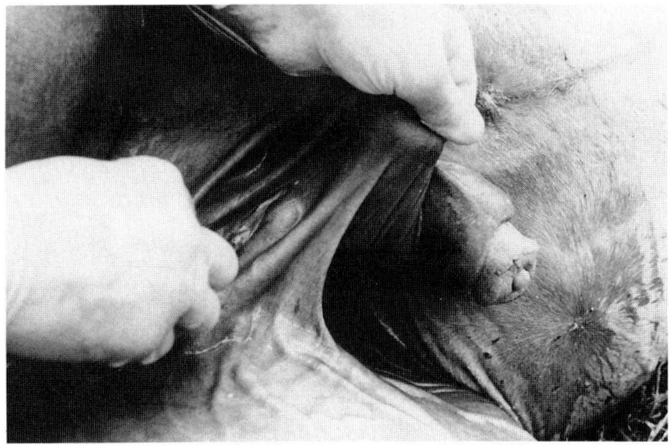

Figure 1. Two longitudinal incisions are made in the scrotum after it is tensed by pulling the sheath craniad and upward.

close to the superficial inguinal ring with an emasculator. The common vaginal tunic is not removed when an open castration is performed.

If a "closed" castration technique is used, the common vaginal tunic is not incised except at the point of spermatic cord transection. The common vaginal tunic, its contents (testicle, epididymis, spermatic cord), and attached external cremaster muscle are freed from surrounding scrotal fascia by blunt dissection and removed by transection close to the superficial inguinal ring with an emasculator. The closed technique of castration can be modified by making a 3- to 4-cm longitudinal incision in the vaginal tunic proximal to each testicle (Fig 2). The left thumb is inserted through the incision into the vaginal cavity and ventral traction is applied while the fingers of the left hand force the

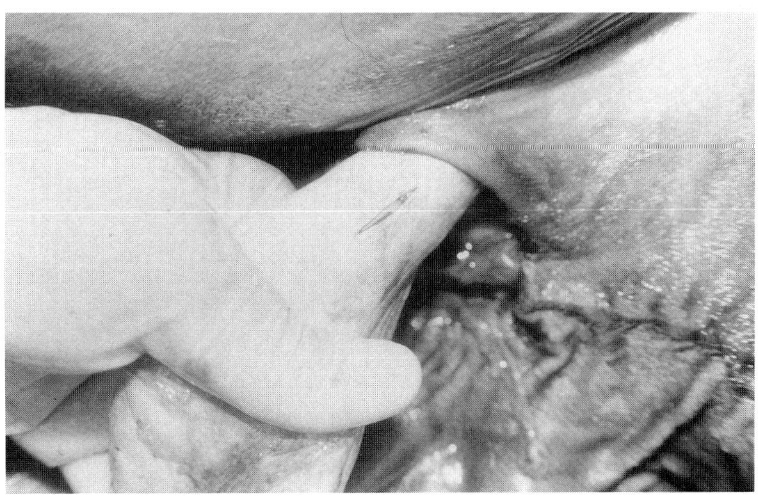

Figure 2. A small longitudinal incision is made through the parietal tunic proximal to the testis in preparation for modified-closed castration.

epididymis and testis through the incision (Fig 3). Because the caudal ligament of the epididymis affixes the fundus of the common vaginal tunic to the epididymis and attached testicle, the fundus inverts and follows the testicle through the incision when it is exteriorized. The left index and middle fingers are placed into the inverted fundus to maintain ventral tension on the vaginal tunic (Fig 4), and the left thumb is wrapped around the spermatic cord firmly to assist in traction. The spermatic cord and attached cremaster muscle are bluntly dissected free from scrotal fascia, and then transected near the superficial inguinal ring with an emasculator. By opening the vaginal tunic,

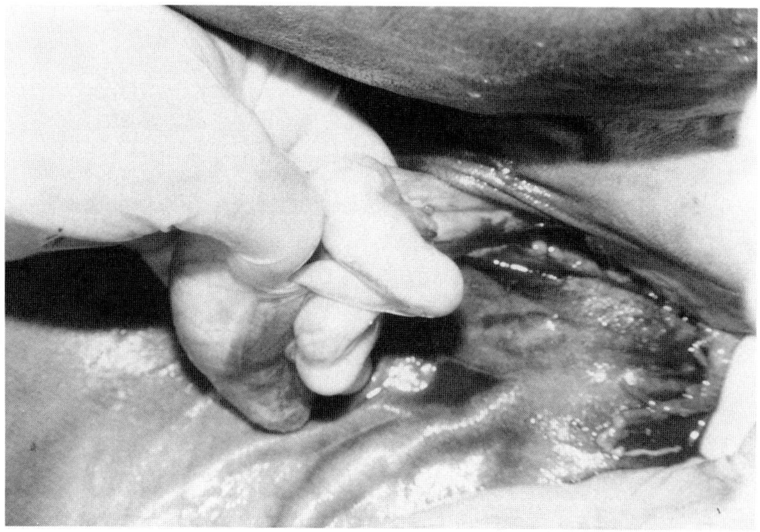

Figure 3. The surgeon's thumb is inserted through the incision of parietal tunic and into the vaginal cavity. The incision is stretched with the thumb so the contained testis can be exteriorized.

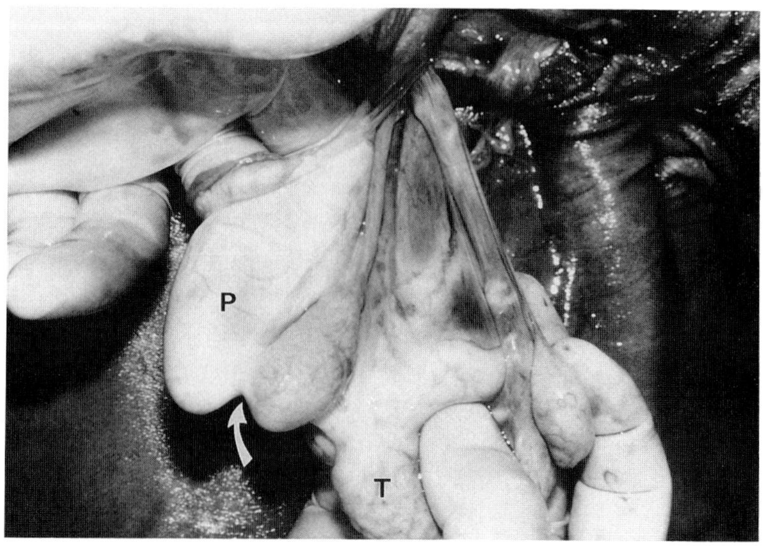

Figure 4. Exteriorizing the testis (T) inverts the parietal tunic (P) because the caudal ligament of the epididymis (arrow) is attached to its internal surface. Fingers are inserted into the sac produced, allowing tension to be easily maintained on the parietal tunic.

this "modified-closed" or "half-closed" castration technique allows observation of all enclosed structures (testes, epididymis, ductus deferens, spermatic vessels).[3]

Because the vaginal tunic is removed with closed and modified-closed castrations, the likelihood of infection or hydrocele formation is decreased. If the horse has a scrotal or inguinal hernia, eventration can be prevented by using the closed technique of castration and placing a ligature around the spermatic cord proximal to the site of transection. The closed technique is indicated in conditions that involve the vaginal tunic, such as neoplasia, periorchitis or torsion of the spermatic cord.

Proper emasculation is crucial to successful castration. The jaws of the emasculator are placed distally around the spermatic cord (or spermatic cord contents if an open castration is performed). The jaws are closed sufficiently to allow proximal movement of the emasculator to the site of transection near the superficial inguinal ring and to prevent inclusion of skin or other tissues in the emasculator's jaws. The emasculator must be applied with the crushing portion of the instrument positioned toward the abdomen. That is, the wing nut of the emasculator is positioned toward the testicle (the so-called "nut to nut" configuration, Fig 5). Tension on the spermatic cord is released before transection. The spermatic cord should be divided transversely, rather than tangentially, because severing the vessels tangentially interferes with the natural hemostatic mechanism of segmental vasospasm. To promote satisfactory hemostasis, the emasculator should be left in place for 30-60 seconds, depending on the size of the cord or its contents. If the

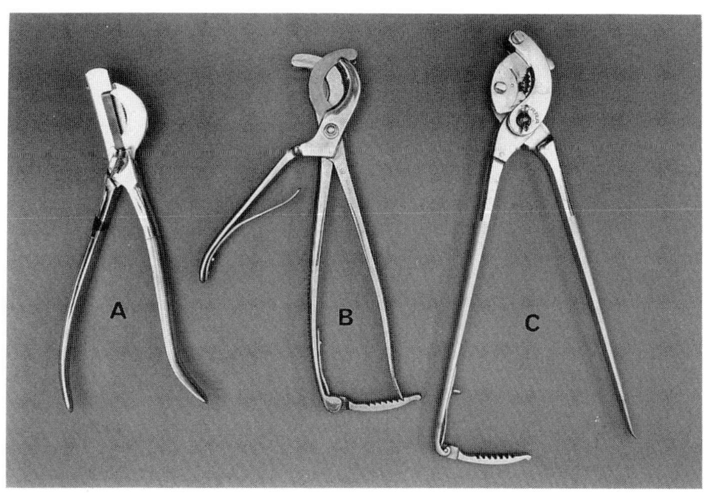

Figure 5. Emasculators for equine castration: A. Improved White. B. Reimer. C. Serra.

cord is large, the ductus deferens and spermatic vessels can be separated from the common vaginal tunic and cremaster muscle, and the 2 components separately transected.

Following removal of the testes and attached epididymides, the skin between the 2 scrotal incisions may be removed (Fig 6). Any fascia or tunics that may protrude from the scrotal incision sites when the horse stands should be removed using emasculators or scissors (Fig 7). The incisions usually are left unsutured to allow drainage, and may be stretched to enlarge the openings (Fig 8). Primary closure of the scrotal incisions following closed castration has been described.[4] Before division of the spermatic cord with emasculators, a transfixation ligature is placed in the cord proximal to the intended point of transection. The skin

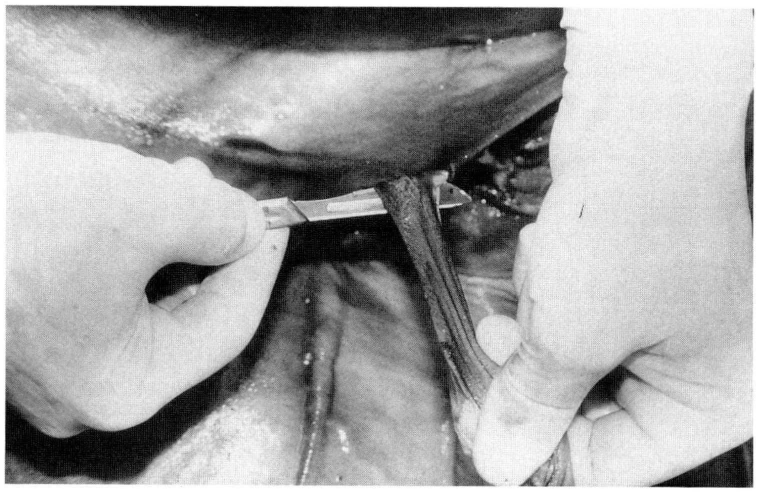

Figure 6. The skin between the 2 scrotal incisions may be removed for better drainage.

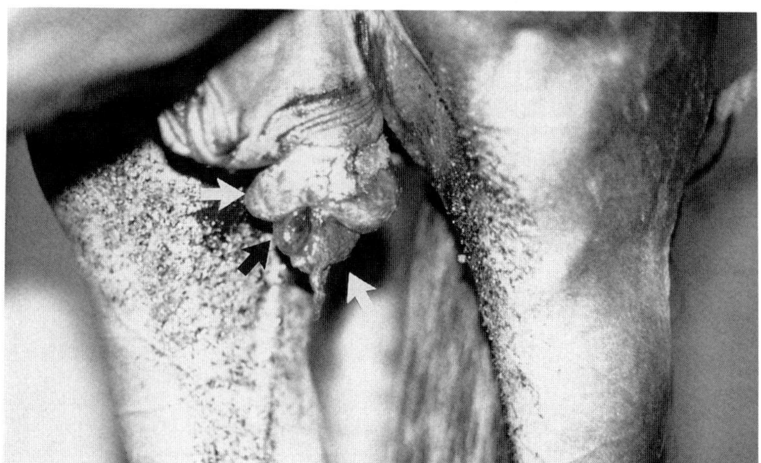

Figure 7. Parietal tunic (arrows) protruding through the scrotal incision following open castration.

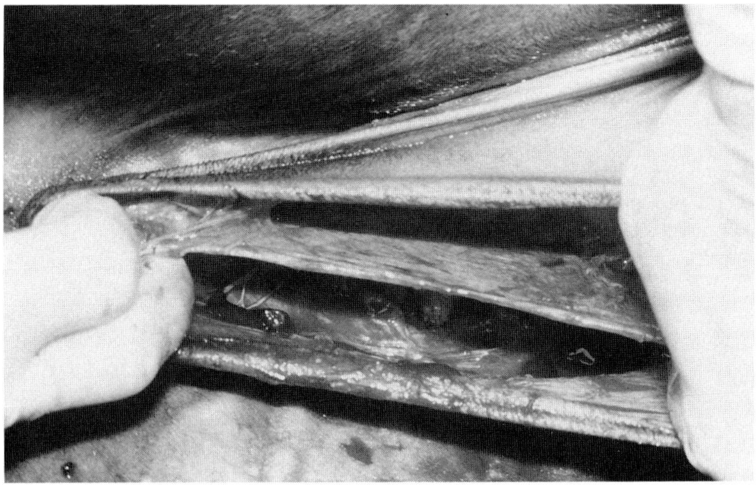

Figure 8. The scrotal incisions may also be stretched to allow better drainage.

incisions are closed with a synthetic absorbable suture material in a continuous horizontal mattress pattern. No attempt is made to close deadspace. Asepsis is required for good results when using a primary closure technique.

Castration in the Standing Position

Sedation or tranquilization for standing castration is optional but strongly recommended. Suitable drugs include chloral hydrate-magnesium sulfate preparations, xylazine, butorphanol tartrate (Torbugesic: Bristol), acepromazine maleate and pentazocine lactate (Talwin-V: Sterling). These drugs often are used in various combinations. The surgical site is anesthetized by SC infiltration with 10-15 ml of local anesthetic, such as 2% lidocaine HCl, along the lines of the scrotal incisions, followed by deposition of 10-15 ml into each spermatic cord (Figs 9, 10). Injection directly into the spermatic cord occasionally causes hematoma formation, which may interfere with cord transection. Alternatively, 15-30 ml of local anesthetic can be injected into the parenchyma of each testis and allowed to diffuse proximally up the cord (Fig 11).

Before injection, the scrotal and inguinal areas should be scrubbed thoroughly and the tail may be wrapped to prevent contamination of the surgical site. If the horse has not been tranquilized or sedated, a twitch should be applied to the muzzle to prevent movement when the surgical site is infiltrated with local anesthesia. The surgeon generally works from the left side

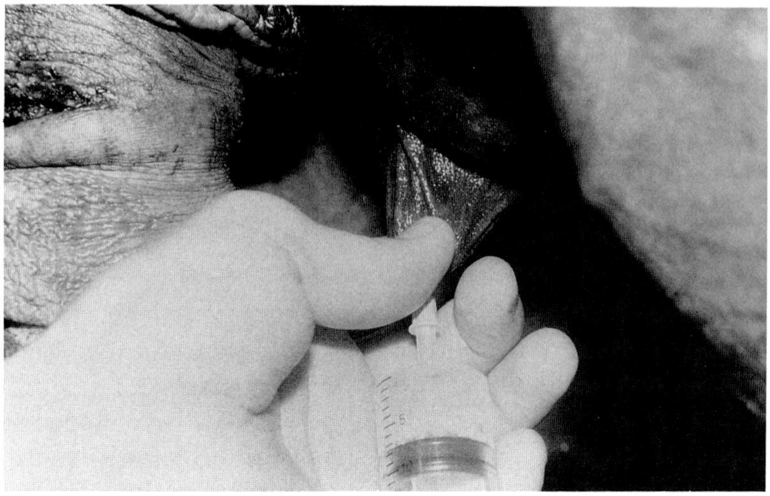

Figure 9. The scrotum may be infiltrated on each side of the median raphe with 10-15 ml of local anesthetic before making skin incisions.

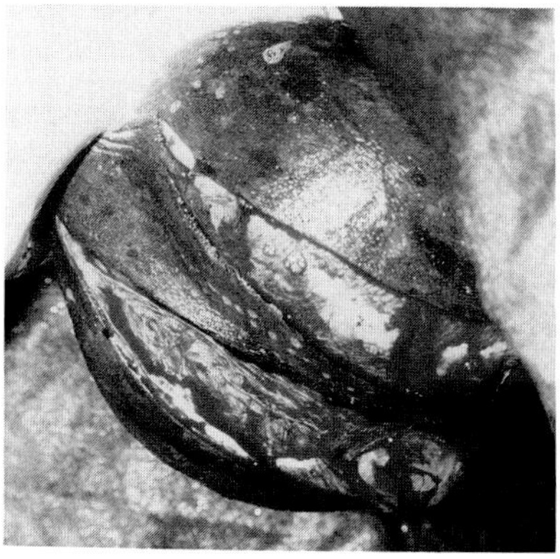

Figure 10. Two longitudinal incisions are made on each side of the scrotal raphe following instillation of local anesthetic.

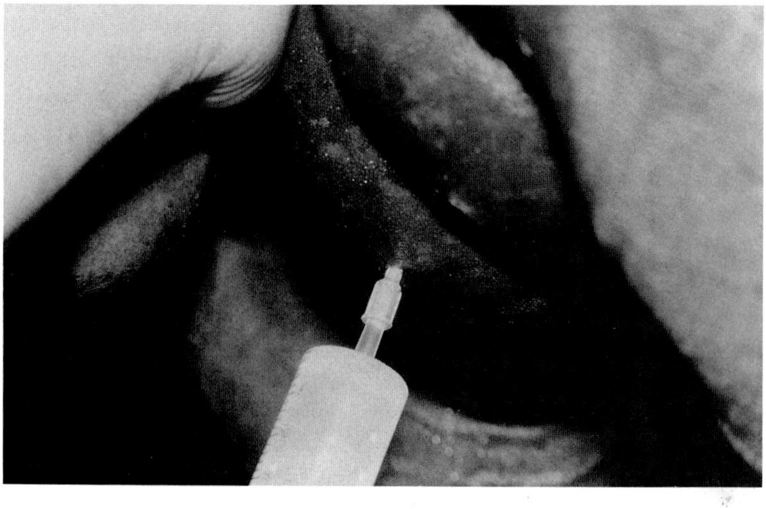

Figure 11. After inserting an 18-ga, 1 1/2-inch needle into the testicular parenchyma, 15-30 ml of local anesthetic are injected.

of the horse, leaning into the horse's side and avoiding the horse's kicking range. After the scrotum and spermatic cord are anesthetized, a final scrub is applied to the operative site.

Standing castration can be done using an open, closed or modified-closed technique, as described for the recumbent horse. By performing the castration with the horse standing, the risks of general anesthesia are avoided. Drug expense generally is less, and the procedure is shorter, as no recovery time from general anesthesia is required. Risks to the surgeon are greater, however, unless the candidates for the procedure are selected carefully. Standing castration should be reserved for well-mannered stallions with well-developed scrotal testicles and no history of recurrent scrotal swellings. If the testes cannot be palpated easily and safely within the scrotum, the horse should be anesthetized and castrated in the recumbent position. Burros, mules and small ponies are castrated more easily and safely under general anesthesia.

Immediately before or after castration, both tetanus antitoxin and tetanus toxoid should be given to all horses not previously immunized with tetanus toxoid.[5] A tetanus toxoid booster should be given to previously immunized horses. Prophylactic systemic antibiotics generally are unnecessary.

The castrated horse should be confined to a clean stall for the first 24 hours after surgery to avoid hemorrhage from the severed spermatic vessels. Thereafter, the horse should be exercised at least 15 minutes twice daily for 2 weeks; this helps prevent excessive edema in the scrotal and preputial areas. To avoid mating and possible mare impregnation in the early postoperative period, the horse should be isolated from mares for a minimum of 1-2 weeks after castration.[6]

Postoperative Complications

Excessive Hemorrhage

Excessive hemorrhage is the most common immediate postoperative complication of castration and often is caused by an improperly applied or malfunctioning emasculator. The spermatic vessels, especially the spermatic artery, may not be crushed sufficiently if scrotal skin is included accidentally in the jaws of the emasculator or if the spermatic cord is exceptionally large. The spermatic cords of older stallions often require double emasculation. In these horses, the spermatic vessels and deferent ducts are isolated from the common vaginal tunic and cremaster muscle and transected separately.

Severe hemorrhage occurs if the emasculator is applied upside down, as the cord is severed proximal to the crushing site. If the blade of the emasculator is too sharp, the spermatic vessels may be severed and the ends retracted before being crushed properly. When hemorrhage occurs, it is difficult to know the source without examination of the area. However, when hemorrhage is severe, it should be assumed it is from the spermatic artery.

The scrotal vessels can be lacerated when incising the scrotum or excising scrotal fascia. This hemorrhage usually is not serious and stops spontaneously. However, an excited horse often has increased blood pressure that could result in excessive hemorrhage. For this reason, horses caught with difficulty or after a long pursuit should be allowed to cool down before surgery. Similarly, frightened horses should be calmed before the operation. Excessive estrogens produced by some lush pastures also may interfere with hemostasis.[7]

If blood flow from the spermatic cord does not diminish after the horse stands quietly for 20-30 minutes, the severed end of the cord can be grasped with the fingers and stretched, and a crushing forceps, ligature or emasculator applied. If the horse was castrated in the recumbent position, the cord will not be anesthetized when the horse stands. The horse likely will resist attempts to grasp the severed spermatic cord. In this case, sedation and analgesia, as with xylazine or butorphanol tartrate, are indicated before exploration. Intractable horses may have to be placed under general anesthesia again.

If the end of the severed spermatic cord is inaccessible, sterile gauze (available in rolls) can be packed tightly through the scrotal incision into the inguinal and scrotal cavities. The skin incision then is closed with closely placed sutures or towel clamps. The pack can be removed the following day if hemostasis is achieved. If hemorrhage continues, the horse must be anesthetized and the hemorrhaging vessel(s) found and ligated.

Intravenous administration of 10-15 ml of 10% formalin in 1 L of physiologic saline solution through an IV catheter promotes hemostasis. In one experiment, this formalin dose decreased coagulation time by 67%.[8] However, another evaluation of hemostasis, including coagulation time, revealed no differences after IV formalin administration.[9] Though we have noted a dramatic reduction of hemorrhage immediately following administration of formalin in clinical cases, the safety and efficacy of this treatment have not been established.

Preputial/Scrotal Swelling

Swelling of the prepuce and scrotum is expected following castration and, unless excessive, is no cause for alarm. Insufficient exercise after castration results in poor drainage from the open scrotal incisions and promotes excessive scrotal swelling. Beginning the day following surgery, the horse should be exercised vigorously every day to promote drainage and discourage premature closure of the scrotal wound. Turning the horse into a large clean field is beneficial but does not ensure sufficient exercise.

Manual massage of the swollen tissue is beneficial for excessive swelling, if the horse will tolerate it. If the scrotal wounds seal prematurely, they should be opened by gentle massage or dilation with a gloved finger to remove blood clots or serum from the scrotal cavity. Hydrotherapy helps prevent the wounds from resealing prematurely and decreases edema in the scrotum and prepuce.

Postoperative swelling may be caused by bacterial infection of the surgical site. Sepsis of the scrotal cavity can occur easily, as the open incisions expose injured tissue to the environment. Forced exercise ensures drainage of the cavity and wound healing without serious complications. Local and systemic antibiotic administration, hydrotherapy and proper scrotal drainage usually correct this problem.

Clostridial infections of castration wounds are particularly catastrophic because they cause severe tissue necrosis and toxemia. Systemic signs vary with the clostridial species involved. Treatment consists of large doses of systemic penicillin, nonsteroidal antiinflammatory and analgesic agents, supportive therapy, and radical debridement of all necrotic tissue from the scrotal wound.

Funiculitis

Infection of the spermatic cord, or funiculitis, is an extension of a scrotal infection stemming from inadequate scrotal drainage. Postoperative infection of the spermatic cords is more likely if the cord stumps are long. Nonsterile surgery, repeated crushing of the spermatic cords, and contaminated ligatures can lead to funiculitis.[10] Signs of funiculitis include scrotal swelling, pain and fever. Antimicrobial treatment, drainage and hydrotherapy may resolve the infection, but removal of the infected stump may be necessary, especially if the cord has been ligated. "Champignon" is a French term for spermatic cord abscessation caused by *Streptococcus* species. The most common cause of champignon is thought to be ligation of the spermatic cords with contaminated suture material.[11]

If funiculitis is not treated, the scrotum may heal but the stump of the cord is likely to remain infected. The stump may reach large dimensions due to formation of excessive granulation tissue. This granulation tissue contains abscesses of various sizes that may communicate with the exterior by fistulous tracts. A chronically infected spermatic cord stump is called a "scirrhous cord" and can be caused by any pyogenic bacterium. Fungi also have been recovered from affected spermatic cords. Scirrhous cord caused by *Staphylococcus* species is sometimes termed botryomycosis. The scirrhous cord adheres to the scrotal skin, and draining tracts usually are present. The mass may elicit only mild pain upon palpation, and affected horses usually are afebrile. Large scirrhous cords may cause rear limb lameness, and in extreme cases may be palpable per rectum.

Surgical removal of a scirrhous cord usually results in uncomplicated recovery. The operation is performed with the horse under general anesthesia and in dorsal recumbency. An incision is made over the mass, and the affected cord and a section of normal cord are exposed. Isolation of the scirrhous cord may be difficult in long-standing cases because of numerous large vessels that have invaded the area. The spermatic cord is resected proximal to the mass with an ecraseur or emasculator, and the wound is left open to heal by second intention. Postoperative management is as for routine castration.

Peritonitis

Though reported infrequently, septic peritonitis can occur following castration, as the cavity of the vaginal process communicates with the peritoneal cavity. Extension of infection from the vaginal to the peritoneal cavities is rare because the funicular portion of the vaginal process is collapsed as it courses obliquely through the abdominal wall.[12]

Signs of septic peritonitis include fever, depression, weight loss, tachycardia, hemoconcentration, colic, and constipation or diarrhea.[13] Development of any of these signs following castration may warrant collection and examination of peritoneal fluid. Results of peritoneal fluid analysis must be interpreted carefully, as nonseptic peritonitis occurs in many horses as a result of castration.[14] Nonseptic peritonitis may be related to postoperative intraabdominal hemorrhage, as free blood within the peritoneal cavity causes peritonitis. A nucleated cell count in the peritoneal fluid >10,000/μl indicates peritoneal inflammation.[15] Counts >10,000/μl commonly occur for 5 or more days after uncomplicated castration, and counts >100,000/μl occasionally are detected.[14] A diagnosis of septic peritonitis should not be based on a high peritoneal nucleated cell count alone. The presence of toxic or degenerative neutrophils or intracellular bacteria in the peritoneal fluid is more indicative of peritoneal sepsis.[16] When this is accompanied by clinical signs, antimicrobial therapy and perhaps peritoneal lavage are indicated.

Hydrocele

A hydrocele, also referred to as a vaginocele or "water seed," may appear several months after castration as a circumscribed, fluid-filled, painless swelling in the scrotum. The swelling may resemble a scrotal testis or even a scrotal hernia, except that most of the swelling is confined to the most ventral part of the scrotum. If neglected, the fluid-filled vaginal tunic can become as large as a football. Sterile amber-colored fluid is obtained by needle aspiration. The swelling is due to a slowly increasing collection of fluid within the vaginal cavity. The condition is uncommon and the specific cause is unknown.

Hydrocele can occur in stallions as well as castrated horses, but the highest incidence appears to be in castrated mules. Open castration predisposes to the condition, as the vaginal tunic is not removed using this castration method. Therefore, the vaginal tunic should always be removed when castrating a mule. Surgical isolation and removal of the vaginal tunic is the indicated treatment for hydrocele.

Evisceration

Evisceration following castration of horses with normally descended testicles is an uncommon but potentially fatal complication. It may occur up to 1 week postcastration but usually happens within 4 hours after castration and may be precipitated by the horse's attempt to rise from general anesthesia. Horses that eviscerate following castration probably have a preexisting inapparent inguinal hernia that preoperative examination fails to reveal.[17,18] If intestine appears in the scrotal incision following castration, the horse should be anesthetized immediately. If not, the prolapsed intestine soon becomes contaminated and damaged during violent struggling due to the pain accompanying evisceration. A balanced electrolyte solution should be given IV in amounts adequate to combat hypotensive shock. The horse should be positioned in dorsal recumbency and the intestine cleaned meticulously with copious amounts of normal saline. Damaged mesentery and intestine should be repaired or resected and the prolapsed intestine reduced as soon as possible to prevent vascular damage. Luminal aspiration facilitates reduction of gas-distended intestine. Intraabdominal traction on the intestine at the vaginal ring through a paramedian or ventral midline celiotomy may be necessary to reduce the prolapsed intestine.

If the fundus of the vaginal sac has not been shredded during reduction of the prolapse, it is ligated with absorbable suture and transfixed to the edge of the superficial inguinal ring. Then the superficial ring is closed with doubled absorbable suture (No. 2 or 3) in a continuous pattern. The superficial layers of the wound are left unsutured if the wound is grossly contaminated. Sterile gauze can be packed into the inguinal canal and scrotum rather than suturing the superficial inguinal ring. Care should be taken to avoid introducing the gauze into the abdomen. The gauze is held in position for 48-72 hours by suturing the scrotal incision. The vaginal ring should be palpated per rectum before the packing is removed to confirm that intestine is not adhered to the pack.

Parenteral antimicrobial treatment should be initiated. If signs of peritonitis develop, abdominal fluid should be obtained and evaluated. Peritoneal lavage is indicated for horses that develop septic peritonitis.

Omentum occasionally may prolapse through the scrotal incision after castration (Fig 12). If this is noted, the vaginal ring should be palpated per rectum to identify any accompanying inapparent intestine. Exposed omentum is removed with emasculators, usually with the horse standing. The horse should not be exercised for 48 hours to prevent further prolapse.

Persistent Stallion-Like Behavior

Continued stallion-like behavior is a frequent complication of castration.[19,20] Such geldings, sometimes referred to as "false rigs," may display masculine behavior ranging from genital investigation and squealing, to mounting and even copulation. False rigs are often said to have been "proud cut," indicating that some epididymal tissue was left in the horse at the time of castration. It is improbable that the epididymis would be partially excised during castration of scrotal testes because the testis is closely attached to the epididymis. In fact, very few false rigs have epididymal tissue. The epididymis is incapable of androgen production, and geldings with epididymal tissue are endocrinologically and behaviorally indistinguishable from geldings without epididymal tissue.[21] Spermatic cord remnants have been removed from false rigs to abolish sexual behavior. However, because the cords contain no androgen-producing tissue, the efficacy of this procedure is doubtful.

The plasma concentration of luteinizing hormone is increased after castration in response to a falling plasma concentration of testosterone.[21] It has been postulated that the rise in luteinizing hormone may stimulate production of androgens by the adrenal cortex. False rigs, however, have no higher circulating concentration of testosterone than do normal quiet geldings, and administration of adrenocorticotropic hormones to false rigs has no effect on plasma concentration of testosterone.[21,22]

Stallion-like behavior in geldings has been attributed to learned response, as it has been noted that some sexually experienced stallions castrated late in life continue to display mas-

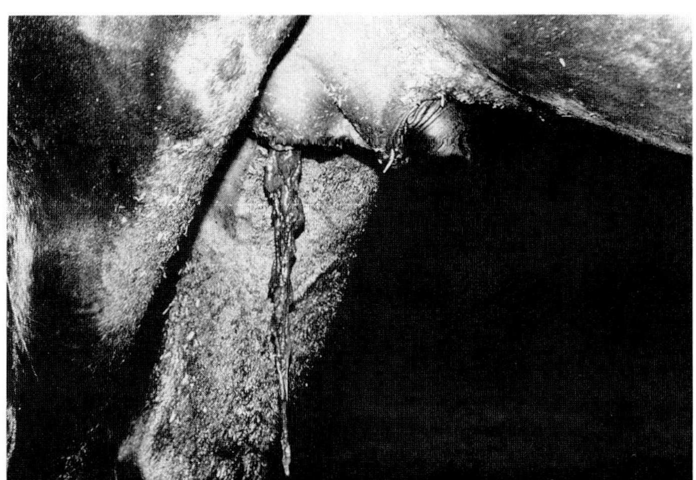

Figure 12. Omentum may occasionally prolapse through the vaginal ring and scrotal incision following castration.

culine behavior.[22] Many false rigs, however, have been castrated as juveniles. A retrospective survey found no difference in the prevalence of continued sexual behavior between horses castrated before or after puberty.[19] In this study, 20-30% of each group displayed stallion-like behavior at least 1 year after castration, and these percentages were considered to be similar to the prevalence of stallion-like behavior in geldings. Therefore, persistent sexual behavior in geldings may be part of the normal social interaction between horses and may be completely independent of sexual stimulation. Changes in management or stricter discipline may alleviate sexual behavior or reduce it to a tolerable level.

References

1. Geiser DR: Practical equine injectable anesthesia. *JAVMA* 182:574-577, 1983.

2. Leahy JR and Barrow P: *Restraint of Animals*. 2nd ed. Cornell Campus Store, Ithaca, New York, 1953. pp 72-80.

3. Kersjes AW *et al: Atlas of Large Animal Surgery*. Williams & Wilkins, Baltimore, 1985. pp 51-82.

4. Cox JE: Castration of horses and donkeys with first intention healing. *Vet Record* 115:372-375, 1984.

5. Liefman CE: Active immunisation of horses against tetanus including the booster dose and its application. *Aust Vet J* 57:57-60, 1981.

6. Shideler RK *et al:* Disappearance of spermatozoa from the ejaculates of geldings. *J Reprod Fertil* 27:25-29, 1979.

7. Johnson JH: Postcastration complications. *MVP* 54:49-51, 1973.

8. Roberts SJ: The effects of various intravenous injections on the horse. *Am J Vet Res* 4:226-238, 1943.

9. Morris DL: Unpublished data, 1986.

10. Wintzer HJ: *Equine Diseases*. Springer Verlag, New York, 1986. pp 194-213.

11. Wright JG: Champignon and scirrhous cord. *JAVMA* 144:402, 1964.

12. Shively MJ: *Veterinary Anatomy*. Texas A&M University Press, College Station, 1984. p 345.

13. Dyson S: Review of 30 cases of peritonitis in the horse. *Eq Vet J* 15:25-30, 1983.

14. Schumacher J and Schumacher J: Effects of castration on peritoneal fluid constituents in the horse. *J Vet Int Med* 2: In press, 1990.

15. Ricketts SW, in Robinson NE: *Current Therapy in Equine Medicine 2*. Saunders, Philadelphia, 1987. pp 79-81.

16. Adams SB *et al:* Cytologic interpretation of peritoneal fluid in the evaluation of equine abdominal crises. *Cornell Vet* 70:232-246, 1980.

17. Hutchins DR and Rawlinson RJ: Eventration as a sequel to castration of the horse. *Aust Vet J* 48:288-291, 1972.

18. Goetz TE *et al:* Inguinal and scrotal hernias in colts and stallions. *Compend Cont Ed Pract Vet* 3:S272-S276, 1981.

19. Line SW *et al:* Effect of prepubertal versus postpubertal castration on sexual and aggressive behavior in male horses. *JAVMA* 186:249-251, 1985.

20. Cox JE: Behavior of the false rig: causes and treatments. *Vet Record* 118:353-356, 1986.

21. Crowe CW *et al:* Plasma testosterone and behavioral characteristics in geldings with intact epididymides. *J Eq Med Surg* 1:387-390, 1977.

22. Cox JE *et al:* Testosterone in normal, cryptorchid and castrated male horses. *Equine Vet J* 5:85-90, 1973.

6

Sexual Behavior Dysfunction

Sexual behavior denotes all events and expressions related to sexual union and consists of precopulatory (courtship) and copulatory phases. Normal sexual behavior depends on proper operation and coordination of numerous psychophysiologic processes involving several body systems (endocrine, nervous, cardiovascular, musculoskeletal systems). Because the specific mechanisms surrounding sexual behavior are complex and not clearly understood, the cause of sexual behavior disorders often can be difficult to diagnose and the response to treatment difficult to predict.

Lack of Libido

The term "libido" refers to sexual drive or the psychic energy directed toward copulation. The intensity of libido varies among individual stallions and is governed by genetic composition, sensory capability (visual, olfactory, auditory), and environmental factors (positive and negative). Upon exposure to a mare in behavioral estrus, a postpubertal stallion should promptly display a high level of libido, manifested by vocalization, sexual curiosity, development of an erection, and a strong urge to copulate (Fig 1).[1] Any deviation from this pattern may be abnormal and should be investigated.

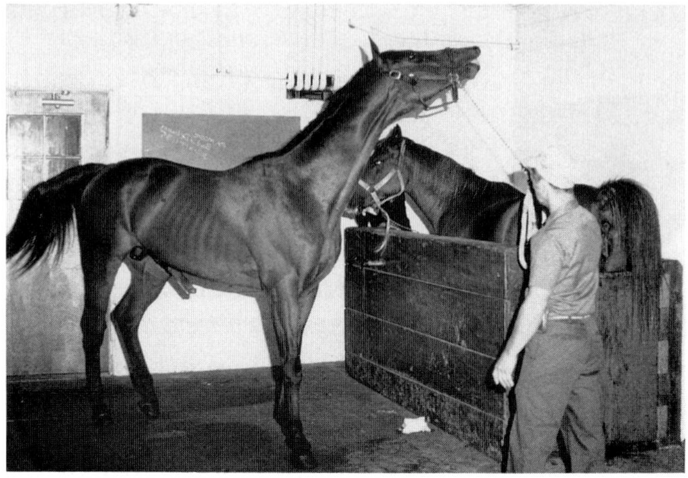

Figure 1. Exposure of a stallion to mare in estrus, resulting in penile erection, vocalization, and display of the "Flehmen" reaction.

Suppression or absence of libido in a mature stallion that is sexually provoked may be of unknown origin, or an obvious response to a negative experience (such as a breeding accident or sexual overuse). Low libido is observed commonly in young "maiden" stallions during their first encounter with a mare in estrus, after retiring to stud from a performance career. The libido of these stallions usually intensifies if they experience positive interactions with mares and handlers during their first few breeding sessions. Stallions may have difficulty in assuming "studdish behavior" in the breeding environment if sexual arousal has been forcefully discouraged by verbal and physical reprimand on previous occasions. Solitary rearing may also result in deficient libido in mature stallions because of inadequate interaction with other horses during their formative years. Occasional stallions are sexually aroused by the presence of their handler, thus indicating that aberrant behavioral patterns can be established, especially through inappropriate social interaction.

Clinical examination of a stallion with low libido always should be preceded by procurement of a detailed history. A historical review includes the stallion's social environment, handling and training techniques, changes in environment, previous reproductive experiences, breeding procedures used, onset of the behavioral problem, and events surrounding the deviation in sexual behavior. Critical investigation into a stallion's background often discloses events that may have contributed to the behavioral disturbance.

The quality and temporal course of sexual preparation should be monitored closely when the stallion is placed near a mare in behavioral estrus. An appropriate sexual stimulus must be offered to the stallion. Ovariectomized mares or breeding dummies sometimes do not serve as a suitable stimulus. Ideally, a docile ovary-intact mare exhibiting behavioral estrus should be used for sexual stimulation of the stallion. It may be advantageous to let the stallion select a mare through group teasing, as preferences for and aversions to certain mares by some stallions have been observed.

The breeding area should be free of unnecessary personnel and other distractions and, preferably, be familiar to the stallion. Variation in the stallion's response to changes in handlers, handling techniques, stimulus mares and breeding areas should be noted. Physical examination of the stallion should include assessment of visual, olfactory and auditory function, and palpation of external genital organs. The stallion's endocrine profile (plasma concentrations of testosterone, estrogen, luteinizing hormone, follicle-stimulating hormone) also can be studied, though the relationship of these various hormones to intensity of libido remains ambiguous.[2,3]

Patience, persistence and positive reinforcement are indispensable elements of treatment for low libido in stallions. Any underlying perturbations, such as abusive handling or sexual overuse, should be corrected. Specific methods of treatment vary with individual cases. For instance, a change in the breeding environment may bolster libido in stallions that have previously experienced a traumatic episode related to breeding at a certain location. Conversely, movement of a stallion to unfamiliar surroundings may interfere with his breeding performance. Depressed libido produced by sexual overuse often can be corrected by simply increasing the time interval between breedings or semen collections. Provisions for a more natural breeding environment may help overcome the sexual inhibitions of some stallions. Hand-mating outdoors in a secluded, grassy area sometimes initiates a favorable response in timid stallions that are reluctant to breed in unfamiliar indoor arenas. A pasture breeding situation, where the stimulus mare is cooperative and solicitous, and the stallion is unrestrained, often resolves libido problems in timid stallions.

Permitting shy breeders to observe vigorous-breeding stallions during the act of mating may help invigorate them. Similarly, slow-breeding stallions sometimes are encouraged to breed mares while other stallions are in the immediate vicinity. This therapeutic approach attempts to energize slow breeders by creating a competitive environment. Training sessions to improve libido of stallions may be most productive during the summer, as stallions are more sexually responsive during the summer months than in winter.[4] Alternatively, stallions can be placed on an artificial lighting program to help stimulate libido (see Chapter 3).[5] A lengthy retraining period may be required to reestablish normal libido in stallions experiencing marked libido depression because of a breeding accident or similar negative sexual experience.

Hormonal supplementation is a controversial mode of therapy for low libido in stallions, especially because the relationship of hormonal profiles to sexual behavior is poorly understood. Exogenous administration of androgens is contraindicated as a method of amplifying libido in breeding stallions because of the attendant impairment in spermatogenesis.[6] Though multiple injections of testosterone or anabolic steroids (which also have androgenic activity) are known to adversely affect testicular function, a single injection of testosterone or the anabolic steroid, nandrolone decanoate (Deca-Durabolin: Organan; anabolic steroids also have androgenic activity) has been used anecdotally to help correct low libido in stallions.[6-10] Neither testosterone nor anabolic steroids enhance the libido of stallions with normal breeding behavior.[7,8] Human chorionic gonadotropin (HCG) and gonadotropin-releasing hormone (GnRH) have been given empirically for treatment of low libido in stallions, but the long-term effects of these hormones on spermatogenesis have not been established. The efficacy and clinical safety of these hormones for treatment of low libido in stallions require further study.

One study revealed no improvement in behavioral characteristics of reproductively active horse stallions after pulsatile or continuous treatment with exogenous GnRH.[11] Results of another investigation, however, indicated that pulsatile administration of GnRH to testosterone-treated pony stallions enhanced copulatory behavior.[12]

Psychotropic drugs have been used to help manage libido depression in selected stallions. Slow IV infusion of diazepam (Valium: Roche) at 0.05 mg/kg with a maximum dose of 20 mg, about 10 minutes before breeding sometimes reverses sexual inhibition associated with a novel environment or previous negative sexual experience.[13] Efficacy and safety of other psychotropic drugs (*eg,* imipramine and clomipramine) are under investigation for treatment of sexual inhibition in stallions.[14]

Erection Failure

Impotence, or lack of productive copulatory ability, can be associated with inability to develop and maintain a normal penile erection. This disability may be a repercussion of suppressed libido, as described above, or it may result from an organic dysfunction, rather than a psychogenic disturbance. Inability to develop an erection despite normal libido suggests a neuromuscular or vascular dysfunction. The incidence of non-psychogenic erection failure does not appear to be as common in horses as in men, so the area has received little study. The most common cause of erection failure in horses with good libido is local vascular or neurologic damage from a breeding accident or other genital injury (Fig 2).

Much of our present understanding of mechanisms of penile erection is derived from studies in men. The sequence of events that leads to penile erection is complex and the precise mechanisms involved remain a subject of controversy. Early experi-

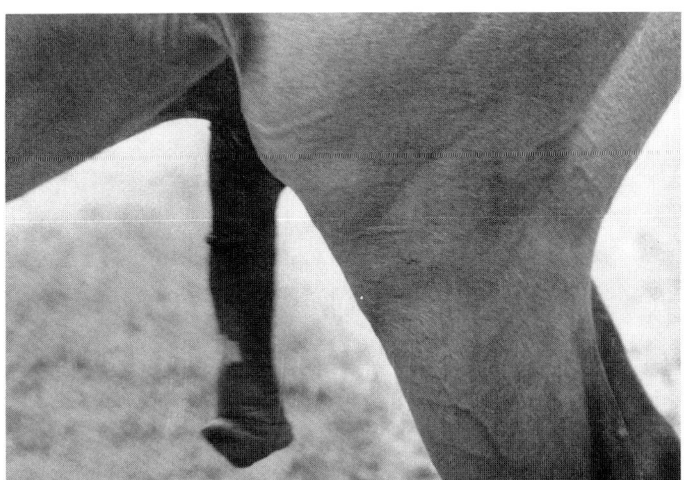

Figure 2. Inability to gain a full erection following reserpine-induced penile paralysis 34 months earlier.

mentation suggested that penile erection was mediated by the sacral parasympathetic pathway, possibly in conjunction with alpha-adrenergic blockade. More recent studies provide convincing evidence that a noncholinergic nonadrenergic neurotransmitter, termed vasoactive intestinal polypeptide (VIP), is a principal mediator of penile erection.[15,16] Penile tumescence is produced by increased local arterial flow (through arterial vasodilation), relaxation of trabecular smooth muscle in the penile cavernous tissue, and restricted venous outflow from the penis.[15] Contraction of the ischiocavernosus and bulbospongiosus muscles is necessary for maximal engorgement of these penile sinuses.[17-20]

Several diagnostic tests, including nocturnal penile tumescence monitoring, pudendal arteriography, corpus cavernography, bulbocavernous reflex latency tests and intracorporeal injection procedures, have been devised for differentiating vasculogenic and neurogenic forms of erectile failure in men with normal libido. However, these techniques have not been adapted for routine use in horses.

A new diagnostic approach to evaluation of impotence in men has been received enthusiastically by urologists worldwide.[21,22] The procedure involves injection of papaverine HCl (a smooth-muscle relaxant) into the corpus cavernosum penis of the conscious patient, followed by observation for penile response. Papaverine serves as a substitute for local neurotransmitters, as it is a potent smooth-muscle relaxant. In normal men, injection results in an erection caused by sinusoidal relaxation and increased arterial flow to the penis. This test evaluates the integrity of the vascular mechanisms associated with erection and, as such, helps distinguish vascular from nonvascular impotence.

Therapeutic management of neurogenic or vascular impotence in men involves either medical or surgical approaches. Medical management consists of intracavernous injection with vasoactive drugs (*eg,* papaverine HCl, phentolamine mesylate, phenoxybenzamine) to induce temporary tumescence.[23,24] This medical approach requires strict supervision because it can lead to serious complications. Surgical management generally involves installation of a penile implant. These treatment regimens have not been reported for use in horses.

Some stallions unable to attain a rigid erection as a result of previous vasculogenic damage to the corpus cavernosum penis (see Chapter 14) can still ejaculate if manual assistance if provided for penile intromission into the mare's vagina, or an artificial vagina.

Mounting or Intromission Difficulty

Despite demonstration of good libido and erectile capability, some stallions are ineffectual breeders because of difficulty in mounting or achieving intromission. Stallions with hind limb or pelvic lamenesses or spinal lesions often are hesitant to mount, even though precopulatory behavior is quite intense. If affected

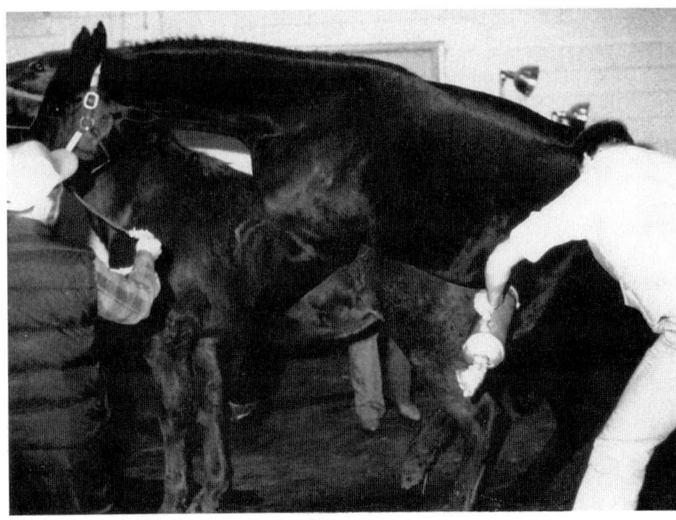

Figure 3. Mating disabilitiy in a stallion, resulting from hind limb lameness.

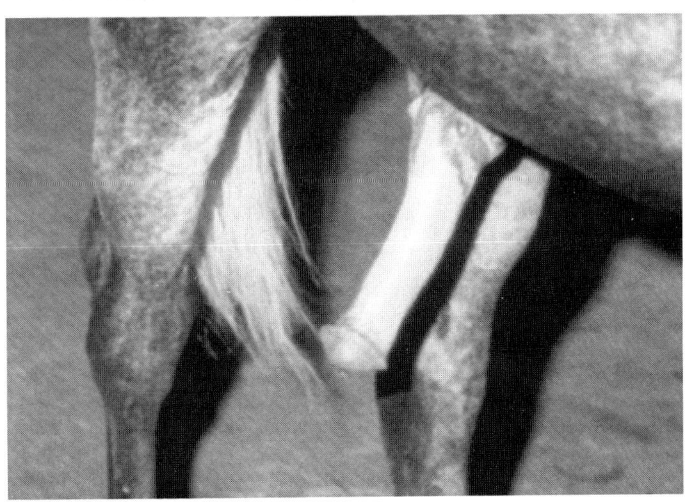

Figure 4. Lateral deviation of the penis in a stallion, resulting from fibrous tissue reaction to previous penile trauma (from a kick by the mare during breeding).

stallions succeed in mounting a mare, they are often unstable during intromission and thrusting efforts, and may collapse during copulation or dismount prematurely (Fig 3). Generally speaking, stallions with forelimb lamenesses are less compromised in breeding activities. Penile injuries may lead to penile deviations during erection that impair intromission (Fig 4).

Treatment should be directed at correction or attenuation of the underlying ailment, when feasible. Nonsteroidal anti-inflammatory medications often are given to provide temporary relief of pain associated with some back and limb problems. Often these injuries do not respond to medical or surgical treatment. Reducing the number of mares such stallions are expected to breed during a season minimizes stress associated with mating. Converting from natural service to artificial insemination provides similar protection. If only natural service is allowed, the stallion manager should select only mares of size proportionate to the stallion, and mares that stand steadily for breeding when in estrus. Artificial insemination permits greater therapeutic latitude. Replacement of a mount mare with a breeding phantom for semen collection provides a more reliable mounting device. The breeding phantom is rigid and can be lowered to ease mating ability. Some stallions can be trained to ejaculate while standing. Semen has been collected successfully in this fashion, using a condom and manual penile massage, or an artificial vagina.[25]

Penile deviations caused by local trauma often are attributed to extracorporeal scar tissue formation from contusions and/or lacerations. Such problems often can be circumvented by semen collection at regular intervals, concentrating on thorough massage and strategic maneuvering of the erect penis into a normal position before its insertion into an artificial vagina. Similar efforts facilitate breeding of stallions with minor penile deviations by natural service.

Ejaculatory Dysfunction

Ejaculation represents the culmination of activities involved in productive coitus. Various components of the ejaculate are discharged from their respective glandular ducts into the lumen of the pelvic urethra. Semen accumulated in the pelvic urethra is expelled by strong contractions of the musculature enveloping the pelvic and penile segments of the urethra (see Chapter 1).

Induction of ejaculation requires the coordinated interaction of several local and central neural pathways. Discharge of semen components into the urethral lumen probably is under the direct control of the sympathetic arm of the autonomic nervous system; this is through stimulation of alpha-adrenergic receptors and suppression of beta-adrenergic receptors. Conversely, propulsion of semen through the urethral lumen is regulated by the somatic nervous system, primarily through branches of the paired pudendal nerves, which innervate the urethralis, bulbospongiosus and ischiocavernosus muscles.[26,27]

The degree of involvement of the central nervous system in the ejaculatory process has not been determined completely. Ejaculation depends on stimulation of the afferent nervous pathway of the genital region during copulation, primarily via impulses carried by the dorsal nerve of the penis the ejaculatory process has been heavily investigated recently. Evidence is strong that serotoninonergic and dopaminergic pathways, originating in the brain, play a role in erection, ejaculation and the postejaculation refractory period to copulation.[28-30] Stimulation of serotonergic receptors is considered responsible for triggering semen emission, suppressing penile erection and curtailing sexual arousal in the postejaculatory period. Dopamine appears to assume an opposing role by initiating copulatory behavior and restoring sexual interest after ejaculation.

Nonejaculatory coitus is a relatively common disorder of breeding stallions and represents a very challenging problem. The condition often is manifested by normal to heightened libido and normal copulatory behavior without a corresponding ejaculation. Outward signs consistent with ejaculation (rhythmic twitching of the tail or rhythmic urethral pulsations) may be observed despite lack of ejaculation. Penile stimulation during the intravaginal thrusting phase may be minimal to marked, as evidenced by the degree of filling of the corpus spongiosum penis with arterial blood. The outcome may include either complete lack of ejaculation or delayed ejaculation that occurs only after several breeding attempts. Discharge of seminal fluid that is free of spermatozoa (azoospermia) also may occur. Often, the numerous unproductive breeding attempts associated failure to ejaculate result in physical exhaustion or extreme frustration that can incite aggressive behavior in the affected stallion.

Because of the complex nature of the ejaculatory process, the cause and pathogenesis of ejaculatory dysfunction often are difficult to establish. Diagnosis of ejaculatory disturbances initially is directed at differentiating psychogenic from organic causes. Psychogenic disorders that produce ejaculatory incompetence can be precipitated by several environmental factors. Abusive handling, previous breeding accidents, an unfamiliar environment and sexual overuse can produce negative effects on supraspinal centers associated with ejaculation.

Organic causes of ejaculatory dysfunction are quite varied. Inadequate stimulation of the afferent ejaculatory reflex pathway can result in failed or retarded ejaculation. Damage to the dorsal nerve of the penis from penile trauma, insufficient penile friction during mating due to incomplete penile erection, inadequate copulatory thrusts or pneumovagina can interfere with transmission of sensory impulses to the central nervous system.[31] While cutaneous sensation of the glans penis is not required for some stallions to ejaculate, loss of sensation may lead to failure of ejaculation in others. The glans penis fails to engorge ("flower") and urethral pulsations and tail-flagging do not occur in affected stallions. Pinching the skin of the glans penis fails to elicit a reaction.

Malfunction of the sympathetic nervous system or antagonism by the parasympathetic nervous system also have been suggested as causes of ejaculatory failure in stallions exhibiting normal copulatory activity that does not culminate in ejaculation.[32,33] Occluded ejaculatory ducts, aspermatogenesis or retrograde ejaculation should be considered if normal copulatory efforts end in azoospermia with sexual satiety. In this circumstance, behavioral signs consistent with ejaculation are followed by a postcoital period of sexual disinterest. Retrograde ejaculation (semen emission followed by expulsion into the urinary bladder) has not been documented in stallions but is a relatively common disorder in men (usually as a secondary complication of diabetes mellitus or bladder neck/prostate surgery). Diagnosis is based on postcoital catheterization of the urinary bladder in an attempt to recover spermatozoa from the urine.

Clinical management of psychogenic ejaculatory dysfunction includes establishment of an optimal breeding environment. The affected stallion should experience only pleasant sexual contacts. Negative encounters should be avoided and positive reinforcement provided. Specific treatment methodologies have been discussed in the section on libido dysfunction.

Treatment of suspected organic ejaculatory dysfunction can take physical or chemical forms, depending on the specific type of ailment. Azoospermia resulting from occluded ejaculatory ducts sometimes can be managed effectively with repeated semen collection attempts in conjunction with intermittent massage of the ampullae by rectal palpation. With positive response to treatment, numerous spermatozoa appear in ejaculate, and are often clumped together in "plugs" and have degenerative changes and head-tail separations. Continued semen collection eventually results in return of normal spermatozoal quantity and quality.

Commonly used drugs that result in smooth muscle contraction, *eg,* oxytocin or prostaglandins, have not been helpful in most cases of ejaculatory dysfunction associated with duct occlusion. We are investigating potential use of beta-adrenergic blocking agents for stimulating contractions of smooth muscle in the epididymis and deferent ducts to aid correction of duct occlusion. Refractory cases of ejaculatory duct occlusion have been corrected by catheterization and luminal flushing of the deferent ducts.[34] Azoospermia resulting from aspermatogenesis may be temporary or permanent. Removal of the inciting factor (such as increased testicular temperature) may improve testicular function in some cases.

Pharmacologic manipulation of ejaculation has been attempted in stallions displaying signs of disruption of the neural mechanisms that control seminal emission. Preliminary results have been encouraging. Specific drug therapy generally consists of alpha-adrenergic agonists, beta-adrenergic antagonists or anticholinergic agents. The potent neurotransmitter, L-norepinephrine, given IM at 0.01 mg/kg 15 minutes before breeding, aids stimulation of alpha-adrenergic receptors. This induces contraction of musculature enveloping the deferent ducts and accessory genital glands. This treatment should be combined with use of the beta-adrenergic receptor blocker carazolol, given IM at 0.015 mg/kg 10 minutes before breeding, to improve the likelihood of semen emission. This combination was effective in correcting organic ejaculatory failure in 17 of 24 stallions.[32] Carazolol is not yet available in the United States. Administration of beta-adrenergic antagonists, alone or in combination with alpha-adrenergic agonists, also increases the number of sperm in ejaculates.[33] This treatment regimen is contraindicated in stallions with chronic obstructive pulmonary disease.

When the tricyclic antidepressant, imipramine hydrochloride (50-100 mg PO or IV), was given to stallions (400-500 kg) receiving no sexual stimulation, the drug induced penile erection and masturbation, sometimes culminating in ejaculation.[14] The drug was effective in treating ejaculatory failure in a 5-year-old stallion. The action of imipramine is thought to be potentiation of peripheral alpha-adrenergic activity by blocking uptake of norepinephrine at sympathetic nerve terminals. The drug also may have anticholinergic properties. Preliminary studies with another tricyclic antidepressant, clomipramine, indicate that its actions on reproductive performance of stallions are similar to those of imipramine.

Our current knowledge of various drug actions on stallion copulatory behavior is quite deficient. As more information becomes available regarding specific drug effects on the stallion reproductive tract, we will be better equipped to formulate a rational approach to chemical treatment of maladies related to breeding performance.

Aggressive Behavior

Excessive aggression in breeding stallions generally takes the form of dominance or irritable aggression or self-mutilation.

Though displays of dominance are a normal testosterone-linked, behavioral characteristic of stallions, these actions can become excessive and may be directed toward mares or handlers when the stallion is in a breeding environment. When uncorrected, overly aggressive behavior can lead to catastrophic injuries. The stallion may savage mares during mating or may attack the handler. Overly aggressive behavior may have a consistent predictive pattern or may surface only intermittently. Such misconduct cannot be tolerated because of its potentially devastating consequences.

Treatment of very aggressive stallions sometimes is quite difficult, especially if the behavior has not been corrected for a long time. Of foremost importance is establishing stallion respect for the handler. Chain shanks strategically placed over the nose, through the mouth, or over the gingiva of the upper front teeth of the stallion usually provide adequate restraint so the

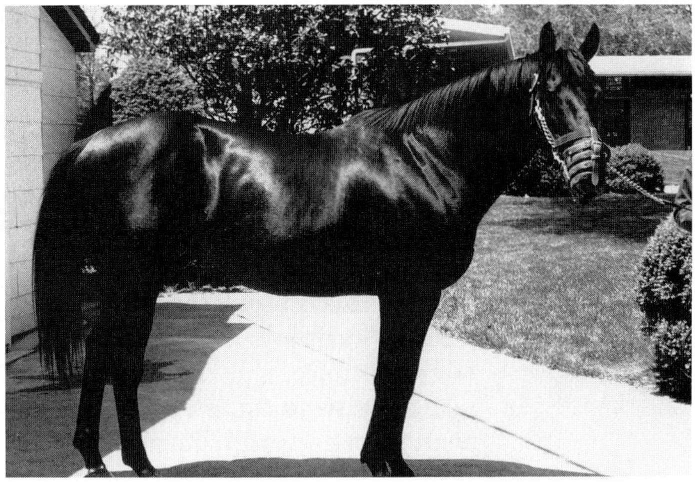

Figure 5. Muzzle applied over the mouth of a stallion to prevent biting of mares during the act of mating.

stallion obeys a handler's wishes without becoming timid from overzealous discipline. Severity of disciplinary measures depends on the type and persistence of aggression demonstrated. The objective is to assert sufficient control over the stallion so that the stallion's energy is directed only toward productive coitus.

Muzzling a stallion before handling eliminates one source of injury to mares and handlers and may help divert the stallion's attention to breeding rather than conflict (Fig 5). Securing a leather breeding shield to the neck of mares to be bred protects them against excessive biting by some stallions (Fig 6). Exogenous progestin therapy is purported to suppress sexual aggres-

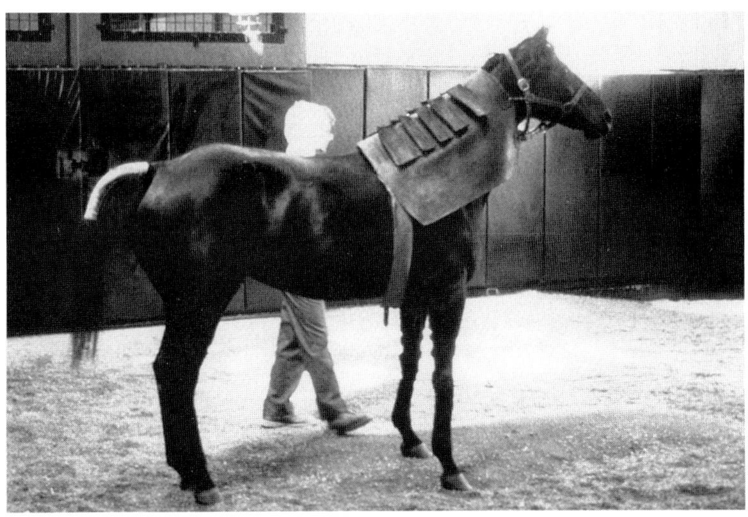

Figure 6. Breeding shield applied over the neck of a mare before breeding to prevent injury from bites of an aggressive stallion.

siveness of stallions. However, the potential antispermatogenic effect of this hormonal regimen should be considered. Short-term progestin therapy may be indicated in the early retraining period for stallions with aggressive behavioral disorders, though the effect of this treatment on testicular function has not been investigated. Castration may effectively control unrelenting aggressive behavior in stallions; however, this usually is not considered a viable treatment option for valuable breeding stallions. This operation or euthanasia may be the most appropriate action for stallions displaying violent and life-threatening aggressiveness.

Aggressiveness sometimes develops in stallions experiencing ejaculatory failure. These stallions typically have good libido and mating ability, but mating does not end in ejaculation. These stallions may become quite aggravated after repeated unsuccessful mating attempts and resort to indiscriminate aggressive behavior to help relieve their frustration. Treatment is directed at correcting the ejaculatory disturbance (see above discussion on Ejaculatory Dysfunction). Stallions may exhibit similar behavioral patterns if they have normal libido but cannot copulate because of limb, pelvic or spinal cord problems.

Behavioral aberrations sometimes are manifested by self-mutilation. The reasons for this bizarre conduct usually are unclear, so corrective measures often are unrewarding. Boredom associated with stall confinement may contribute to a variety of stable vices, that can produce injury, such as wall-kicking. Daily exercise programs or confinement exclusively to an outdoor paddock may eliminate or reduce such undesirable behavior.

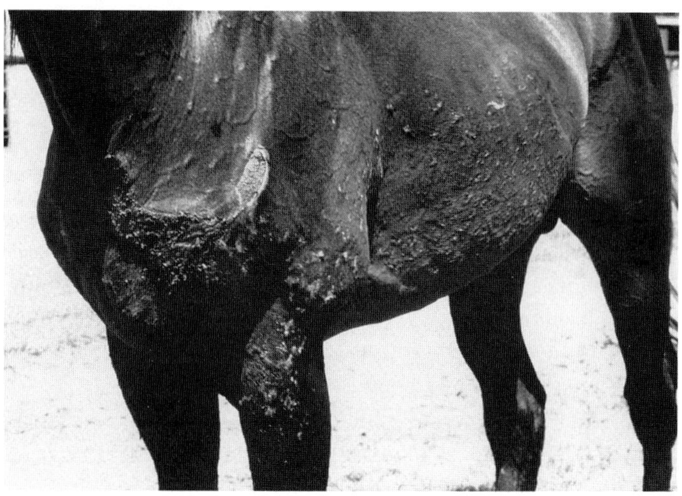

Figure 7. Numerous self-inflicted wounds in a breeding stallion.

Providing a stallion with a goat as a stallmate has been used to divert attention away from the vices; however, the stallion may direct his aggression toward the goat.

Some stallions are obsessed with deliberate self-abuse, characterized by insatiable biting of the shoulders, flanks and hips (Fig 7). Such behavior is not always related to stall confinement, and the underlying causes generally defy detection. There may be a genetic predisposition to this behavior. Though regular exercise programs, dietary (*ie,* energy) restriction and stress-reduction management have been used to suppress self-mutilation, physical restraint usually is essential. Crossties, neck cradles, side poles or muzzles can prevent self-mutilation. These devices may need to be used for the remainder of the horse's life. Because of their antianxiety properties, progestins and diazepam have been proposed for use in affected stallions.[35] The effects of these drugs have not been studied fully in this clinical syndrome. The neurosis appears to be a chronic problem and, despite treatment efforts, few stallions revert to a normal tranquil state.

References

1. McDonnell S, in Crowell-Davis SL and Houpt KA: Reproductive behavior of the stallion. *Vet Clin No Am* (Equine Practice) 2:535-555, 1986.

2. Wallach SJR *et al:* Sexual behavior and serum concentration of reproductive hormones in impotent stallions. *Theriogenology* 19:833-840, 1983.

3. Irvine CHG *et al:* Sexual behavior and serum concentration of reproductive hormones in normal stallions. *Theriogenology* 23:607-617, 1985.

4. Pickett BW *et al:* Reproductive physiology of the stallion. VI. Seminal and behavioral characteristics. *J Anim Sci* 43:617-624, 1976.

5. Clay CM *et al:* Influences of season and artificial photoperiod on stallions: testicular size, seminal characteristics and sexual behavior. *J Anim Sci* 64:517-525, 1987.

6. Squires EL *et al:* Restoration of reproductive capacity of stallions after suppression with exogenous testosterone. *J Anim Sci* 53:1351-1359, 1981.

7. Berndtson WE *et al:* Influence of exogenous testosterone on sperm production, seminal quality and libido of stallions. *J Reprod Fertil* (Suppl) 27:19-23, 1979.

8. Squires EL *et al:* Effect of anabolic steroids on reproductive function of young stallions. *J Anim Sci* 54:576-582, 1982.

9. Blanchard TL *et al:* The effects of stanozolol and boldenone undecycenate on scrotal width, testis weight, and sperm production in pony stallions. *Theriogenology* 20:121-131, 1983.

10. Blanchard TL: Some effects of anabolic steroids - especially on stallions. *Compend Cont Ed Pract Vet* 7:S372-S380, 1985.

11. Squires EL *et al:* Effect of pulsatile and continuous administration of GnRH on reproductive function of stallions. *Proc Intl Symp Equine Reprod,* 1990. pp 60-61.

12. Pozor MA *et al:* GnRH facilitates copulatory behavior in testosterone-treated geldings.

13. McDonnell SM: Stallion sexual behavior dysfunction: experimental models and clinical considerations. *Proc Ann Mtg Soc Theriogenol,* 1986. pp 11-12.

14. McDonnell SM *et al:* Pharmacological manipulation of sexual behavior in stallions. *J Reprod Fertil* 35:45-49, 1987.

15. Lue TF and Tanagho EA: Physiology of erection and pharmacological management of impotence. *J Urol* 137:829-836, 1987.

16. Adaidan PG *et al:* Is vasoactive intestinal polypeptide the principal transmitter involved in human penile erection? *J Urol* 135:638-640, 1986.

17. Karacan I *et al:* Erectile mechanisms in man. *Science* 220:1080-1082, 1983.

18. Beckett SD *et al:* Corpus spongiosum penis pressure and penile muscle activity in the stallion during coitus. *Am J Vet Res* 36:431-433, 1975.

19. Beckett SD *et al:* Blood pressures and penile muscle activity in the stallion during coitus. *Am J Physiol* 225:1072-1075, 1973.

20 Bartels JE *et al:* Angiography of the corpus cavernosum penis in the pony stallion during erection and quiescence. *Am J Vet Res* 45:1464-1468, 1984.

21. Virag R *et al:* Intracavernous injection of papaverine as a diagnostic and therapeutic method in erectile failure. *Angiology* 35:79-87, 1984.

22. Sidi AA *et al:* Intracavernous drug-related erection in the management of male erectile dysfunction: experience with 100 patients. *J Urol* 135:704-706, 1985.

23. Orvis BR and Lue TF, in Howards SS and Lipshultz: Male Infertility. *Urol Clin No Am* 16:569-581, 1987.

24. Zorgniotti AW and Lefleur RS: Auto-injection of the corpus cavernosum with a vasoactive drug combination for vasculogenic impotence. *J Urol* 133:39-41, 1985.

25. Crump J and Crump J: Stallion ejaculation induced by manual stimulation of the penis. *Theriogenology* 31:341-346, 1989.

26. Lipshultz LI *et al:* Current concepts of the mechanisms of ejaculation: normal and abnormal states. *J Reprod Med* 26:499-507, 1981.

27. Thomas AJ: Ejaculatory dysfunction. *Fertil Steril* 39:445-454, 1983.

28. McIntosh TK and Barfield RJ: Brain monoaminergic control of male reproductive behavior. I. Serotonin and the post-ejaculatory refractory period. *Behav Brain Res* 12:255-265, 1984.

29. McIntosh TK and Barfield RJ: Brain monoaminergic control of male reproductive behavior. II. Dopamine and the post-ejaculatory refractory period. *Behav Brain Res* 12:267-273, 1984.

30. Mas M *et al:* Stimulation of spinal serotonergic receptors facilitates seminal emission and suppresses penile erectile reflexes. *Brain Res* 342:128-134, 1985.

31. Rasbech NO: Ejaculatory disorders of the stallion. *J Reprod Fertil* 23:123-128, 1975.

32. Klug E, in Robinson NE: *Current Therapy in Equine Medicine 2.* Saunders, Philadelphia, 1987. pp 562-563.

33. Klug E *et al:* Effect of adrenergic neurotransmitters upon the ejaculatory process in the stallion. *J Reprod Fertil* 32:31-34, 1982.

34. Hughes JP: Significance of fertility evaluation of the stallion. *Proc Ann Mtg Soc Theriogenol,* 1983. pp 167-175.

35. Beaver BV: Aggressive behavior problems. *Vet Clin No Am* 2:635-644, 1986.

7

Diseases of the Scrotum

Diagnostic and Therapeutic Considerations

The equine scrotum is less pendulous than that of ruminants and is well concealed between the hind limbs. This anatomic position provides protection from physical injury except during breeding. Though shielded by the hind limbs, the scrotum is examined easily when the horse is properly restrained. Most stallions tolerate examination with only minimal physical restraint. Sedation rarely is required.

Thorough palpation coupled with visual examination yields much information about scrotal integrity. The scrotum normally is thin walled, soft and pliable, with easily identified and freely movable scrotal contents. Abnormalities should be noted and investigated further. Ultrasonographic examination of suspicious scrotal lesions provides more complete evaluation of their identity, degree of involvement, and amount of compromise to adjacent tissues. Skin biopsies or needle aspirations of selected lesions also may be warranted. Scrotal thermography has been used as a noninvasive diagnostic technique in bulls.[1] By measuring infrared radiation emission from the surface of the scrotum, local thermal patterns are defined. Abnormal increases or decreases in surface temperature, asymmetry of temperature patterns or abnormal temperature gradients indicate underlying pathologic changes. Because normal spermatogenesis and epididymal function are heavily dependent on scrotal temperature, the technique has obvious prognostic value. The procedure certainly would be applicable to stallions and should be investigated.

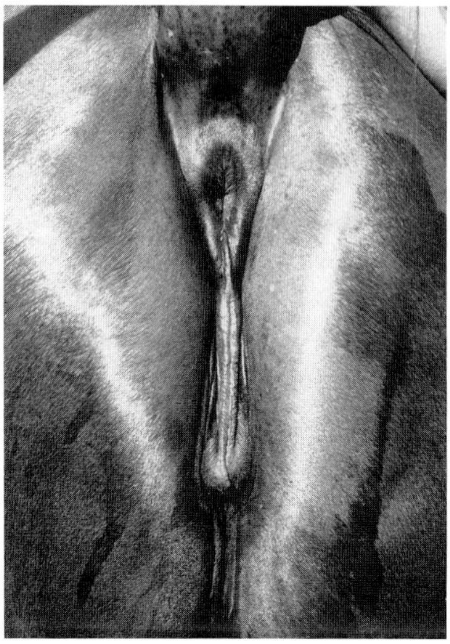

Figure 3. External genitalia of a horse with testicular feminization.

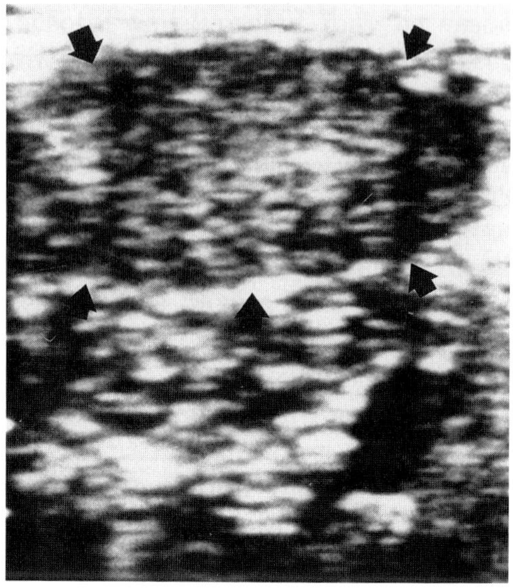

Figure 4. Ultrasonic image of an abdomial testis (arrows) in a horse with testicular feminization.

tubercle of the fetus develop into a vestibule, vulva and clitoris (Fig 3). The condition is considered heritable.

The X-Y sex reversal syndrome also is heritable but differs from testicular feminization in that it produces horses with a male (XY) karyotype but strictly female genitalia.[4] They have small inactive ovaries and a hypoplastic tubular genital tract. These horses are typically sterile, though 1 affected horse was fertile.[5]

Tentative diagnosis of intersexuality is based on external and internal physical examination. Confirmation requires cytogenetic studies and documentation of gonadal sex.

Bilateral Cryptorchidism

Bilateral cryptorchidism prevents full scrotal development. Chapter 8 (Diseases of the Testes) contains a discussion of cryptorchidism.

Diseases With Physical Causes

Scrotal Trauma

Scrotal trauma usually is associated with a breeding accident, such as blunt trauma from a kick during mating, when the scrotum is relatively unprotected. Scrotal contusions and lacerations also occur when stallions unsuccessfully hurdle fences or similar barriers.

Blunt trauma to the scrotum can produce an array of local disturbances, including scrotal edema, dartos or scrotal hemorrhage, hematocele (blood accumulation in the cavity between the visceral and parietal vaginal tunics), orchitis or rupture of the tunica albuginea (which encapsulates each testis). Rupture of the tunica albuginea results in extensive testicular hemorrhage. Any local trauma may incite bilateral scrotal and preputial edema. More severe blows can cause the lesions described above, but usually these are unilateral. Inflammation always ensues. Secondary bacterial infection is possible, especially when the skin is broken by lacerations or puncture wounds.

Blunt scrotal injury usually can be diagnosed from the history (*eg,* verification of a breeding accident), but the specific lesions often are difficult to identify. Initial examination of the scrotal area may require mild sedation and physical restraint, as the area usually is quite painful. Phenothiazine tranquilizers should be avoided because of their peripheral vasodilatory action and propensity to induce penile paralysis or priapism. The extent of scrotal and preputial edema should be recorded. Injury to the scrotum causes rapid local edema. Extensive edema interferes with evaluation of scrotal contents. The scrotal surface should be examined thoroughly for injuries, including abrasions, lacerations, puncture wounds and foreign bodies, such as thorns.

The scrotal contents should be evaluated next. If the testes and attached epididymides are readily palpable, the swelling is probably unassociated with scrotal edema, dartos hemorrhage or hematocele, but originates in the testis(es), as with orchitis. Conversely, inability to manually define the testes and epididymides suggests one of the above, *ie,* excessive scrotal edema, dartos hemorrhage or hematocele (Fig 5). Rupture of the tunica albuginea also may preclude identification of the involved testis and adjacent epididymis because of extreme hemorrhage from the rent (Fig 6).

It sometimes is difficult to differentiate massive scrotal edema from hemorrhage of scrotal, spermatic cord or testicular origin. Needle aspiration of the affected scrotum helps make this distinction. It is mandatory, however, that the external and internal inguinal rings first be palpated thoroughly to ensure that the scrotal swelling is not associated with a scrotal hernia. The needle-aspiration technique should be performed aseptically, and care should be taken to avoid laceration of vessels. Torsion of a spermatic cord also should be included in the differential diagnosis of acute scrotal swelling.

Ultrasound examination of an enlarged scrotum may also help establish the underlying cause. Fresh blood which accumulates in the vaginal space (*ie,* hematocele) or scrotal wall typically has a homogeneous anechoic (black) appearance, even if freshly clotted. Conversely, a thickened scrotal wall resulting from edema usually has a more heterogeneous (or mottled) pattern, *ie,* an intermixture of anechoic and echoic areas.

Intrascrotal hemorrhage, whether from the scrotal wall, spermatic cord or testis, becomes organized to form fibrous tissue. Fibrin deposition in the scrotal fascia and vaginal cavity leads to adhesions and immobilization of the testicle within the scrotum. The fibrous tissue can interfere with thermoregulation of spermatogenesis, especially when it envelops the testes (Fig 7). Degeneration of the seminiferous epithelium and progressive testicular atrophy result. Persistent scrotal edema also can promote tissue fibrosis; however, if arrested in the acute phase,

Figure 5. Diffuse swelling of the scrotum associated with dartos hemorrhage.

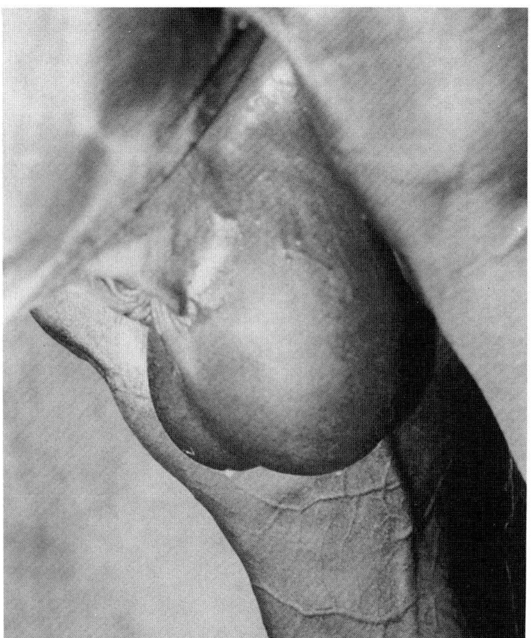

Figure 6. Extreme swelling of the prepuce and scrotum of a jack as a result of a breeding accident. The scrotal enlargement was due primarily to testicular hemorrhage through a rent in the tunica albuginea.

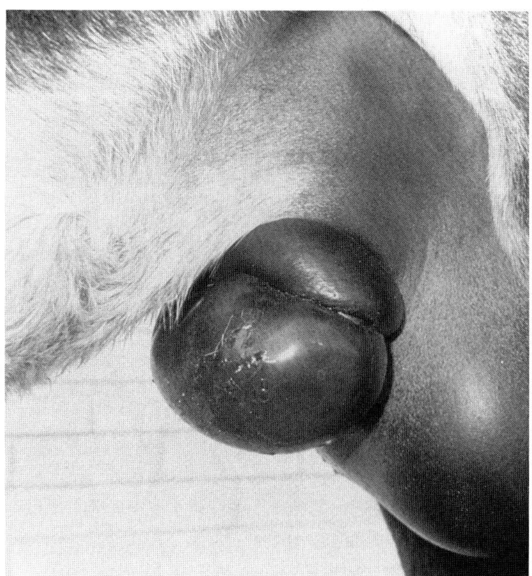

edema generally subsides without this complication. Another consequence of uncorrected edema is local hypoxia and malnutrition, causing cell death and sloughing of scrotal tissues (Fig 8).

Treatment of acute scrotal trauma initially is aimed at controlling local inflammation, edema and hematoma formation. Cryotherapy (therapeutic use of cold temperature) probably is the most important yet inexpensive therapeutic method. However, awareness of cryotherapeutic principles is critical. Indiscriminate cold application to tissues (excessively cold or prolonged applications) can accentuate edema and produce additional tissue damage.[6,7] Cold application sessions should not exceed 20 minutes and should be applied at 1- to 3-hour intervals. Local blood flow is reduced by using this cold application strategy, thus minimizing tissue edema and hemorrhage. Short-term (20 minutes) topical cold application offers beneficial cooling effects lasting up to several hours and also a degree of analgesia. However, continuous application of cold temperature increases local blood flow and lymphatic permeability. These changes negate beneficial effects and enhance inflammation and swelling. These negative effects are most dramatic when tissue temperature drops below 5 C. Skin damage also occurs.

Figure 7. Exposed vaginal cavity (solid arrow) and surrounding subcutaneous tissue (open arrow), demonstrating pronounced fibrous tissue formation after dartos hemorrhage. The resulting disturbance to the scrotal thermoregulatory mechanism negatively affects spermatogenic function of the contained testis.

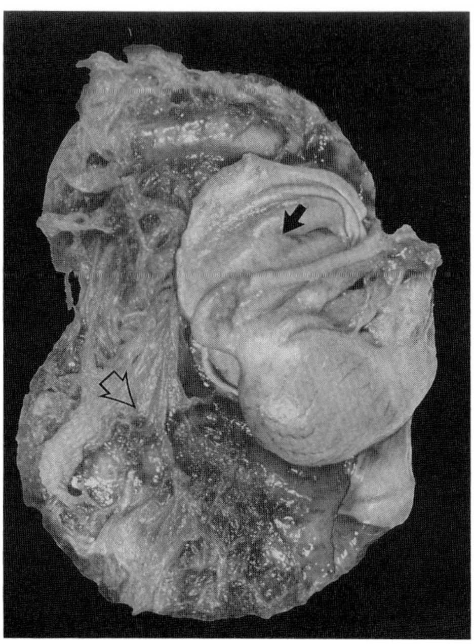

Figure 8. Necrosis of scrotal skin subsequent to long-standing scrotal (and preputial) edema.

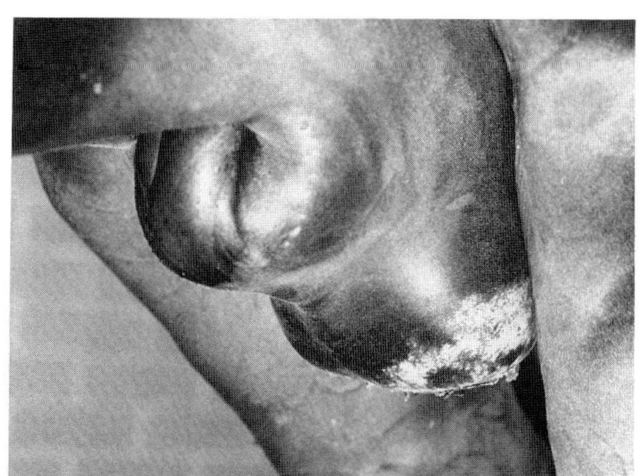

Icepack application (*eg,* crushed ice in plastic bags), or scrotal immersion in cold water or icewater baths are the most common forms of cryotherapy. Simultaneous gentle massage of the scrotum helps cool affected tissues and mechanically reduces edema. Refrigerant sprays should be avoided, as they can induce frostbite. Coldwater sprays are not recommended because they can cause additional skin damage if tissue has been compromised.[8]

Systemic antiinflammatory and diuretic medications are useful adjuncts to local therapy for controling inflammation and edema. Prophylactic antibiotic therapy also should be instituted to prevent secondary infection. A tetanus toxoid booster is recommended if the horse has not been vaccinated against tetanus within the past year. Emollients should be applied to the skin intermittently to protect it against maceration.

Significant intrascrotal hemorrhage leads to permanent testicular damage due to the insulating effect of secondary fibrous tissue formation. To save the compromised testis, surgical removal of the organized blood clot can be attempted 4-5 days after injury. The testis need not be removed unnecessarily, but if a rent in the tunica albuginea has caused the intrascrotal hemorrhage, unilateral castration is recommended. Hemorrhage into one scrotal pouch can result in fibrous tissue formation that can interfere with thermoregulation of the contralateral testis. Surgical removal of the fibrous tissue may be indicated under these circumstances. If the condition is chronic, with pronounced atrophy of the ipsilateral testis, the affected testis could be removed along with the fibrous tissue. This may promote some compensatory hypertrophy (and increased sperm production) of the remaining testis.[9]

The inflammatory reaction associated with scrotal trauma interferes with thermoregulatory function, and the temperature of intrascrotal contents becomes elevated, thus disturbing spermatogenesis and probably epididymal function.[10-13] This damage is clinically recognizable in ejaculates within days of the injury by reduced spermatozoal quantity, altered spermatozoal motility, increased incidence of morphologic defects in spermatozoa, and occasionally the presence of immature germ cells. Azoospermia may occur within 2-4 weeks. If significant adhesions do not develop between the testes, their overlying tunics and the scrotal wall (*ie,* if the normal thermoregulatory mechanism is restored), spermatozoal quantity and quality in ejaculates generally begin to improve within 40-60 days after the insult is corrected. Affected testes may return to normal size and spermatogenic capacity within 2-5 months following correction of the problem. Uncorrected disruption of the thermoregulatory mechanism often results in irreparable testicular damage.

Scrotal lacerations generally incite marked tissue swelling, so proper measures should be taken to neutralize the inflammatory response (described above). The wound should be cleaned thoroughly, then treated locally to control bacterial infection and progressive cellulitis. Lacerations in this area generally do not heal by first intention after surgical closure, even if attempted within 6-8 hours after injury. First-intention healing is compromised by pronounced tissue swelling. Nevertheless, wound closure always is indicated to cover exposed testes and their tunics. When lacerated, the parietal vaginal tunic should be sutured to protect the testis, after thoroughly cleansing the vaginal cavity with a balanced salt solution containing antibiotics. Surgical debridement of subcutaneous tissues should be followed by skin closure with nonabsorbable nonreactive suture material. If a seroma forms in the subcutaneous tissue, drainage should be established. Systemic antibiotics, antiinflammatory drugs, and a tetanus toxoid booster also are advised.

Temperature-Induced Scrotal Edema

Scrotal frostbite, resulting in scrotal edema, tissue necrosis and reduced spermatogenic function, has been described in bulls, rams and boars exposed to extremely low ambient temperature. The location of the scrotum between the hind limbs of the horse lends much more protection against this form of injury; hence, scrotal frostbite is unlikely in stallions.

During the hot summer months, scrotal edema has been noted in some stallions.[14] The pathophysiology of this condition is not known, but affected horses often respond to daily exercise and diuretic therapy. Hot weather also may induce hydrocele in stallions, though the mechanism is unknown. This condition must be distinguished from scrotal edema. See Chapter 10 for a discussion of hydrocele.

Varicocele

Varicoceles, which are abnormally distended and tortuous veins of the pampiniform plexus and/or varicosities of superficial scrotal vessels, have been proposed as causes of idiopathic scrotal edema.[15] Chapter 11 contains a discussion of varicoceles.

Scrotal Contact Dermatitis

The delicate scrotal skin is susceptible to injury from many topical substances tolerated by skin of other body regions. Various chemicals, such as fly spray, disinfectants, detergents and solvents, can cause local inflammation. Scrotal edema, a common feature of acute irritant-induced inflammation, can temporarily disrupt spermatogenesis by insulating the testes. Repeated scrotal contact with chemical irritants can produce chronic skin reactions, such as hyperkeratosis with fissure formation, that permanently interfere with the thermoregulatory action of the scrotum. Spermatogenic dysfunction results.

Treatment of contact dermatitis includes preventing further contact with the irritant and suppressing the local inflammatory reaction. Cryotherapy (discussed in the section on Scrotal Trauma) helps curtail acute inflammation and its consequences. Systemic and topical corticosteroid therapy is indicated for both acute and chronic inflammation. Systemic antibiotics are advised if secondary bacterial infection is present or likely.

Inflammatory, Infectious and Immune Diseases

Systemic disorders, particularly those that result in anemia or hepatic disease, may cause scrotal edema.[16] Systemic infections may also disseminate to include the scrotum and its contents.[17] Discussions of specific disorders that may affect the scrotum follow.

Dourine

Dourine is a chronic systemic disease caused by the trypanosome, *Trypanosoma equiperdum.* The disease, presently eradicated from the United States, is transmitted venereally. Scrotal or preputial edema is a consistent manifestation of the disease in its early stages. Urticarial skin plaques, paralysis and emaciation become apparent as the disease progresses. The section entitled Examination for Venereal Diseases in Chapter 2 contains a discussion of dourine.

Scrotal Infection

Scrotal infections usually are a sequel to breaks in the protective scrotal skin. Castration, scrotal lacerations, blunt scrotal trauma and puncture wounds can damage skin integrity sufficiently to permit invasion by microorganisms. Uncommonly, scrotal infections represent extensions of septic orchitis or peritonitis via the inguinal canal (Fig 9). Conversely, infections of the testes and abdominal cavity can be secondary to progressive scrotal infections. Septic peritonitis is an uncommon sequel to castration, perhaps because the funicular portion of the vaginal process is collapsed as it courses obliquely through the abdominal wall, and because the vaginal process is lined by phagocytic mesothelial cells. A draining scrotal lesion has also been reported secondary to surgical insertion of a human mammary prosthesis into the scrotum of a cryptorchid stallion (Figs 10, 11).[18]

Infections of scrotal lacerations or incisional wounds (*eg*, postcastration wounds) can result from impaired immune function due to malnutrition, corticosteroid therapy or overwhelming wound contamination with virulent bacteria. Both aerobic and anaerobic bacteria can invade scrotal wounds, causing progressive soft tissue necrosis.

Infected scrotal wounds are characterized by unrelenting local pain and swelling, in conjunction with fever and malaise. Purulent exudate often exudes from the wound surface. Tissue crepitus strongly suggests gaseous cellulitis caused by a clostridial infection.

Aerobic and anaerobic bacteriologic culture of these infected wounds is very important. A Gram stain should be performed on the wound exudate to help identify the causative bacteria so

Figure 9. Scrotal infection secondary to peritonitis.

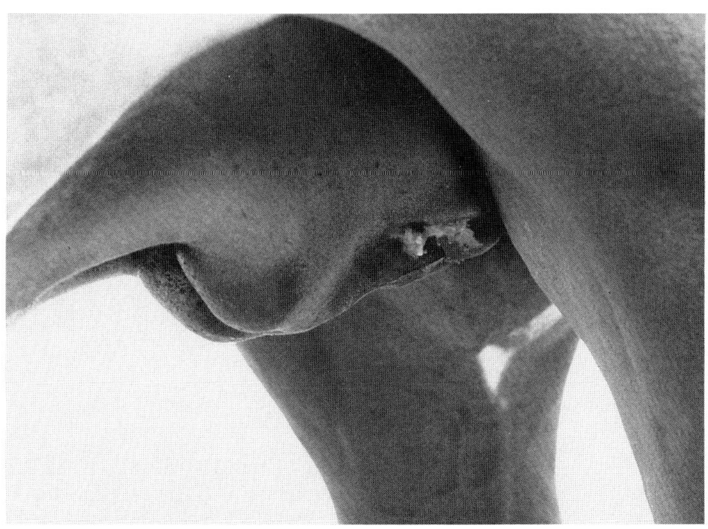

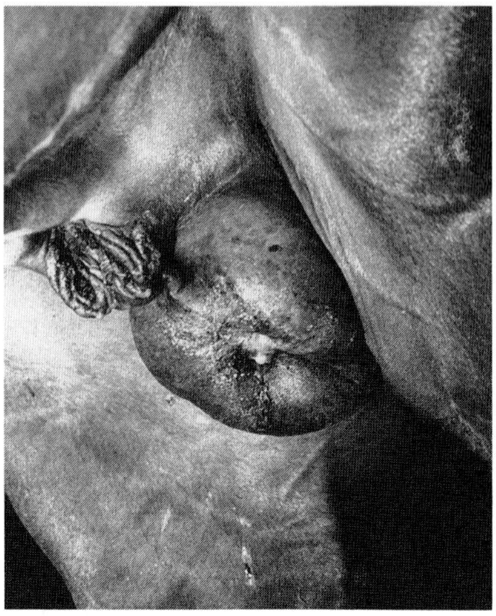

Figure 10. Draining scrotal lesion secondary to surgical insertion of a testicular prosthesis.[18]

that appropriate antimicrobial therapy can be instituted promptly.

The wound should be examined thoroughly to establish its extent and to identify and remove any foreign bodies. Infected scrotal lacerations or incisional wounds then should be cleansed thoroughly by irrigation with large volumes of sterile physiologic saline solution, or other balanced salt solution. Grossly contaminated wounds can be cleansed with tap water initially, followed by ample irrigation with physiologic saline solution. Pulsating irrigators may improve mechanical removal of bacteria and tissue debris from the wound surface. Care should be taken, however, to avoid additional tissue trauma and to prevent

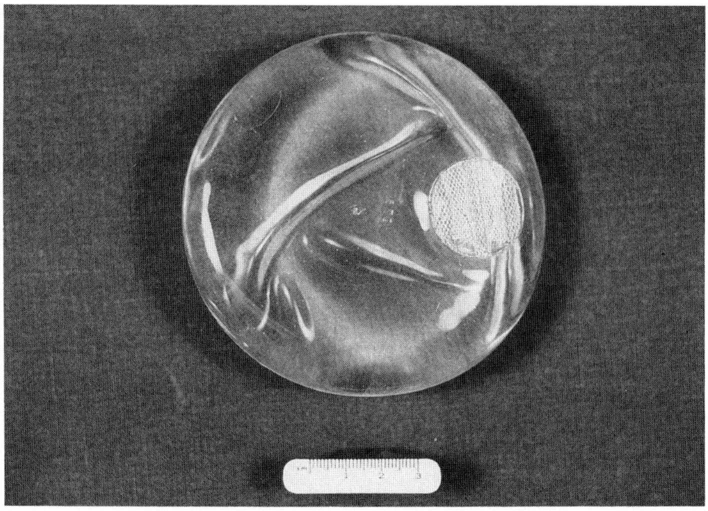

Figure 11. Testicular prosthesis recovered at surgery from the stallion in Figure 10.[18]

bacteria from being driven deeper into the tissues. Addition of antimicrobial drugs to the lavage fluid may improve its efficacy. Dilute povidone-iodine solution helps control bacterial growth but may simultaneously cause tissue damage and interfere with wound healing.

Thorough surgical debridement of the wound should follow irrigation to remove all devitalized and contaminated tissue. Extension of scrotal infections to a testis usually necessitates its removal. Ventral scrotal drainage must be established. Infected wounds should not be sutured.

Antibiotic-impregnated sterile gauze can be placed in the deadspace of the scrotum to help control infection. If this technique is used, daily dressing changes are recommended, using aseptic technique. Topical ointments have questionable value in controlling bacterial growth. Frequently bathing the tissue surface with antibiotic-containing aqueous solutions probably is more beneficial. Systemic antibiotics should be used to control bacterial growth and should be continued for at least 5-7 days. Initial antibiotic therapy is based on results of Gram stains of wound exudate, and should be effective against clostridial organisms. Antibiotic selection can be modified during the course of therapy if indicated by bacterial culture results. Antibiotic therapy should only supplement local wound management, not replace it. As is true with all wounds, tetanus prophylaxis is essential. Puncture wounds or severe contusions of the scrotum can lead to secondary infection, occasionally with abscessation. Puncture wounds always should be examined meticulously for evidence of retained foreign bodies. The opening of the wound may need to be enlarged to allow adequate examination of the tract. Ultrasonic examination of the scrotum may help identify foreign objects. Occasionally, radiographic examination may be performed to identify radiodense objects, but this technique can disrupt spermatogenesis.

Flushing of draining tracts or fistulas sometimes removes foreign bodies. If a puncture wound or contusion results in scrotal infection, the ventral scrotal wall can be liberally incised made to allow drainage. The other therapeutic principles applied to infected scrotal lacerations (described above) also should be followed. Extension of scrotal infection into the abdominal cavity necessitates additional therapeutic measures.

Adhesions often develop between visceral and parietal tunics secondary to scrotal inflammation. The adhesions are usually thin fibrinous strands initially, but tend to become thickened over time.[17] In such cases, the testis and its tunics are not freely movable within the scrotum, and semen quality deteriorates from disruption of the local thermoregulatory mechanism.

Superficial Scrotal Dermatitis

Unlike rams, bulls and boars, stallions rarely develop superficial scrotal dermatitis. In horses, the condition usually is associated with contact chemical irritants (see Scrotal Dermatitis), but may occur if unclean bedding (due to buildup of manure and urine) scalds the scrotal skin, predisposing to secondary infection with environmental bacteria or fungi.[19] Such occurances are unlikely except in debilitated or injured horses that are managed poorly. Lesions are usually not restricted to the scrotal skin, and are present on other areas in frequent contact with contaminated bedding. Treatment is seldom necessary once environmental sanitation is corrected.

Microfilariae of the filarid parasite, *Onchocerca cervicalis,* can produce mild scrotal dermatitis and associated depigmentation (Fig 12).[15] Affected stallions are usually >4 years of age. Lesions are commonly crusted, and may become scaly and depigmented in advanced cases. Bites of the *Onhocherca* vector, *Culicoides* spp, also may evoke mild scrotal dermatitis and edema. Examination of biopsies or deep skin scrapings of affected skin may reveal microfilariae, confirming diagnosis. Though treatments have been devised for parasite-induced skin lesions (see Chapter 14), the most successful has been ivermectin. Administration of this parasiticide to horses 2-4 times per year has greatly reduced frequency and severity of *Onchocerca* and *Habronema* lesions.[20]

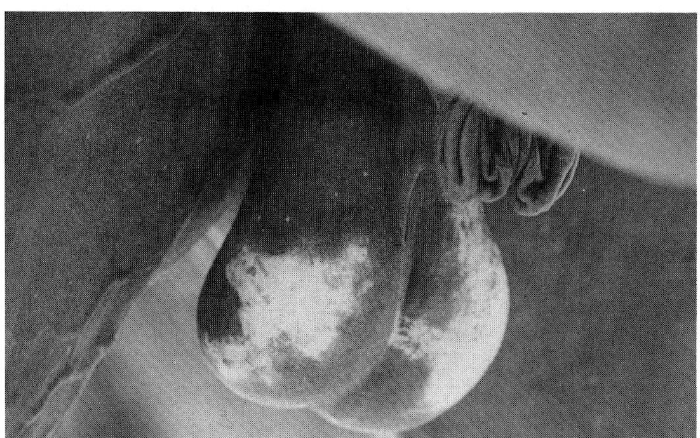

Figure 12. Depigmentation of the scrotum caused by *Onchocerca* microfilariae.[15]

Ivermectin use may result in transient edematous swelling of the scrotal wall, edema along the ventral midline of the abdomen and, possibly, pruritus.[21] Tissue reaction is thought to be associated with microfilarial death.[22] Though ivermectin does not appear to kill adult *Onchocerca,* regular use seems to have decreased the incidence of reactions. Concurrent use of corticosteroids may reduce severity of tissue reaction associated with ivermectin use.[23] If tissue reactions are expected, it is advisable to delay treatment until the end of the breeding season to avoid transient adverse effects on fertility. Insect populations should be controlled to diminish transmission of *Onchocerca* or *Habronema* larvae.

Scrotal irritation may occur in conjunction with fly-bite dermatitis, though other areas of the skin are more commonly involved. Bites by the black fly (*Simulium*) on the scrotum results in swelling and pruritus, similar to skin reactions on other areas. Fly-bite dermatitis is diagnosed by identifying a large population of flies, as well as involvement of other animals and other body surfaces. Though fly repellents may be useful if applied frequently (2-3 times per day), treatment of scrotal lesions is seldom necessary if fly populations are controlled with proper sanitation. Stall protection during heightened fly activity is helpful. Short-term corticosteroid therapy during acute outbreaks may relieve discomfort.[15]

Scrotal dermatitis rarely occurs as an extension of generalized forms of dermatitis.

Cutaneous Habronemiasis

(Summer Sores)

Cutaneous habronemiasis is a parasitic skin disease caused by infective larvae of the stomach worm, *Draschia megastoma, Habronema muscae* and *Habronema microstoma.* Larvae are transmitted to various cutaneous locations by fly vectors, *Musca domestica* (housefly) or *Stomoxys calcitrans* (stable-fly), as they feed. Typical larval deposition sites include wounds and moist body surfaces, such as eyes, prepuce and penis (especially the urethral process). The scrotum is affected infrequently. Deposited larvae produce a mildly pruritic granulomatous tissue reaction. Primary differential diagnoses are neoplasms and sarcoids. For a thorough discussion of cutaneous habronemiasis, refer to Chapter 14.

Equine Infectious Anemia

Equine infectious anemia (EIA) can produce scrotal edema in stallions. Diagnosis of EIA is confirmed by a positive agar-gel immunodiffusion (Coggins) test; therefore, serum should be tested in stallions with scrotal edema of unknown origin.

Equine Viral Arteritis

Scrotal edema is a characteristic clinical finding of viral arteritis during the acute phase. Infected stallions can become long-term asymptomatic carriers once the acute phase of the disease has subsided. The virus sequesters in the genital tract and is shed in the semen (see Chapter 2).

Neoplasia

Melanoma

Melanomas are potentially metastatic tumors arising from melanocytes. They are most common in older gray horses. Primary melanotic tumors typically arise from the skin of the perianal area. These are found occasionally on the prepuce or scrotum as dermal or subcutaneous lesions. They vary in size, and may be firm or soft. The overlying epidermis generally remains intact but may ulcerate. Melanomas are mostly seen in aged horses, typically grow slowly and can remain benign. These tumors are rapidly fatal, however, following metastasis with vital organ involvement. Diagnosis is based on gross and histologic apearance.[15] See Chapter 15 for a discussion of melanomas.

Sarcoid

Sarcoids are nonmetastatic cutaneous tumors peculiar to horses. Common sites are the head, limbs and ventral abdomen, including the prepuce and scrotum. See Chapter 15 for a discussion of sarcoids.

Multifactorial Disease

Noninflammatory Scrotal Edema

Noninflammatory scrotal edema often is noted in diseases causing generalized edema. The force of gravity leads to accumulation of fluid in the scrotum, as well as in the ventral abdomen and limbs (Fig 8). Hypoproteinemia commonly results in noninflammatory scrotal edema. Potential causes include protein-losing enteropathies, malnutrition, liver disease and kidney disease. Local venous and/or lymphatic obstruction also may produce localized and protracted noninflammatory scrotal edema.

References

1. Purohit RC *et al:* Thermography of the bovine scrotum. *Am J Vet Res* 46:2388-2392, 1985.

2. Hare WCD and Singh EL: Equine cytogenetics. *Compend Cont Ed Pract Vet* 2: S111-S118, 1980.

3. Kieffer NM *et al:* Male pseudohermaphroditism of the testicular feminizing type in a horse. *Equine Vet J* 8:38-41, 1976.

4. Kent MC *et al:* XY sex-reversal syndrome in the domestic horse. *Cytogenet Cell Genet* 42:8-18, 1986.

5. Sharp AJ *et al:* H-Y antigen in a fertile XY female horse. *J Reprod Fertil* 58:157-160, 1980.

6. Ivers T: Cryotherapy: an in-depth study. *Equine Pract* 9(10):17-19, 1987.

7. Meeusen R and Lievens P: The use of cryotherapy in sports injuries. *Sports Med* 3:398-414, 1986.

8. Walker DF and Vaughan JT: *Bovine and Equine Urogenital Surgery.* Lea & Febiger, Philadelphia, 1980. pp 105-182.

9. Hoagland TA *et al:* Effects of unilateral castration on morphologic characteristics of the testis in one-, two-, and three-year-old stallions. *Theriogenology* 26: 397-405, 1986.

10. Gerona GR and Sikes JO: Effects of elevated scrotum temperature on spermatogenesis and semen characteristics. *J Dairy Sci* 53:659, 1970.

11. Ross AD and Entwistle KW: The effect of scrotal insulation on spermatozoal morphology and the rates of spermatogenesis and epididymal passage of spermatozoa in the bull. *Theriogenology* 11:111-121, 1979.

12. Ashdown RR, in Hafez ESE: *Reproduction in Farm Animals.* 5th ed. Lea & Febiger, Philadelphia, 1987. pp 17-34.

13. Ewing LL and Chang TSK, in Walsh PC *et al: Campbell's Urology.* 5th ed. Saunders, Philadelphia, 1986. pp 200-233.

14. Neely DP, in Morrow DA: *Current Therapy in Theriogenology.* Saunders, Philadelphia, 1980. pp 694-706.

15. McMullan WC, in Mansmann RA and McAllister ES: *Equine Medicine and Surgery.* 3rd ed. American Veterinary Publications, Goleta, CA, 1982. pp 789-883.

16. Kenney RM *et al: Manual for Clinical Fertility Evaluation of the Stallion.* Soc for Theriogenol, Hastings, NE, 1983. pp 3-100.

17. Ladds PW, in Jubb KVF *et al: Pathology of Domestic Animals.* 3rd ed. Vol 3. Academic Press, New York, 1985. pp 409-459.

18. Hinrichs K *et al:* Complications of a testicular prosthesis in a stallion. *JAVMA* 186:390-391, 1985.

19. Roberts SJ: *Veterinary Obstetrics and Genital Diseases.* David & Charles, North Pomfret, VT, 1986. pp 826-827.

20. Karus PA and Kuther DG: A survey of adverse effects associated with ivermectin use in Louisiana horses. *JAVMA* 185:782-783, 1984.

21. Herd RP and Donham JC: Efficacy of ivermectin against *Onchocerca cervicalis* microfilarial dermatitis in horses. *Am J Vet Res* 44:1102-1105, 1983.

22. Bello TR: Ivermectin from a researcher-clinician viewpoint. *Proc Ann Mtg AAEP,* 1983. pp 328-331.

23. Cotchin E: Tumours of farm animals: A survey of tumours examined at the Royal Veterinary College, London, during 1950-60. *Vet Record* 69:816-822, 1960.

24. Stannard AA and Pulley LT, in Moulton J: *Tumors of Domestic Animals.* 2nd ed. Univ of California Press, Berkeley, 1978. pp 16-74.

25. Schumacher J and Vaughan JT: Surgery of the penis and prepuce. *Vet Clin No Am* (Equine Pract) 4:473-491, 1988.

domen but a portion of the epididymis lies within the inguinal canal, the horse is called a partial abdominal cryptorchid.[8]

Retained testes are aspermic because spermatogenesis is inhibited by temperature elevation; therefore, bilateral testicular retention results in sterility. Because the androgen-producing Leydig cells of cryptorchid testes remain functional, cryptorchid horses develop secondary sexual characteristics and male sexual behavior.

Cryptorchidism is a sex-limited, complex developmental condition, the cause of which is not understood completely. It is the most common disorder of sexual differentiation in male horses and one of the most common congenital abnormalities in mammalian males. Of every 6 colts, aged 2-3 years, referred to 16 North American veterinary university teaching hospitals for medical attention, 1 was cryptorchid.[9] The condition was most prevalent in Percherons and least prevalent in Thoroughbreds. Quarter Horses ranked third, behind the Palomino, in relative risk. The mechanisms of testicular differentiation and descent in domestic animals and men are similar.[10] The details of this process have been studied for horses but remain incompletely understood.[11,12] Chapter 1 contains a review of testicular descent.

Cause: Testicular descent is a very complex process, so causes for abnormal descent can be varied, and are often difficult to document. Reported mechanical causes for abnormal testicular descent in stallions include: overstretching of the gubernacular cord; insufficient abdominal pressure to cause expansion of the vaginal process; inadequate growth of the gubernaculum and related structures, resulting in inadequate dilation of the vaginal ring and inguinal canal for passage of the testis; and displacement of the testis into the pelvic cavity, where abdominal pressure precludes its passage through the inguinal canal.[11,12]

Several reports suggest a genetic basis for cryptorchidism in horses. One of the most widely cited studies revealed that a dominant factor was responsible for cryptorchidism in horses.[7] Another investigator believed the transmission of cryptorchidism was due to a simple autosomal recessive gene.[13] One German study concluded that at least 2 genetic factors are involved, one of which is located on the sex chromosomes. A second German study suggested that cryptorchidism in horses is transmitted by an autosomal dominant gene.[13]

Of 58 colts sired by a cryptorchid Quarter Horse at Texas A&M University, 56 had normally descended testes.[14] The 2 remaining foals were unavailable for evaluation when the data were compiled. If cryptorchidism of the above Quarter Horse was heritable, transmission of the trait by an autosomal dominant gene is highly unlikely, unless the gene has extremely low penetrance. It also is difficult to support autosomal recessive inheritance unless the frequency of the recessive gene in the mates of the stallion was near zero.[14]

In men and horses, cryptorchidism has been reported as a feature of abnormal karyotypes. In men, 18 different autosomes have been involved, with trisomy and partial trisomy the most frequent karyotypic abnormalities.[15] Cryptorchidism has been associated with intersexuality in horses; in most cases, the intersexual phenotype resulted from an abnormal sex chromosome complement. These observations suggest that, at least in some cases, normal descent of the testes is not a simple trait controlled by a single gene. Rather, it is a complex developmental condition sensitive to abnormal numbers of large blocks of genes located on many different chromosomes.[16]

All of the published studies dealing specifically with genetic aspects of cryptorchidism in horses suffer from the same weakness: the data presented are not adequate to support the models advocated for genetic transmission. Difficulty in determining patterns of inheritance in cryptorchid stallions arises from an insufficient number of critical test breedings, and an inability to obtain accurate information (*eg*, incidence and specific pathologic findings) in males born from such breedings. Most colts, including cryptorchids, are castrated before puberty and have no opportunity to sire offspring. The occurrence of abnormally located testes often is not recorded, particularly because inguinal testes can often be retrieved during castration without using special surgical approaches. Owners frequently may believe that keeping records of this defect is unjustified because of its low incidence in most herds. Also, bilateral cryptorchids are infertile, and use of unilateral cryptorchids for breeding stock is discouraged. The likelihood of perpetuating the defect in a sufficient number of offspring to ascertain patterns of inheritance is therefore quite low. While it is likely that many cases of cryptorchidism have a genetic basis, a definitive study detailing a plausible genetic mechanism has yet to be performed. Perhaps more than one pattern of inheritance exists.

Retrospective studies of large numbers of cryptorchid horses indicate that right and left testicular retention occurs with nearly equal frequency, but that unilateral retention occurs about 9 times more frequently than bilateral retention.[17,18] Most retained left testes are located abdominally (75%), whereas most retained right testes are located inguinally (60%).[17] Bilateral abdominal retention of testes is nearly 2.5 times as prevalent as bilateral inguinal retention, but the occurrence of both abdominal and inguinal testes in the same horse is relatively uncommon.

During testicular development and descent, the left testis tends to be larger than the right one.[5,6] This anatomic difference supports the finding that the left testis is more likely to resist access to the inguinal canal (and thereby be retained in the abdomen), whereas the right testis is predisposed to inguinal retention.[12]

One survey of cryptorchidism showed that the tendency for abdominal retention in left-sided cryptorchid horses does not apply to ponies.[19] This study found an equal distribution between right-sided and left-sided abdominal testes in ponies. Because this distribution differed from that found by other investigators, these workers postulated that there are breed differences in the incidence of right and left abdominal cryptorchids. Right-sided inguinal retention predominated in young ponies. In older ponies, right and left inguinal retention of testes occurred with equal frequency. Right-sided inguinal retention is considered to become less common with advancing age because the inguinal testis can descend into the scrotum between 2 and 4 years of age. The investigators theorized that there are 2 types of inguinal cryptorchids. One type occurs predominantly on the right side in ponies and is temporary. The second type occurs equally on the right and left sides and is not affected by age.

Diagnosis: If no attempt has been made to castrate a horse, cryptorchidism is easily diagnosed. External palpation of the scrotal contents reveals absence of one or both testes. If the history is reliable, the retained testis is most likely to be in an ectopic, inguinal or abdominal position, as gonadal agenesis is extremely rare. Horses purchased as geldings but displaying stallion-like behavior pose more of a diagnostic challenge. One must determine if the horse is a cryptorchid and, if so, whether one or both testes are retained.

Examination of a suspected cryptorchid begins with palpation of scrotal contents and external inguinal ring. If both testes cannot be palpated, a tranquilizer should be given and the genital area palpated again. Tranquilization may relax the cremaster muscles, thereby making a subcutaneous or inguinal testis more accessible. Because the average length of the inguinal canal is about 10 cm, testes high within this canal cannot be palpated in most horses. Inguinal testes lie in the canal with their long axis in a vertical position. Testicular entry into the inguinal canal is preceded by that of the adjoining epididymal tail; hence, the latter structure sometimes is mistakenly identified by palpation as the testis.[20,21] One should palpate and visually inspect the scrotum for scar tissue that might indicate previous surgery. However, a scrotal scar indicates only that an incision has been made, not that a testis has been removed.

If external palpation fails to reveal both testes, rectal palpation can be performed in an attempt to locate an abdominal testis. Male horses probably present a greater risk for rectal tears from palpation than do mares, as they seldom are palpated rectally and may resist more violently. Most cryptorchids are presented at a young age, and young horses are more prone to rectal tears due to their more nervous dispositions, increased straining and smaller rectums. Caudal epidural anesthesia or sedation can facilitate palpation per rectum. The risks of rectal injury must be measured against the diagnostic value of the information gained from rectal examination.

By palpation per rectum, an attempt is made initially to trap the testis between the hand and abdominal wall just beyond the brim of the pelvis, or to grasp the testis while sweeping the caudal abdominal cavity.[22]. Actual palpation of an abdominal testis is difficult, as abdominal testes are small and flaccid, and may have great mobility. Locating the vaginal ring on the side of suspected testicular retention may be informative. The left vaginal ring can be palpated with the right hand and the right vaginal ring with the left hand.[23] The lateral aspect of the wrist should be positioned on the pubic brim near the pelvic symphysis. The fingertips are pressed against the abdominal wall. The middle finger is flexed and extended in a cranioventral direction until it enters the slit-like vaginal ring. Moving caudally, the finger slides over the vaginal ring because the ring opens dorsally. Some examiners can identify both vaginal rings equally well using only one hand for palpation. If the vaginal ring can be identified, the testis, or at least the epididymis, probably has descended into the inguinal canal.

Structures converging at the vaginal ring can sometimes be identified by palpation per rectum. The ductus deferens is the most readily palpable structure, and can usually be felt as it enters the caudomedial aspect of the vaginal ring if the testis or epididymis has descended.[23] Using this diagnostic approach, it is difficult to differentiate partial abdominal cryptorchids from horses in which both the epididymis and testis have descended through the vaginal ring.[17] In horses with complete abdominal testicular retention, the vaginal ring usually is difficult to identify by rectal palpation.

Ultrasonography was reported to be a more useful diagnostic method than palpation for locating and sizing retained testes, in either the inguinal canal or abdominal cavity.[24] Inguinal canals were scanned from the external inguinal rings outward. Transrectal scans were initiated at the pelvic brim, and continued cranially using a to-and-fro scanning pattern between the midline and lateral abdominal wall(s). The ultrasonic image of retained testes was found to be less dense (less echogenic) than that of normally descended testes, but retained testes were still identified easily and measured accurately in this study. A 5-mHz transrectal transducer was used for ultrasonic examinations.

When the castration history is incomplete and external and/or internal genital examinations are inconclusive, hormonal assays are of considerable diagnostic value. Testosterone and/or estrogen levels can be measured in the serum to help differentiate geldings from cryptorchids. Comparison of testosterone concentration in plasma samples taken before and 30-100 minutes after IV injection of 6000 or 12,000 IU of human chorionic gonadotropin (hCG) has been reported to be superior to evaluation of only baseline testosterone concentration for differentiating cryptorchids and geldings.[25] Concentrations of testosterone <40 pg/ml indicated the absence of testicular tissue, and values >100 pg/ml indicated its presence, whereas concentrations of 40-100 pg/ml were nondiagnostic. Young colts (<18 months of age) usually had a testosterone concentration in serum <100 pg/ml. Serum concentration of testosterone during the winter can be as low as 200 pg/ml in normal stallions.[26]

Human chorionic gonadotropin injection is used to elevate testosterone concentrations in suspected cryptorchids above a baseline (prestimulation) level in an effort to enhance the diagnostic accuracy of this test. Paired plasma samples (pre- and poststimulation) may be necessary to distinguish geldings with relatively high basal testosterone concentrations from cryptorchids with relatively low concentrations. In a study measuring testosterone concentrations in paired plasma samples taken before and after hCG stimulation, 6.7% of the tests were inconclusive.[26] If only the prestimulation testosterone concentration was used, the percentage of tests that were inconclusive rose to 14%. The investigators concluded that the hCG stimulation test was 94.6% accurate in diagnosing cryptorchidism.

Other workers reported that baseline testosterone concentration in serum was more reliable than the hCG stimulation test for differentiating geldings from cryptorchids (mean testosterone concentration in geldings ranged from 30 to 150 pg/ml, whereas testosterone concentration in horses with testicular tissue had means ranging from 620 to 800 pg/ml).[27] Baseline testosterone concentration was found to be 95% accurate for diagnosing the presence of testicular tissue in horses. These workers also reported that better results can be achieved with the HCG stimulation test if post-hCG serum samples are taken at 1 hour (200% increase) or preferably at 24 hours (400% increase), as opposed to 30-60 minutes. An additional study revealed that the rise in serum testosterone of stallions following hCG stimulation is highest 2- 3 days later, and that this may be the most appropriate time to collect the post-hCG serum sample.[28] It becomes obvious that more studies are needed to verify the most appropriate time for collection of the posttreatment serum sample in an hCG stimulation test.

Single-sample assays for conjugated estrogen (*eg,* estrone sulfate) are reported to be 95-96% accurate for diagnosis of cryptorchidism in horses >3 years of age, but can produce a high incidence of false-negative results in both donkeys and young horses (<3 years of age).[26,27] Though cryptorchids tended to produce less conjugated estrogen than normal stallions, estrone sulfate concentration in plasma of geldings was markedly lower than that of cryptorchids and normal stallions. One study revealed that total estrogen concentration was higher, and total androgen concentration lower, in bilaterally cryptorchid stallions than in unilaterally cryptorchid or normal stallions.[29] Donkeys had no detectable estrogens in their serum,[26] and normal stallions <3 years of age produced much less estrogen than mature stallions.[26,27] Therefore, baseline testosterone concentration and/or the hCG stimulation test should be employed for diagnosis of cryptorchidism in donkeys of all ages, and horses <3 years of age.

Much variation exists among laboratories regarding serum concentrations of estrogens (estrone sulfate) or androgens (testosterone) in horses. These individual laboratories should therefore state the serum concentrations of either hormone that they consider to be consistent with geldings or cryptorchids. It may be necessary to compare laboratory values from known geldings and stallions with the suspected cryptorchid to interpret results of assays if the laboratory has not established standards.

Treatment: For horses with one retained testis and one scrotal testis, a search for, and removal of, the retained testis should precede emasculation of the descended testis. If the cryptorchid testis cannot be found, removing the descended testis gives an unscrupulous owner the opportunity to unethically sell the horse as a gelding. Removal of the scrotal testis only may cause growth of the cryptorchid testis, due to interference with the testicular feedback mechanism, which may in turn lead to increased gonadotropin secretion by the pituitary gland.[6,12]

A retained testis can be removed through an inguinal, flank, paramedian or parainguinal approach.[6,20,30-34] For the inguinal approach, the horse is anesthetized and placed in dorsal recumbency. Depending on the size of the horse, an 8- to 14-cm skin incision is created directly over the superficial inguinal ring, or over the scrotum parallel to the median raphe. Using digital dissection, the subcutaneous inguinal fascia then is separated down to the level of the superficial inguinal ring. If the incision is centered over the superficial inguinal ring, care must be taken not to lacerate the branches of the external pudendal vein. If the incision is through the scrotum, these veins are less likely to be encountered, but the superficial inguinal ring is not exposed as easily.

Testes in an inguinal position are enveloped by the tunica vaginalis (vaginal process), and are usually identified readily in the area of the superficial inguinal ring. The parietal (common) vaginal tunic is incised with a scalpel and its contents examined completely to avoid mistaking the epididymal tail for the testis, especially in a partial abdominal cryptorchid. If the testis has previously been removed, the partially excised spermatic cord is found within the inguinal canal. The remaining deferent duct usually can be located near the superficial inguinal ring and traced toward the scrotum to search for any epididymal or testicular tissue inadvertently left behind during a previous operation. The effect of shortening the spermatic cord on alleviation of stallion-like behavior is discussed in Chapter 5.

The vaginal process and enclosed epididymis of the partial abdominal cryptorchid are everted into the inguinal canal. These structures should be identified readily during exploration of the inguinal canal by this approach. The vaginal process, with its contents, may resemble a very small testis. The vaginal process should be stripped of surrounding fascia and incised longitudinally (1 cm long). The body or tail of the epididymis often protrudes through this incision site. The proper ligament of the testis then is identified where it attaches to the epididymal tail (Fig 1), and grasped with hemostat forceps. By simultaneously applying traction to this ligament and dilating the vaginal ring with a finger inserted into the abdomen (via the incision in the vaginal process), the testis gradually is pulled through the vaginal ring and into the inguinal canal. There, it and the attached epididymis can be emasculated. On rare occasions, it may be difficult to exteriorize the testis sufficiently to apply an emasculator. In this event, the cord can be ligated and severed, or crushed with a chain ecraseur.

The vaginal process of the complete abdominal cryptorchid is inverted within the abdomen, but can be everted into the ingui-

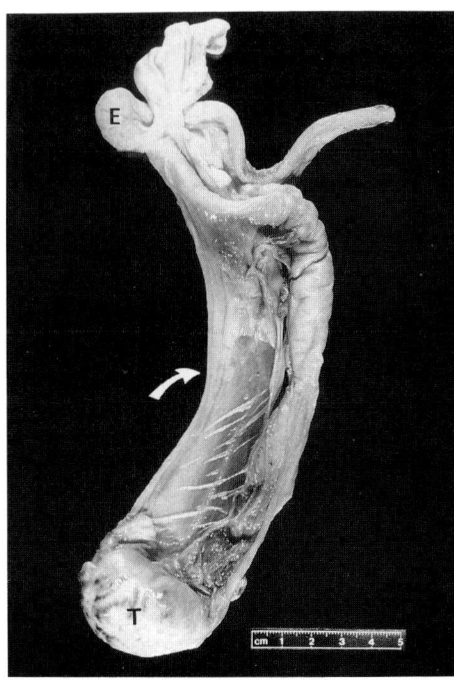

Figure 1. Cryptorchid testis (T), with an elongated proper ligament of the testis (arrow) connecting the testis with the cauda epididymidis (E).

nal canal by traction on the inguinal extension of the gubernaculum, which attaches the vaginal process to the scrotum, also called the scrotal ligament.[30] This portion of the gubernaculum is identified as a 0.5- to 2.0-cm-diameter fibrous band, running into the inguinal canal at the craniomedial or craniolateral edge of the superficial inguinal ring. The superficial inguinal ring is stripped of fat and loose connective tissue to aid identification of the gubernaculum. Locating the gubernaculum may be facilitated by gathering and retracting fascia at the edge of the superficial inguinal ring with the thumb and forefinger. If the gubernaculum is identified, traction should be placed on this structure to evert the vaginal process. If the gubernaculum cannot be located, the inverted vaginal process can be everted by inserting a 10-inch curved sponge forceps through the vaginal ring and grasping the apex of the vaginal process. The vaginal process is then retracted gently into the inguinal canal. Once exteriorized, the vaginal process should be incised, and the epididymis and attached testis exteriorized and excised, as described above. The vaginal ring should be repalpated after the testis and epididymis are removed. If no more than the tips of the index and middle fingers can be inserted through the vaginal ring, the superficial inguinal ring can be left unsutured.

If techniques to evert the vaginal process fail, a finger can be inserted into the abdomen by perforating the internal abdominal oblique muscle and peritoneum cranial to the vaginal ring. The area surrounding the vaginal ring then is explored and the proper ligament of the testis or the scrotal ligament hooked with a finger. If this technique fails, the opening should not be enlarged further; rather, the surgeon should resort to the parainguinal approach. It is much easier to suture the aponeurosis of the external abdominal oblique muscle than to suture the internal abdominal oblique muscle through the inguinal canal.

When a peritoneal opening >2 fingers in diameter has been created, the superficial inguinal ring should be sutured to prevent evisceration. Alternatively, the inguinal canal can be packed with gauze. The gauze pack should be maintained in the canal for 24-36 hours by placing a suture through the edges of the skin incision and the gauze. Insertion of the gauze through the vaginal ring should be avoided. Before removing the pack, the vaginal ring should be examined per rectum to determine if gauze is in the abdominal cavity. Gauze in the abdomen prevents contraction of the ring and may adhere to viscera. Placing gauze in the inguinal canal generally is considered a poor alternative to surgical closure of the superficial inguinal ring. Suturing the superficial inguinal better prevents evisceration than packing the canal with gauze. It also avoids visceral adhesions to the gauze.[22] The edges of the superficial inguinal ring are fibrous, support sutures well, and are easily accessible. The superficial inguinal ring can be sutured with absorbable sutures, using an interrupted or continuous pattern. The inguinal fascia and skin can be left as an open wound or sutured; these tissues should be sutured only if the surgical technique was aseptic.

For a parainguinal approach, an 8- to 14-cm skin incision is made medial and parallel to the superficial inguinal ring.[34] With digital dissection, the subcutaneous inguinal fascia is separated from the superficial inguinal ring. The inguinal canal is examined for the testis or epididymis and everted vaginal process. If these structures cannot be found, or if an inverted vaginal process cannot be everted using the techniques described above, the aponeurosis of the external abdominal oblique muscle is penetrated with scissors medial to the vaginal ring, at the ring's cranial aspect. The underlying internal abdominal oblique muscle is separated in the direction of its fibers to allow the introduction of 1-2 fingers into the abdomen. The peritoneum is penetrated with a sharp thrust of the index finger, and the region of the vaginal ring explored for the gubernaculum, epididymis or deferent duct. Each of these structures can be followed to the tail of the epididymis, which is connected to the testis by the proper ligament of the testis. The testis can be exteriorized through the abdominal incision by placing traction on this ligament. If necessary, the opening can be enlarged to accommodate the entire hand. After removal of the testis and epididymis, the incision in the aponeurosis of the external oblique muscle is closed with an interrupted or continuous suture pattern using absorbable material. The subcutis and skin are closed routinely.

For a paramedian approach, an 8- to 15-cm skin incision is made 5 cm lateral to and parallel with the midline, 10-12 cm cranial to the pubis.[32,33] The outer sheath of the rectus abdominus muscle is incised in the same direction as the skin incision, and the fibers of the rectus abdominis muscle are bluntly separated. The inner rectus sheath is incised longitudinally or transversely, according to the surgeon's preference, and the peritoneum is perforated with a finger. After locating and removing the testis and attached epididymis, the inner and outer layers of the rectus sheath, the subcutis and skin are closed separately with an interrupted or continuous suture pattern.

For the flank approach, a 10- to 15-cm vertical skin incision is made over the paralumbar fossa in the standing or laterally recumbent horse.[33,139] The peritoneum is exposed by a muscle-splitting grid technique and perforated with a finger. After the testis and epididymis have been removed, each muscle layer, the subcutis and skin are closed separately with a continuous or interrupted suture pattern.

The flank and suprapubic paramedian approaches to cryptorchid testis removal require prior location of the testis, as retraction of an inguinal testis back into the abdomen may not be possible. Because the location of the missing testis cannot always be determined reliably, it may be necessary to explore the inguinal canal to rule out the presence of an inguinal testis before performing a flank or paramedian approach. If inguinal or parainguinal approaches are used, it is not necessary to determine the location of the testis before surgery. It is sufficient to determine the existence of cryptorchidism and which testis is retained. Because an abdominal testis generally can be removed by an inguinal or parainguinal approach, a flank or paramedian approach usually is unnecessary. An abnormally large abdominal testis such as a neoplastic testis, may require removal through a flank or paramedian incision. A standing flank approach can sometimes be used if general anesthesia is economically unfeasible.

Testicular Hypoplasia

Testicular hypoplasia often occurs in association with chromosomal aberrations. See Multifactorial Diseases for a discussion of testicular hypoplasia.

Ectopic Testes

Infrequently, one or both testes undergo bizarre excursions during the course of testicular descent, with final residence in the extrascrotal subcutis of the inguinal area. The genetic or mechanical factors resulting in testicular maldescent are not understood. Affected individuals should be distinguished from intersexes. Horses with ectopic testes unassociated with an intersex condition always have an XY sex chromosome complement. Testes that do not reside in the scrotum undergo spermatogenic arrest because of disruption of the thermoregulatory mechanism crucial to normal spermatogenesis.

Diseases With Physical Causes

Testicular Laceration

Testicular lacerations generally occur as a result of a severe blow to the scrotum that ruptures the tunica albuginea (Figs 2, 3) or from lacerations of the scrotum. Testicular lacerations are readily detectable if the scrotum is lacerated, but testicular lacerations without associated scrotal lacerations are much more difficult to identify. Generally, the latter state is manifested clinically as acute and pronounced scrotal enlargement. It must be differentiated from other causes of scrotal enlargement (see Chapter 7). An anechoic (black) or hypoechogenic ultrasonic appearance is initially present as blood is released into the surrounding tissues, but this gradually changes to contain echoic densities as the blood organizes into fibrin clots. Visualization of the ruptured tunica albuginea is unlikely during ultrasonic examination. Definitive diagnosis generally requires surgical exploration.

Testicular lacerations produce extensive hemorrhage. The sperm-producing potential of lacerated testes is poor. Unilateral castration generally is the treatment of choice, to maximize the probability of salvaging the contralateral testis. Unilateral castration should be done before fibrin organization of the blood

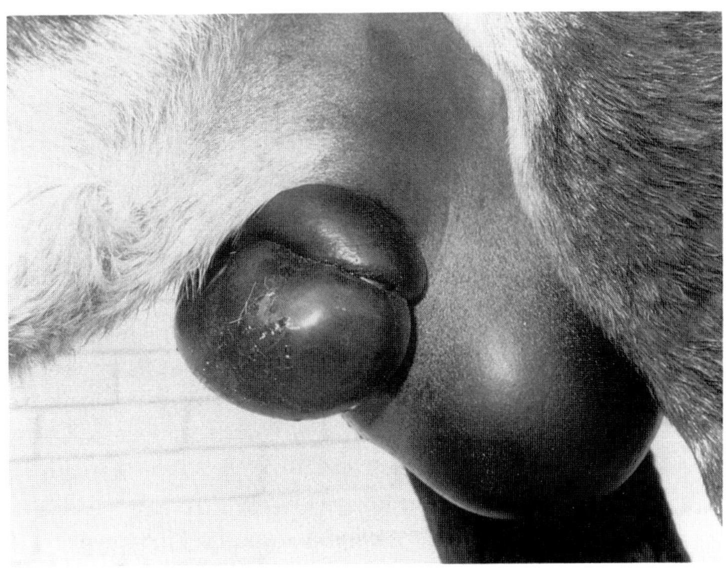

Figure 2. Extreme swelling of the prepuce and scrotum of a jack as a result of a breeding accident. The scrotal enlargement was due primarily to testicular hemorrhage through a rent in the tunica albuginea (see Figure 3).

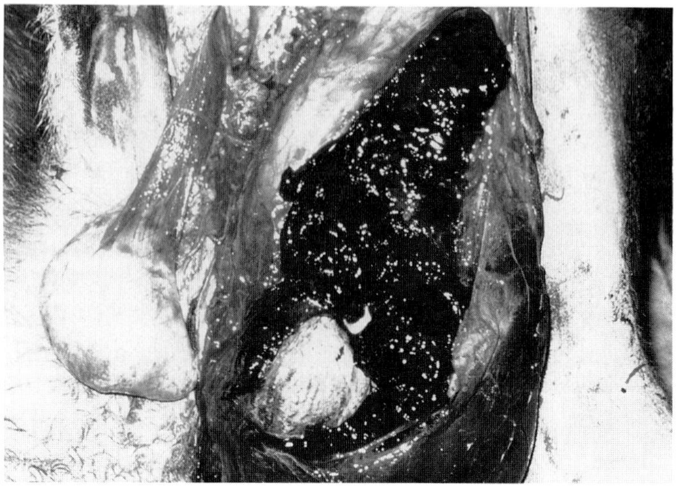

Figure 3. Massive bleeding into the vaginal space of a jack emanating from a ruptured tunica albuginea and testicular hemorrhage (see Figure 2).

clot becomes too extensive (generally 5-7 days). Removal of extravasated blood and primary skin closure also are indicated to minimize interference with thermoregulation of the contralateral testis. Aseptic surgical technique is critical to healing. Surgical repair of testicular rupture has been attempted in men to salvage the testis, but the technique has not been described for stallions.[35]

Testicular Hematoma

Testicular hematomas are caused by extravasation of blood into the testicular parenchyma. Integrity of the testicular capsule (tunica albuginea) usually is maintained. Testicular hematomas can be caused by blunt trauma or as a sequel to locally invasive testicular tumors or testicular biopsies. Testicular tissue is very vascular, and considerable hemorrhage can result from rupture of testicular vessels. Extensive necrosis of testicular parenchyma ensues, often ending in complete loss of testicular function. The testis eventually becomes small and atrophic.

Diagnosis of testicular hematomas by physical examination is difficult. High-resolution real-time ultrasonography is the most reliable noninvasive diagnostic method and is used frequently in the human field.[36] On ultrasonograms, normal testicular parenchyma is homogeneous, with medium-level echogenicity and distinct borders. Recent intratesticular hemorrhage produces focal anechoic or hypoechogenic areas, whereas regional scar formation associated with previous hemorrhage causes increased echogenicity.

The need for surgical intervention is debatable. If hemorrhage is contained within the tunica albuginea, development of adhesions between the surrounding tunics and scrotum may not occur, thus preserving the local thermoregulatory mechanism. Hemicastration often is performed if massive hematomas are detected. It is unknown whether surgical removal of the affected testis hastens or delays recovery of the contralateral testis. If left untreated, the affected testis probably undergoes irreversible degeneration and atrophy. We have examined a number of stallions with a history of blunt scrotal trauma that resulted in an atrophied, firm testis unassociated with overlying scrotal adhesions. Given time, the contralateral testis may undergo some compensatory hypertrophy. Prophylactic antimicrobial therapy may be indicated to prevent development of hematogenous septic orchitis.

Radiation Injury

Ionizing radiation has a devastating effect on the germinal epithelium because rapid cell division, a constant feature of the postpubertal testis, increases radiosensitivity. Late-generation type-A spermatogonia and all type-B spermatogonia are the most radiosensitive germinal cells.[37] The relatively inactive stem spermatogonia are remarkably resistant to irradiation. These refractory cells may permit eventual repopulation of the seminiferous epithelium if the source of irradiation is removed, and if Sertoli cells and Leydig cells are not irreparably damaged. The long-term effect of ionizing radiation on fertility of stallions has not been investigated.

Thermal Degeneration (Heat Injury)

Normal spermatogenesis of domestic animals depends on a temperature differential between the testis/epididymis and the body proper (see Chapter 1). These reproductive organs function normally only when maintained at a temperature several degrees below core body temperature. The scrotum and regional vascular system normally provide this proper thermal environment, but a variety of mishaps can disrupt the thermoregulatory mechanism that is critical to normal spermatogenesis. The consequence of elevated testicular temperature is spermatogenic arrest and testicular degeneration. The section entitled Testicular Degeneration contains a discussion of heat-related injury.

Traumatic Orchitis

Blunt scrotal trauma can produce acute noninfectious orchitis, characterized by hot, tense, painful testes. One or both testes may be involved. Swelling of affected testes may not be perceptible clinically because of the investing nonexpansive tunica albuginea. Testicular and scrotal edema invariably are present. Extensive testicular edema may be identified as hypoechoic areas within the testis parenchyma during ultrasonic exam.

Increased intratesticular pressure, produced by interstitial edema, and increased testicular temperature lead to marked testicular degeneration. Severe cases usually result in irreversible atrophy of the seminiferous epithelium with replacement fibrosis.

Treatment is directed at counteracting local inflammation with scrotal cryotherapy, nonsteroidal antiinflammatory drugs and perhaps prophylactic antimicrobial therapy. Chapter 7 contains a discussion of medical management, including cryotherapeutic techniques. Sexual rest is indicated. Serial (monthly) determinations of testicular size and texture, and semen quantity and quality, help assess permanence of testicular damage.

Torsion of the Spermatic Cord

Extensive and protracted torsion of the spermatic cord can interfere with the vascular supply to the ipsilateral testis, resulting in ischemic necrosis. Chapter 11 contains a discussion of spermatic cord torsion.

Inflammatory, Infectious and Immune Diseases

Bacterial Orchitis

Bacterial orchitis is rare in stallions. It reportedly occurs through hematogenous spread of *Streptococcus zooepidemicus, Streptococcus equi, Actinobacillus equuli, Pseudomonas mallei, Salmonella abortus equi* and *Brucella abortus.* Local bacterial invasion of the testes also can be secondary to infectious peritonitis (via the inguinal canal) or, more commonly, penetrating wounds of the scrotum. A variety of bacterial organisms, including *Streptococcus* spp, *Staphylococcus* spp and *Escherichia coli* can produce bacterial orchitis by this route. Retrograde transmission of pathogenic bacteria to the testes via the extragonadal duct system is quite rare, though bacterial orchitis can be accompanied by corresponding epididymitis. Unilateral or bilateral bacterial orchitis can develop, depending on the route and extent of infection.

Affected testes are hot, tense, slightly swollen and acutely painful. Testicular enlargement, due to inflammation and edema, is limited by the inelastic overlying tunica albuginea. Edema may be apparent during ultrasonic examination. The testes remain freely movable within the scrotum unless periorchitis also is present. Fever and scrotal edema also are common.

Increased testicular temperature, congestion and circulatory interference often lead to localized ischemia or infarction. Physical restriction to expansion by the overlying tunica albuginea also results in pressure necrosis of testicular parenchyma. Suppurative and necrotizing lesions can develop in affected testes. Abscessation sometimes occurs in infectious orchitis, occasionally culminating in purulent liquefaction of the entire parenchyma.[38] Granulomas may form as a result of spermatozoal extravasation into the interstitial tissue. Marked testicular degeneration, the usual sequel to bacterial orchitis, is manifested clinically by oligospermia or azoospermia, and eventual decrease in testicular size (see Testicular Degeneration). Horses with acute orchitis may refuse to breed. If obtained, ejaculates may contain numerous leukocytes, sometimes incorporated into clots. Deterioration of spermatozoal quality is evident through decreased spermatozoal motility and increased morphologic abnormalities. Premature germ cells (*ie,* spermatogonia, spermatocytes or spermatids) may also be present in ejaculates.

Medical management of bacterial orchitis should always include appropriate systemic antimicrobial therapy against the causative organisms(s). Nonsteroidal antiinflammatory drugs and local cryotherapy may help reduce interstitial edema of the testes, which contributes to degeneration in the seminiferous epithelium. Associated problems, such as scrotal infection or peritonitis should be treated expeditiously. Bacterial orchitis often necessitates orchiectomy, as well as medical management. Prompt excision of a unilaterally affected testis may curtail or minimize damage to the contralateral gonad.

Viral Orchitis

Orchitis can result from viral infections, such as equine infectious anemia, viral arteritis or influenza.[37] Local vascular lesions may be the cause of virus-induced orchitis. Degenerative and inflammatory lesions of the tunic vasculature causes degeneration of the seminiferous tubules supplied by these vessels. Severe vascular lesions may cause focal testicular infarction.

Parasitic Orchitis

Migrating larvae of the nematode, *Strongylus edentatus,* can produce focal inflammatory lesions in the testes of horses.[39] Most lesions probably are subclinical. Larva-induced lesions are most commonly seen in the testes, testicular tunics and epididymides of young horses. Larvae become covered by fibrin as they die, which may result in adhesions between the testes and their overlying tunics. Larvae occasionally penetrate the testis, resulting in hemorrhage within the migration tract(s).[38] Another common location for strongyle larvae to lodge is the appendix testis, a remnant of the paramesonephric duct located on the cranial aspect of the testis. Treatment with ivermectin eliminates strongyle larvae.

Ehrlichiosis has been reported to sometimes cause testicular swelling, presumably orchitis, that results in testicular atrophy.[40]

Autoimmune Orchitis

The immune system of an animal recognizes and tolerates antigens to which it was exposed in late fetal life. The antigenic determinants of spermatozoa, however, are not established until puberty, so they are perceived as foreign to the immune system. Spermatozoal maturation is completed in an immunologically privileged site, the adluminal compartment of the seminiferous tubules, to circumvent immunologic attack. The blood-testis barrier, comprised of tight junctional complexes between adjacent Sertoli cells, forms during the prepubertal period, coincident with the onset of spermatogenesis.[41,42] Thus, developing spermatozoa are normally sequestered from the immune system. Additional protection against rampant immunologic attack of spermatozoa may be provided by immunosuppressive factors intrinsic to spermatozoa, and immunosuppressive properties of the testicular interstitium, epididymal epithelium and seminal plasma.[43]

Escape of highly antigenic spermatozoa (or their haploid precursors) from the adluminal compartment of the seminiferous tubules likely incites an immune response, with formation of antisperm antibodies. Precipitating factors for this immunologic attack of spermatozoa might include lacerations, biopsies, neoplasms, trauma or degeneration of the testes. Localized granulomatous reactions and degenerative changes in the testicular parenchyma are likely consequences of extravasation of spermatozoa.

Infertility associated with formation of antisperm antibodies has been experientially induced in domestic animals, but its impact under natural circumstances is unknown. Antibody-mediated causes of infertility are well documented in men.[43,44] Complement-dependent spermatozoal immobilizing factors have been suggested as the underlying cause of infertility in 2 stallions, though the association of antisperm antibodies and infertility was questioned in these 2 cases.[43,45,46] Closer study of this process in horses is warranted.

Toxic Diseases

Adverse Effects of Anabolic Steroids

Anabolic steroids often are used to improve muscle mass and performance of equine athletes. Though no beneficial effects have been substantiated with use of these drugs, negative effects on reproductive function as well as nonreproductive systems have been documented.[47] Testicular degeneration, decreased sperm production and quality and diminished testicular size are the most obvious sequelae to anabolic steroid use in stallions.[47-50] The volume of testicular parenchyma decreases due to atrophy of Leydig cells and reduction in diameter of seminiferous tubules (Fig 4).[48,49]

The negative effect of anabolic steroids on testicular function probably results from interference with endogenous gonadotropin production and release. Aggressive behavior often is intensified in treated stallions due to testosterone-like qualities of anabolic steroids. The effects of anabolic steroids on reproductive performance are considered temporary in adult stallions, but the effects on the prepubertal testis are unknown.[47,51,52] Administration of exogenous androgens to young postpubertal stallions results in histologic changes consistent with testicular hypoplasia or degeneration.[48] Stallions of this age group may take longer to reestablish normal spermatozoal output than older, more mature stallions.[48,52] Testicular growth is delayed when endogenous anabolic steroids are given to colts during the prepubertal period (beginning at 12-16 months).[53]

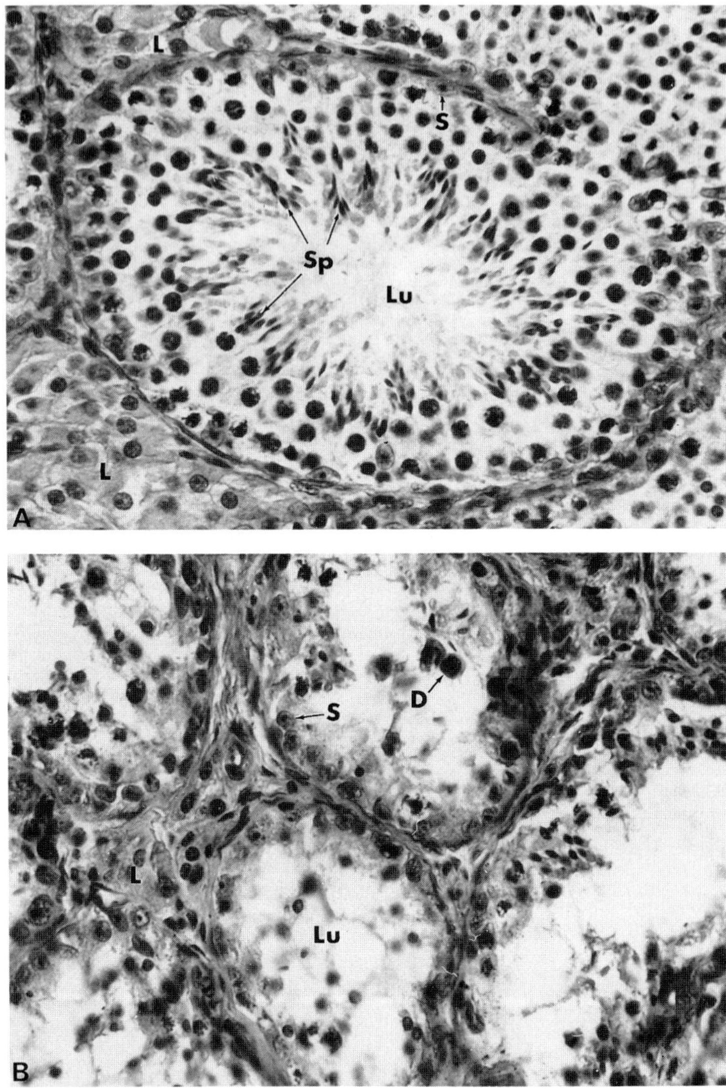

Figure 4. Seminiferous tubules of an untreated pony stallion (A) and a pony stallion receiving anabolic steroids (B).[47] Leydig cells (L), Sertoli cells (S), lumina of the seminiferous tubules (LU), elongated spermatids (Sp) and desquamated germ cells (D) are abbreviated.

Adverse Effects of Miscellaneous Drugs

The drugs used in veterinary practice are quite diverse and little data exist regarding their effects on testicular function. The relatively high incidence of idiopathic subfertility/infertility in horses, coupled with our ignorance of most drug effects on spermatogenesis/sperm maturation, leads one to suspect that use of drugs may play a role in this syndrome. This subject certainly warrants intensive investigation. In any event, indiscriminate use of drugs is discouraged, and the prescriber should be especially cognizant of the potential side effects of all drugs administered to breeding stock.

Neoplasia

General Considerations

Testicular neoplasia of stallions is uncommon, but its actual incidence cannot be measured because most male horses are castrated when young. Because testicular neoplasms of horses are rare, much of their biologic behavior must be inferred from similar neoplasms of men or dogs. Primary testicular neoplasms occur more frequently than secondary neoplasms. Primary testicular neoplasms are classified as germinal or somatic (nongerminal), based on their cellular origin.[54] The tumors are further classified by histologic features. Germinal neoplasms originate from germ cells of the seminiferous epithelium.

Reported germinal neoplasms of the horse are the seminoma, teratoma, teratocarcinoma, and embryonal carcinoma. Germ cells may give rise to a seminoma, representing gonadal differentiation, or may transform into neoplastic pluripotential cells capable of producing any tissue found in the body. These neoplastic pluripotential cells are primitive embryonic cells indistinguishable from those of an early blastula. Cells that proliferate in this state of undifferentiation form an embryonal carcinoma. If the pluirpotential tumor cells differentiate and proliferate into somatic tissues, a teratoma is formed and, if some pluripotential cells remain undifferentiated while others differentiate into somatic tissues, a teratocarcinoma is formed. Other parenchymatous neoplasms, such as Leydig-cell tumors and Sertoli-cell tumors, and all nonparenchymatous neoplasms, such as lipomas, fibromas and leiomyomas, have a nongerminal derivation; hence, they are categorized as somatic tumors. Most equine testicular tumors are of the germinal type.[38]

Environmental and/or genetic factors involved in testicular tumor formation are unknown. Many tumor types, including seminomas, teratomas, Leydig-cell tumors and Sertoli-cell tumors, have been found in cryptorchid testes of stallions.[54] Factors that may promote neoplasia of the cryptorchid testis are abnormal morphology of the seminiferous epithelium, increased temperature, interference with blood supply, hormonal dysfunction, and gonadal dysgenesis.[54] Though the predisposition of cryptorchid testes to neoplasia has been documented in men and dogs, the specific cause-and-effect relationship between testicular maldescent and tumor formation has not been firmly established firmly for horses.[37,54,56] Factors that eventually initiate neoplastic transformation of the testis may also contribute to maldescent of the testis.

The growth characteristics and metastatic behavior of various equine testicular tumors have been studied insufficiently, owing to their uncommon occurrence. Metastasis of germinal tumors has been well documented in stallions.[37,55,57-61] Because of the possibility of metastasis, all testicular tumors are regarded as potentially malignant and treated accordingly. Nearly all reported testicular tumors have been unilateral.

A thorough physical examination of scrotal contents is the obvious starting point for diagnosis of neoplasia in scrotal testes. Tumors arising from cryptorchid testes usually are not discovered until associated systemic illness ensues (weight loss, colic, dyspnea) or routine cryptorchidectomy is performed. Because most tumors of cryptorchid testes are teratomas (which are benign), most tumors involving abdominal testes are discovered during routine cryptorchid castration.[62]

Examination of a horse with a suspected testicular neoplasm should start with evaluation of the normal contralateral testis as a reference guide. A normal testis should feel smooth, compliant and free of nodules. The head, body and tail of the attached epididymis should be smooth and discrete. The dimensions, consistency and sensitivity of the suspect testis should be compared to those of the normal contralateral testis. Small testicular tumors are not likely to be clinically detectable by palpation alone. As neoplasms expand locally, testicular enlargement occurs. Uncommonly, pain may accompany the increase in testicular size. Abnormal testicular contour also may be detected. The affected testis is usually heavier and harder than the normal testis. The history often reveals information on the growth rate of an enlarged testis. Testes harboring tumors tend to remain freely movable within the scrotum, unless the tumor has crossed the testicular capsule and invaded surrounding tissues. Testicular neoplasms must be differentiated from other causes of scrotal enlargement, such as orchitis, periorchitis, hydrocele, testicular/scrotal hematomas and scrotal hernia. A detailed history and a careful genital examination aid in this differentiation. Swelling and pain that develop acutely in the scrotal region are more likely a result of inflammation or ischemia than neoplasia.

Real-time ultrasound instruments are rapidly becoming an indispensable diagnostic tool. Their usefulness extends to examination of the scrotum and its contents. High-resolution ultrasonography may reveal some testicular masses that are undetectable by palpation. Intrascrotal masses may be identified as intra- or extratesticular, and characterized as solid or cystic.[63] Normal testicular parenchyma is homogeneously echogenic, but testicular tumors tend to have areas of decreased echogenicity.[64]

Palpation per rectum, and possibly transrectal ultrasonography, should be incorporated into the diagnostic protocol, especially if tumor dissemination is suspected, or for evaluation of an undescended testis. Both pelvic and abdominal organs should be evaluated thoroughly. When metastasis from equine testicular tumors occurs, it can often be palpated rectally as lymphadenopathy of the medial iliac lymph nodes, located at the origins of the deep circumflex iliac arteries and the external iliac arteries.[65] Unless the scrotum is involved, the superficial and deep inguinal lymph nodes are unlikely to enlarge.

Semen examination may reveal no abnormalities and fertility may be acceptable, as a significant amount of normal testicular parenchyma may remain. However, swelling of the affected testis may interfere with thermoregulation of the contralateral testis, resulting in decreased spermatozoal output.[38,66]

Microscopic evaluation of a suspect testicular mass by testicular biopsy or aspiration cytology can aid in its identification. The suitability of these diagnostic methods is questionable, however, because of the dangers of intratesticular hemorrhage, attendant necrosis of parenchyma, and increased potential for dissemination of the tumor. Needle aspiration is less likely to result in complications.

General anesthesia may be required before performing a punch biopsy of the equine testis. The biopsy site is prepared for aseptic surgery, and a small incision is made in the scrotal skin and parietal tunic to facilitate introduction of a 12-ga Vim-Silverman biopsy instrument. The cutting prongs and cannula are inserted through the visceral tunic and tunica albuginea, then manipulated toward the center of the testicular mass. The cannula is withdrawn and the cutting prongs are advanced. The cannula is then slid over the cutting prongs, and the entire instrument is removed. Digital pressure is applied over the biopsy site for 1-2 minutes to minimize hemorrhage. The incisions in the parietal tunic and scrotal skin can be left unsutured. To minimize artifacts, either Bouin's or Cleland's medium is recommended as a fixative for the biopsy specimen.

To perform a needle aspiration of a testicular mass, the area is first prepared as if for aseptic surgery; infiltration of the scrotal skin with a local anesthetic is unnecessary. The testis is immobilized, and a 23- or 25-ga needle is introduced into the testicular mass. A 5-ml syringe is attached to the needle, and the plunger of the syringe is retracted as 2 or more passes are made into the mass. The plunger is released, then the needle is withdrawn and the aspirate is expressed onto glass slides and smeared. Digital pressure is maintained on the biopsy site for 1-2 minutes to control hemorrhage. After drying, slides are stained with new methylene blue or Giemsa stain. The cytologist must be able to recognize cells of the testis, as normally developing spermatocytes have cytologic characteristics that could lead to erroneous diagnosis of neoplasia.[67]

Many methods used to diagnose and stage neoplasms in men, such as lymphangiography, computed tomography and nuclear magnetic resonance imaging, are not technically feasible in horses. In men, evaluation of biochemical tumor markers, such as alpha-fetoprotein or human chorionic gonadotropin, have proven useful for differentiating germ-cell tumors and evaluating the liklihood of metastasis. Use of similar tests has not been reported in horses.[54,68]

Prompt orchiectomy is the primary treatment for all testicular neoplasms, regardless of type. Unilateral orchiectomy is recommended when only one testis is involved, if the stallion is to remain a breeding animal. The unilateral orchiectomy is likely to result in compensatory hypertrophy of the remaining testis.[69] If semen quality is satisfactory, removal of the affected testis may be delayed until the breeding season is completed. This will avoid the transient decrease in semen quality associated with postsurgical scrotal swelling and resultant thermal effects on the contralateral testis. The owners must be advised, however, that the neoplasm is potentially malignant. If testicular neoplasia is bilateral, surgical removal may be delayed until semen quality deteriorates to the point that the horse is unsuitable for breeding.

During orchiectomy, the proximal spermatic cord should be ligated before emasculation, and the affected testis should be handled minimally during the surgical procedure to reduce the possibility of iatrogenic metastasis. Radical removal of the spermatic cord is advised. The excised spermatic cord should be evaluated histologically for evidence of metastatic lesions.[38]

Hemiorchiectomy incisions can be closed to reduce postoperative swelling and minimize heat-related damage to the contralateral testis. Incisional hemostasis is critical to the success of closure by primary intention. Radical scrotal ablation should accompany orchiectomy if the tumor has invaded peritesticular tissues. Excision of adjacent lymphatic chains is indicated if metastatis is suspected. A parainguinal, paramedian or flank approach may be superior to an inguinal approach for surgical removal of large tumorous cryptorchid testes.

Irradiation and/or chemotherapy often are used in conjunction with surgery to treat men with testicular tumors.[54] This regimen has not been perfected for use in horses.

Seminomas

Seminomas are one of the most commonly reported equine testicular tumors. They have been described in retained and scrotal testes and are more common in older stallions.[60,70] The tumor arises from the germinal epithelium of the seminiferous tubules. Seminomas are locally invasive, spreading by intratubular and extratubular pathways. Progressive testicular enlargement occurs because sheets of neoplastic cells gradually replace normal testicu lar tissue (Fig 5). The tunica albuginea generally restricts the tumor's expansion, but occasionally the tumor breaches the testicular capsule and spreads to adjacent tissues. Metastasis of seminomas to the thoracic and abdominal cavities also has been reported (Fig 6). The cut surface of the

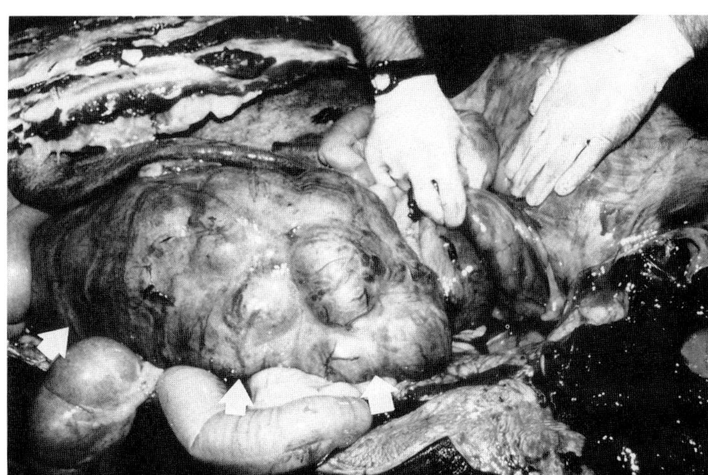

Figure 5. Primary seminoma of a cryptorchid testis (arrows) within the abdominal cavity of a stallion. (Courtesy of Dr. T.S. Ford)

tumor is lobular and soft, with a glistening gray-white appearance, and may exude a milky fluid.

Definitive diagnosis is based on histologic characteristics.[37,61,66] Microscopically, seminomas are comprised primarily of cords or sheets of round or polygonal cells with large nuclei and prominent nucleoli. Normal and bizzare mitotic figures may be present, as may focal lymphocytic infiltrations (Fig 7). Because of their malignant histologic appearance, all seminomas should be considered potentially malignant.[70] Seminomas have been reported to cause feminization of dogs, but this is probably due to inapparent Sertoli-cell tumors in the same or opposite testis. Hormonal changes in horses caused by seminomas have not been reported.

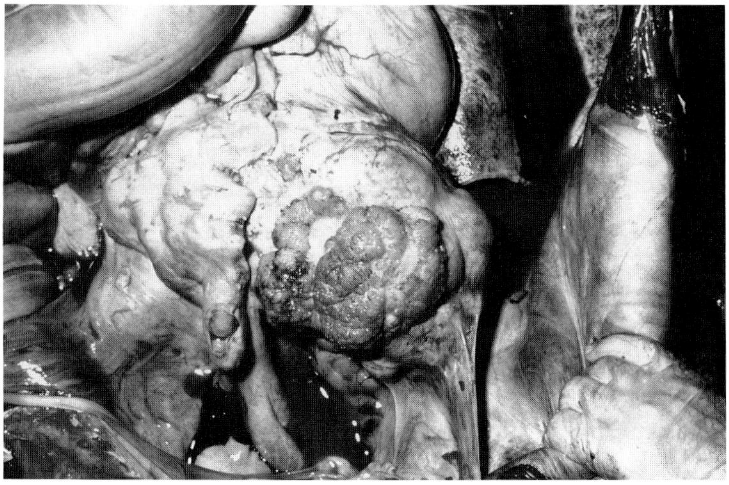

Figure 6. Metastasis of a scrotal testis seminoma to the abdominal cavity.

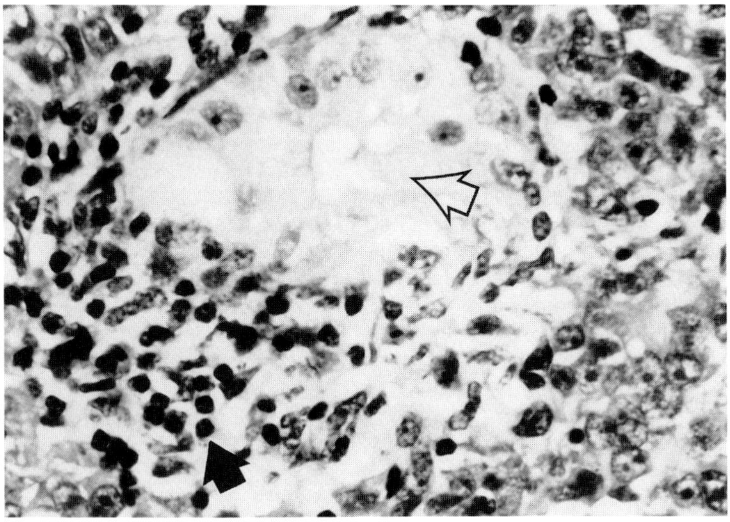

Figure 7. Histologic section of a Sertoli-cell tumor from a stallion's testis. The section contains predominantly neoplastic germ cells, with an isolated seminiferous tubule (open arrow), and occasional lymphocytes (solid arrow). (hematoxylin and eosin, 40X magnification) (Courtesy of Dr. J.F. Edwards)

Teratomas

Though a teratoma can occur anywhere in the body, they are most frequently located in the gonads in horses.[71] This neoplasm constitutes a large percentage of testicular tumors. Teratomas are classified as germinal tumors, as they are derived from pluripotential germ cells. They are complex tumors, composed of a disorderly arrangement of recognizable tissues not native to the testis (bone, cartilage, or skin). Teratomas contain only mature elements and are considered benign.

Tumors are found predominantly in cryptorchid testes but can be found in descended testes.[62,72,73] Of 29 teratomatous testes described in 1 study, 22 were scrotally located.[74] Neoplastic tissue may be present in late fetal life, impeding normal testicular descent into the scrotum. Teratomas usually are recognizable on cross section as multilocular structures containing a variety of ectopic tissues, such as dermal, neural, adipose, respiratory, alimentary and musculoskeletal tissues. These are identified grossly or on microscopic examination (Fig 8).[37]

Embryonal Carcinomas

This tumor is rare but deserves mention because of its malignant characteristics and close relationship to the benign teratoma. Embryonal carcinomas and teratomas both are derived from pluripotential germ cells. However, embryonal carcinomas are composed of poorly differentiated germinal cells, whereas teratomas contain only mature germ-cell tissue.[75]

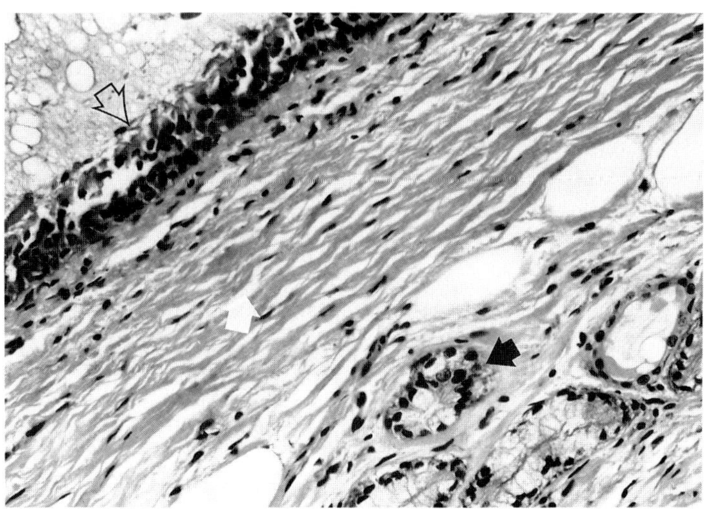

Figure 8. Histologic section of a teratoma of an equine testis. Note the seminiferous tubules (solid black arrow), substantial connective tissue (solid white arrow) and respiratory epithelium (open black arrow). (hematoxylin and eosin, 25X magnification) (Courtesy of Dr. J.F. Edwards)

Teratocarcinomas

These tumors are so classified because of mixed histologic patterns. They contain both mature and primitive germ-cell tissue representative of both teratomas and embryonal carcinomas. Teratocarcinomas are highly malignant because of their primitive germinal component. They are sometimes referred to as malignant teratomas. The teratocarcinoma is a relatively common germ-cell neoplasm of men, but it is rare in stallions.[54,76]

Leydig-Cell Tumors

Leydig-cell tumors arise from the androgen-producing Leydig cells of the testicular interstitium; hence, the synonym interstitial-cell tumor. This tumor is relatively common in dogs and bulls (especially of the Guernsey breed) but is rare in stallions.[37] The tumor typically induces precocious sexual development in children and gynecomastia in men because of excessive steroid production. Such findings are not a feature of Leydig-cell tumors in domestic animals. However, vicious behavior in a stallion with an abdominal Leydig-cell tumor ceased after castration, suggesting that they may be secretory in some cases.[37,77]

Because Leydig-cell tumors are uncommon in horses, their tendency for malignant transformation has not been studied fully. Most Leydig-cell tumors of other domestic animals and men are benign. Similar biologic behavior is likely in stallions. Testes can have either solitary or multiple tumors (commonly 1-2 cm in diameter). Sufficient growth results in clinically detectable testicular enlargement. Tumor growth usually is slow and limited by the unyielding testicular capsule. Local growth of the tumor can result in compression atrophy of surrounding parenchyma. Leydig-cell tumors in other species are usually smaller than other types of testicular tumors.[54,70]

On cut section, Leydig-cell tumors are typically soft, homogeneous, oval or lobulated masses with a thin capsule, characterized by a yellow to brown coloration. Normal parenchyma may remain and produce viable spermatozoa. Definitive identification of the tumor is based on histologic exam. The cells are round or polygonal with small nuclei and voluminous cytoplasm.[37]

Sertoli-Cell Tumors

Sertoli-cell tumors arise from the somatic elements of the seminiferous epithelium (Sertoli or sustentacular cells). Because of its origin, the tumor sometimes is referred to as a tubular adenoma. Though Sertoli-cell tumors are a relatively common testicular tumor of dogs, they are rare in horses. Over one-half of Sertoli-cell tumors in dogs are in cryptorchid testes. Sertoli-cell tumors of dogs usually secrete estrogens that cause feminization.[37] Hyperestrogenism has been reported as a feature of this tumor in men.[54] This feminizing tendency has not been described in stallions. Because the tumor is locally expansive, it can change the size and contour of the affected testis. The metastatic potential of the tumor is unknown but malignancy is possible. Sertoli-cell tumors of dogs and men are infrequently malignant.

On cut section, the tumor is gray to white and unusually firm. Histologic study is required to identify the neoplasm.[37,71,78] Microscopically, most Sertoli-cell tumors display tubules of neoplastic cells separated by thick collagenous septa. Spermatogenic and interstitial cells are rare. Stroma is plentiful and often hyalinized. Mitotic figures are sparse, except when malignancy is obvious.

Nonparenchymatous Tumors

Various mesenchymal testicular neoplasms have been reported in horses, including the lipoma, fibroma and leiomyoma.[37] Their incidence is very low. Lipomas are the most frequently encountered tumors of this group. The metastatic behavior of these tumors has not been critically evaluated. They are considered to be benign space-occupying lesions resulting only in compressive atrophy of adjacent testicular parenchyma.

Multifactorial Diseases

Testicular Hypoplasia

Testicular hypoplasia is considered a relatively common pathologic entity of stallions. However, the true incidence in the equine population and specific breed predilections have not been critically studied. An incidence of 3% was reported in one study of 1000 stallions, in which it was associated with concurrent epididymal hypoplasia.[37] Testicular hypoplasia is characterized by incomplete gonadal development and must be differentiated from testicular degeneration or atrophy, which implies gonadal regression after maturation is completed.

Accelerated development of the testis into a sexually functional organ does not begin until puberty; therefore, derangement of numerous prepuberal events can result in testicular hypoplasia. Testicular hypoplasia is thought to result primarily from congenital aberrations, but it may be acquired.[79] Both genetic and teratogenic causes are suspected. Some types of testicular hypoplasia have a hereditary basis in some species, so genetically induced testicular hypoplasia of horses is possible.[37,79] The pathophysiology of testicular hypoplasia may involve abnormal primordial germ-cell activity during fetal life, such as inadequate proliferation in the yolk sac, improper migration en route to the fetal gonad, or insufficient multiplication/inordinate degeneration after arrival at the gonad; or it may involve postnatal disruption of the germinal epithelium.[78]

Testicular hypoplasia occurs in association with cryptorchidism (both intersex and idiopathic forms) but also occurs as an unexplainable phenomenon of intrascrotal testes. Elevated testicular temperature may contribute to hypoplasia. Small testes are produced when thermoregulation is impaired (*eg,* with abdominal or inguinal cryptorchidism, inguinial herniation, or congenitally short cremaster muscles or excessive intrascotal fat in bulls).[79] While testicular degeneration and atrophy follow impairment of thermoregulation, testicular hypoplasia may occur when such conditions as those above are present before testis growth and development are complete. A high incidence of testicular hypoplasia occurs concurrently with unilateral cryptorchidism in some flocks of sheep, suggesting that the 2 conditions may be related.[37] The testes of male equine hybrids (mules or hinnys) are typically hypoplastic.

In addition to genetic miscues, it is possible that infections, intoxications, malnutrition, endocrinologic disturbances, irradiation or other factors may precipitate testicular hypoplasia. Circumstantial evidence for external influences contributing to hypoplasia includes small testis size frequently noted in young stallions retired from racing. Stallions on the racetrack have smaller testes than stallions of the same age at breeding forms, suggesting that vigorous training and/or drug administration adversely affect testis size.[80]

Testicular hypoplasia can be mild to severe and can involve one or both testes, with the resulting fertility determined by the degree of hypoplasia.[37,38] Clinical findings vary accordingly. Evaluation of testicular size and consistency is a simple noninvasive method of estimating the severity of testicular hypoplasia. Hypoplastic testes are usually small but may occasionally be of normal size.[37] Affected testes vary in texture from normal to soft with mild or moderate hypoplasia, to firm in severely affected testes. The firmness in severely affected testes is due to the disproportionate amount of stromal connective tissue present.[38] The testes of a suspect stallion should be compared with those of similarly aged stallions. The question of unilateral versus bilateral involvement must be addressed. However, one should keep in mind that the left testis tends to be larger than the right one during fetal development, and this size disparity seems to continue after birth.[5,6,81-83]

The examiner must be fully aware that testicular maturation and growth are not triggered until puberty approaches (see Chapter 1). Prepubertal testes are quite small and can be erroneously diagnosed as pathologically hypoplastic. Testicular growth in prepubertal/pubertal stallions usually increases at a fairly rapid and linear rate between 12 and 22 months of age, but testicular growth continues until at least 4-5 years of age.[82-84] Puberty may be delayed because of malnutrition or other factors; therefore, diagnosis of pathologic testicular hypoplasia can be quite difficult before a stallion reaches 2-3 years of age.

Testicular hypoplasia is often suspected when a testis is smaller than normal, particularly in a relatively young postpubertal stallion. Without knowledge of the duration of small testicular size, differentiation between testicular hypoplasia and testicular degeneration (*ie,* atrophy) is difficult. Physical examination findings, testicular histologic findings and semen characteristics are very similar between the 2 pathologic states.[37] If a congenital condition is present, such as inguinal herniation, there is a high likelihood that testicular development was impaired. Because the epididymis is a target organ of testicular products that influence its size, an underdeveloped (*ie,* small) epididymis associated with a small testis provides indirect evidence for testicular hypoplasia. If there is sufficient doubt as to whether reversible testis atrophy (due to degeneration) may exist, reexamination at a later date (in 2-5 months) is indicated.

With mild forms of testicular hypoplasia, most affected seminiferous tubules exhibit active spermatogenesis that progresses to the primary spermatocyte stage or beyond. Isolated tubules remain completely hypoplastic. Hypoplastic seminiferous tubules are interspersed with numerous tubules that appear normal histologically. Individuals that are mildly affected with testicular hypoplasia tend to have slightly small testes with a normally turgid to soft consistency. Mild hypoplasia may be imperceptible by physical examination. Severe testicular hypoplasia is characterized by a preponderance of completely hypoplastic seminiferous tubules. These tubules generally are lined only by Sertoli cells, though some contain a small rim of nondividing spermatogonia or spermatogonial precursors. The basement membrane of affected tubules tends to be thickened and infiltrated with hyaline connective tissue. Connective tissue also accumulates in the interstitial compartment. Because the diameter of the seminiferous tubules is reduced, the testes are smaller than normal. The testes may be soft, but gradual replacement of parenchyma with connective tissue eventually imparts a firm texture to the testes.[37,38]

Depending on the severity of testicular hypoplasia, affected stallions are oligospermic to azoospermic. Libido often is unaffected, and semen volume may be normal. Spermatozoa in ejaculates usually have a high incidence of morphologic defects and poor motility. Round spermatogenic cells often are present in ejaculates, and multinucleated germ cells may also appear as a result of incomplete cytoplasmic divisions during spermatogenesis.[38]

There is no known effective therapy for testicular hypoplasia in stallions. Hypoplastic testes may be predisposed to testicular degeneration. Use of stallions with testicular hypoplasia for breeding should be discouraged because the condition is likely to be hereditary, and the stallions have reduced fertility. However, the value of some stallions encourages owners to breed them. Effective management of affected stallions is predicated on breeding a reduced book of mares, and inseminating mares just before or after ovulation (*ie,* within 6-12 hours of ovulation).

Testicular Degeneration

Spermatogenesis is a very lengthy and delicate process that is easily upset by a variety of extrinsic factors.[85] The susceptibility of the germinal epithelium to damage makes testicular degeneration a major cause of infertility/subfertility in stallions. The responses of the germinal epithelium to assaults are similar, despite the nature of the assault. Histologic changes only vary according to severity of the condition. The specific architectural changes of the testicular parenchyma are usually indistinguishable from those noted with testicular hypoplasia (see above discussion on Testicular Hypoplasia).[37]

Testicular degeneration is strictly an acquired condition as opposed to testicular hypoplasia, which can be congenital or acquired. Hypoplastic testes, however, have an increased susceptibility to degenerative changes.[79,86] Testicular degeneration can affect one or both testes, depending on whether the causative factor is localized, as with a locally aggressive tumor, or generalized, as with fever of variable origin.[38] The condition can be temporary or permanent, depending on the sever ity and duration of the insult. Late-generation spermatogonia, spermatocytes and spermatids are more susceptible to injury than are mature spermatozoa or early-generation spermatogonia, such as undifferentiated and recently differentiated germ cells. Though the germinal epithelium is quite susceptible to injury, the damage created often is temporary because of the more resistant nature of the stem-cell spermatogonia, Sertoli cells and Leydig cells. These refractory cells allow restoration of normal spermatogenic function if the factor responsible for the testicular degeneration is removed.[37]

Testicular degeneration has a multitude of causes. One of the more common causes of testicular degeneration is thermal injury. Any event that disturbs the critical temperature differential of the testis can interfere with normal spermatogenic function. Many conditions can produce such an effect. High environmental temperature, fever, orchitis, periorchitis, hydrocele, scrotal hemorrhage, scrotal edema, scrotal dermatitis and improper scrotal descent all can interfere with the thermoregulatory mechanism necessary for normal spermatogenesis. Testicular degeneration usually results. Systemic and/or local infections often produce testicular degeneration, though the relative damage produced by thermal versus toxic effects is poorly understood. Injury to essential vasculature, as through torsion of the spermatic cord, inflammation of the testicular artery or degenerative changes in testicular arterioles, can result in degeneration of the seminiferous epithelium. Hormonal disturbances, ionizing radiation, malnutrition, ingestion of toxic plants, testicular tumors, efferent/epididymal duct obstruction, production of antisperm antibodies or uncontrolled intratesticular hemorrhage can also lead to testicular degeneration. Age-related testicular degeneration has been documented in other species and may also occur in stallions. Degenerative vascular lesions within the testis have been postulated to be a cause of "senile" changes in testicular parenchyma.[37,38] The effects of various drugs and chemicals on spermatogenic function are largely unexplored. Some drugs produce spermatogenic arrest, particularly systemic chemotherapeutic agents used in the treatment of cancer.[37,38,87] Most drugs are unstudied in this context and should be used as though potentially toxic to the seminiferous epithelium.

To differentiate testicular degeneration from hypoplasia, a good history is essential. Physical examination of general body systems and the genital tract, and specific evaluations of testicular size/consistency and ejaculated spermatozoal quantity/quality are fundamental to assessment of testicular integrity. If an identifiable cause of testicular degeneration is noted, *eg,* adhesions of the testicular tunics, then the acquired nature of degeneration can be confirmed. As discussed above with testicular hypoplasia, testes with only mild degenerative changes tend to be slightly small, with a normally turgid to soft consistency. Severe testicular degeneration results in a marked reduction in testicular size (Fig 9). The enveloping tunica albuginea often becomes wrinkled and has a corrugated texture. Acutely affected testes have a soft, flabby consistency, while chronically affected testes become increasingly firm as testicular parenchyma is replaced by connective tissue stroma. In some instances, the testicular tissue seems to disappear with only the collapsible tunica albuginea remaining palpable. With advanced testicular degeneration, the epididymis may feel dispro-

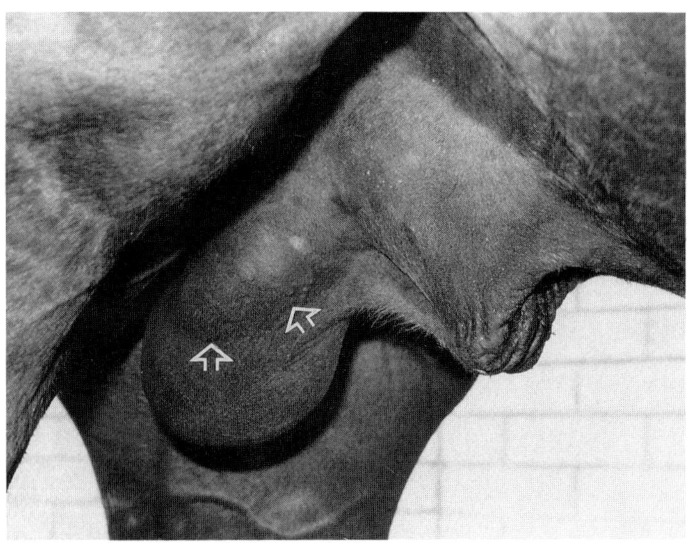

Figure 9. Atrophy (degeneration) and corresponding reduction in size of the right testis (arrows) subsequent to injury.

portionately large and is more readily palpable along its entire course simply because the testis is markedly diminished in size.

Depending on the severity and duration of the insult, oligospermia or azoospermia may be noted during semen evaluation. In the earlier stages of testicular degeneration, daily spermatozoal output may be disproportionately low, based on measurements of testicular size with calipers or an ultrasound instrument. Reduced spermatogenic efficiency produces this inconsistency. As with testicular hypoplasia, libido and semen volume may be normal.

Testicular biopsy can be used to substantiate the presence of testicular degeneration or hypoplasia. However, to obtain sufficient testicular parenchyma for adequate histologic evaluation, wedge biopsies are preferred, using open surgical excision techniques are preferred. Removal of this amount of parenchyma often results in considerable hemorrhage and attendant pressure-induced degeneration and necrosis.[88] Decrease in sperm counts and formation of antisperm antibodies are among the reported complications in men.[89] There has been a recent resurgence of interest in using aspiration cytology or needle biopsies for obtaining testicular parenchyma for histologic evaluation.[90] While these techniques may seem more appealing than open excision for obtaining biopsies, they are discouraged in men because results obtained may not be representative and testicular damage may go unnoticed.[89] More investigation is required before testicular biopsy can be recommended as a routine method for diagnosing testicular degeneration/hypoplasia in-stallions. Nonetheless, histologic evaluation of testicular tissue can confirm testicular degeneration or hypoplasia, especially if the testis is uniformly affected. It is important to remember that testicular degeneration and testicular hypoplasia are virtually indistinguishable on physical examination, semen examination and histologic evaluation of testicular architecture. One possible exception is that on histologic examination the basement membrane of collapsed seminiferous tubules buckles more with testicular degeneration than with testicular hypoplasia.[37]

Unlike testicular hypoplasia, testicular degeneration may be reversible. Treatment is directed at removing the factor(s) responsible for inducing the degenerative changes. These measures might include correcting fever associated with an upper respiratory infection, discontinuing exogenous anabolic steroid medication or eliminating scrotal edema. Treatment with gonadotropin-releasing hormone (GnRH) has reportedly improved semen quality in aged stallions with suspected testicular degeneration.

The efficacy of GnRH therapy is not documented, but this approach is worthy of intensified study. Improvement in fertility has been noted in men with hypogonadotropic hypogonadism following GnRH therapy, but results are inconsistent.[92]

Replacement therapy with GnRH is likely to be of most benefit in stallions with hypogonadotropic hypogonadism in stallions (suggesting a defect originating from the hypothalamic-pituitary axis) rather than stallions with elevated follicle-stimulating hormone (FSH) concentrations (suggesting damage originating within the seminiferous epithelium).[91] Low concentrations of luteinizing hormone (LH) or FSH in the peripheral plasma are used as the criterion for diagnosing hypogonadotropic hypogonadism in men.[93] High FSH concentrations, associated with damage to the seminiferous epithelium, apprars to be relatively common in aged (>20 years) stallions with declining fertility.[94]

The optimal dosage schedule for GnRH remains to be determined. In men, the dosage and frequency of administration must mimic physiologic pulsatile release characteristics to avoid desensitizing the pituitary gland.[95] One report indicated that exogenous GnRH given to reproductively sound or unsound stallions by pulsatile (10 μg GnRH every 2 hours SC via peristaltic pump) or continuous (5 μg via osmotic pump implanted SC) injection did not increase serum testosterone levels or improve sperm output.[96] Continuous use of a potent GnRH analogue suppresses secretion of gonadotropins and testosterone in stallions.[97]

Periodic measurements of testicular size and consistency and serial (monthly) evaluations of semen quality aid evaluation of testicular improvement/deterioration. In cases of temporary testicular degeneration, complete restoration of normal spermatogenic function takes several months after removal of the causative factor. In many instances, the preinjury level of spermatogenic activity is never fully recovered.

References

1. Parks AH *et al:* Monorchidism in the horse. *Equine Vet J* 21:215-217, 1989.

2. George FW and Griffin JE, in Santen RJ and Swerdloff RS: *Male Reproductive Dysfunction*. Marcel Dekker, New York, 1986. pp 127-142.

3. Johnson CA: Role of the fetal testis in sexual differentiation. *Compend Cont Ed Pract Vet* 5:129-132, 1983.

4. Johnson BD *et al:* A horse with one kidney, partially obstructed ureter and contralateral urogenital anomalies. *JAVMA* 169:217-219, 1976.

5. Bishop MWH *et al:* Some observations on cryptorchidism in the horse. *Vet Record* 76:1041-1048, 1964.

6. Arthur GH: The surgery of the equine cryptorchid.*Vet Record* 73:385-389, 1961.

7. Technical Development Committee: Cryptorchidism with special reference to the condition in the dog.*Vet Record* 66:482-483, 1954.

8. Genetzky RM *et al:* Equine cryptorchidism: pathogenesis, diagnosis, and treatment. *Compend Cont Ed Pract Vet* 6:S577-S582, 1984.

9. Hayes HM: Epidemiological features of 5009 cases of equine cryptorchidism. *Equine Vet J* 18:467-471, 1986.

10. Gier HT and Marion GB: Development of mammalian testes and genital ducts. *Biol Reprod (Suppl 1)* 1:1-23, 1969.

11. Bergin WC *et al:* A developmental concept of equine cryptorchidism. *Biol Reprod* 3:82-92, 1970.

12. Smith JA: The development and descent of the testes in the horse. *Vet Annual* 15:156-161, 1975.

13. Leipold HW *et al:* Cryptorchidism in the horse. *Proc Ann Mtg AAEP*, 1986. pp 579-589.

14. Kieffer NM and Webb G: Unpublished data, 1986.

15. de Grouchy J and Turleau C:*Clinical Atlas of Human Chromosomes.* 2nd ed. John Wiley & Sons, New York, 1984. pp 2-369.

16. Kieffer NM: Personal communication, 1987.

17. Stickle RL and Fessler JF: Retrospective study of 350 cases of equine cryptorchidism. *JAVMA* 172: 343-346, 1978.

18. Coryn M *et al:* Clinical, morphological and endocrinological aspects of cryptorchidism in the horse. *Theriogenology* 16:489-496, 1981.

19. Cox JE *et al:* An analysis of 500 cases of equine cryptorchidism. *Equine Vet J* 11:113-116, 1979.

20. Wright JG: The surgery of the inguinal canal in animals. *Vet Record* 75:1352-1363, 1963.

21. Trotter GW and Aanes WA: A complication of cryptorchid castration in three horses. *JAVMA* 178: 246-248, 1981.

22. Walker DF and Vaughan JT: *Bovine and Equine Urogenital Surgery.* Lea & Febiger, Philadelphia, 1980. pp 105-182.

23. O'Connor JP: Rectal examination of the cryptorchid horse. *Irish Vet J* 25:129-131, 1971.

24. Jann HW and Rains JR: Diagnostic ultrasonography of evaluation of cryptorchidism in horses. *JAVMA* 196:297-300, 1990.

25. Cox JE: Experiences with a diagnostic test for equine cryptorchidism. *Equine Vet J*:179-183, 1975.

26. Cox JE *et al:* Comparison of the measurement of plasma testosterone and plasma oestrogens for the diagnosis of cryptorchidism in the horse. *Equine Vet J* 18:179-182, 1986.

27. Arighi M and Bosu TK: Comparison of hormonal methods for diagnosis of cryptorchidism in horses. *J Equine Vet Sci* 9:20-26, 1989.

28. Silberzahn P *et al:* Testosterone response to human chorionic gonadotropin injection in the stallion. *Equine Vet J* 20:61-63, 1988.

29. Ganjam VK and Kenney RM: Androgens and oestrogens in normal and cryptorchid stallions. *J Reprod Fertil* 23:67-73, 1975.

30. Valdez H *et al:* Abdominal cryptorchidectomy in the horse using inguinal extension of the gubernaculum testes. *JAVMA* 174:1110-1112, 1979.

31. Cox JE *et al:* Suprapubic paramedian laparotomy for equine abdominal cryptorchidism.*Vet Record* 97:428-432, 1975.

32. Lowe JE and Higginbotham R: Castration of abdominal cryptorchid horses by a paramedian laparotomy approach. *Cornell Vet* 59:121-126, 1969.

33. Moore JN *et al:* Equine cryptorchidism: pre-surgical considerations and surgical management. *Vet Surgery* 7:43-47, 1978.

34. Wilson DG and Reinertson EL: A modified parainguinal approach for cryptorchidectomy in horses. An evaluation in 107 horses. *Vet Surg* 16:1-4, 1987.

35. Howards SS, in Walsh PC *et al: Campbell's Urology.* 5th ed. Saunders, Philadelphia, 1986. pp 2955-2975.

36. Jeffrey RB *et al:* Sonography of testicular trauma. *Am J Roentgenology* 141:993-995, 1983.

37. Ladds PW, in Jubb KVF *et al: Pathology of Domestic Animals.* 3rd ed. Vol 3. Academic Press, New York, 1985. pp 409-459.

38. McEntee K, in Jubb KVF and Kennedy PC: *Pathology of Domestic Animals.* 3rd ed. Vol 1. Academic Press, New York, 1970. pp 443-481.

39. Smith, JA: The occurrence of larvae of *Strongylus edentatus* in the testicles of stallions. *Vet Record* 93:604-606, 1973.

40. Gribble DH: Equine ehrlichiosis. *JAVMA* 155:462-469, 1969.

41. Setchell BP: The functional significance of the blood-testis barrier. *J Androl* 1:3-7, 1980.

42. Schanbacher BD and Amann RP: Physiology of male reproduction. *J Anim Sci* (Suppl 2) 57:380-403, 1983.

43. Boyle M: Immune related infertility in stallions? *Equine Vet J* 22:67-69, 1990.

44. Haas GG Jr: Antibody-mediated causes of male infertility. *Urol Clin No Am* 14:539-550, 1987.

45. Zhang J *et al:* Antisperm antibodies in the semen of a stallion following testicular trauma. *Equine Vet J* 22:138- 141, 1990.

46. Papa FO *et al:* Infertility of autoimmune origin in a stallion. *Equine Vet J* 22:145-146, 1990.

47. Blanchard TL: Some effects of anabolic steroids - especially on stallions. *Compend Cont Ed Pract Vet* 7:S372-S380, 1985.

48. Garcia MC *et al:* The effects of stanozolol and boldenone undecylenate on plasma testosterone and gonadotropins and on testis hystology in pony stallions. *Theriogenology* 28:109- 119, 1987.

49. Squires EL *et al:* Effect of anabolic steroids on reproductive function of young stallions. *J Anim Sci* 54:576-582, 1982.

50. Blanchard TL *et al:* The effects of stanozolol and boldenone undecylenate on scrotal width, testis weight, and sperm production in pony stallions. *Theriogenology* 20:121-131, 1983.

51. Berndtson WE: Steroids to enhance growth and performance: effects on fertility. *Equine Pract* 8(3):27-30, 1986.

52. Squires EL *et al:* Restoration of reproductive capacity of stallions after suppression with exogenous testosterone. *J Anim Sci* 53:1351-1359, 1981.

53. Koskinen E *et al:* Effect of anabolic steroids on testes of colts. *Proc Intl Symp Equine Reprod,* 1990. pp 230-231.

54. Morse MJ and Whitmore WF, in Walsh PC *et al. Campbell's Urology.* 5th ed. Saunders, Philadelphia, 1986. pp 1535-1575.

55. Peterson DE: Equine testicular tumors. *J Equine Vet Sci* 4:25-27, 1984.

56. Rajfer J, in Walsh PC *et al: Campbell's Urology.* 5th ed. Saunders, Philadelphia, 1986. pp 1947-1968.

57. Becht JL *et al:* Malignant seminoma in a stallion. *JAVMA* 175:292-293, 1979.

58. Vaillancourt D *et al:* Seminoma in the horse: report of two cases. *J Equine Med Surg* 3:213-218, 1979.

59. Metastatic equine seminoma: report of two cases. *Vet Pathol* 21:259-260, 1984.

60. Caron JP *et al:* Equine testicular neoplasia. *Compend Cont Ed Pract Vet* 7:S53-S62, 1985.

61. Smith BL *et al:* Malignant seminoma in a cryptorchid stallion. *JAVMA* 195:775-776, 1989.

62. Stick JA: Teratoma and cyst formation of the equine cryptorchid testicle. *JAVMA* 176:211-214, 1980.

63. Nachtsheim DA *et al:* Ultrasonography of testis tumors. *J Urol* 129:978-981, 1983.

64. Leopold GR *et al:* High resolution ultrasonography of scrotal pathology. *Radiol* 131:719-722, 1979.

65. Schummer A *et al: The Circulatory System, the Skin, and the Cutaneous Organs of the Domestic Mammals.* Paul Parey, Berlin, 1981. pp 410-440.

66. Knudsen O and Chantz B: Seminoma in the stallion: A clinical, cytological and pathologico-anatomical investigation. *Cornell Vet* 53:395-403, 1963.

67. Barton C: Personal communication, 1989.

68. Javadpour N, in Talerman A and Roth LM: *Pathology of the Testis and Its Adnexa.* Churchill Livingstone, New York, 1986. pp 221-230.

69. Hoagland TA *et al:* Effects of unilateral castration on morphological characteristics of the testis in one-, two-, and three-year-old stallions. *Theriogenology* 26:397-405, 1986.

70. Moulton JE: *Tumors of Domestic Animals.* Univ of California Press, Berkeley, 1978. pp 309-320.

71. Smith HA *et al: Veterinary Pathology.* 4th ed. Lea & Febiger, Philadelphia, 1972. pp 190-298.

72. Smyth GB: Testicular teratoma in an equine cryptorchid. *Equine Vet J* 11:21-23, 1979.

73. Parks AH *et al:* Partial obstruction of the small colon associated with an abdominal testicular teratoma in a foal. *Equine Vet J* 18:342-343, 1986.

74. Willis RA and Rudduck: Testicular teratomas in horses. *J Path Bact* 55:165-171, 1943.

75. Valentine BA and Weinstock D: Metastatic testicular embryonal carcinoma in a horse. *Vet Pathol* 23:9296, 1986.

76. Shaw DP and Roth JE: Testicular teratocarcinoma in a horse. *Vet Pathol* 23:327-328, 1986.

77. Smith HA: Interstitial cell tumor of the equine testis. *JAVMA* 174:356-358, 1954.

78. Rahaley RS *et al:* Sertoli cell tumour in a horse. *Equine Vet J* 15:68-70, 1983.

79. Roberts SJ: *Veterinary Obstetrics and Genital Diseases.* David & Charles, North Pomfret, VT, 1986. pp 752-893.

80. Woods GL *et al:* Variations in testicular size of Standardbred stallions. *Proc Ann Mtg AAEP,* 1980. pp 117-121.

81. Nishikawa Y and Horie T: Studies on the development of the testes and epididymides of the horse. 1. Studies on the development of the testes of the horse, with special reference to singularity and the age of sexual maturity. *Natl Inst Agric Sci Jpn Bull Ser G Anim Husb* 10:229-349, 1955.

82. Johnson L and Thompson DL: Age-related and seasonal variation in the Sertoli cell population, daily sperm production and serum concentrations of follicle-stimulating hormone, luteinizing hormone and testosterone in stallions. *Biol Reprod* 29:777-789, 1983.

83. Johnson L *et al:* Establishment of adult levels of spermatogenesis in the horse. *J Reprod Fertil* (Submitted for publication, 1990).

84. Naden J *et al:* Testicular growth, hormone concentration, seminal characteristics and sexual behavior in stallions. *J Reprod Fertil* 88:167-176, 1990.

85. Amann RP: A review of anatomy and physiology of the stallion. *J Equine Vet Sci* 1:83-105, 1981.

86. Veeramachaneni DNR *et al:* Pathophysiology of small testes in beef bulls: relationship between scrotal circumference, histologic features of testes and epididymides, seminal characteristics, and endocrine profiles. *Am J Vet Res* 47:1988-1999, 1986.

87. Paoletti M and Straus FH: *Pathology of the Testis and its Adnexa.* Churchill Livingstone, New York, 1986. pp 243-255.

88. Kenney RM: Personal communication, 1980.

89. Glezerman M, in Bandhauer K and Frick J: *Disturbances in Male Fertility.* Springer-Verlag, New York, 1982. pp 215-223.

90. Threlfall WR and Lopate C: Testicular biopsy. *Proc Ann Mtg Soc Theriogenol,* 1987. pp 65-73.

91. Douglas, RH: Personal communication, 1987, 1990.

92. Sigman M and Vance ML: *Male Infertility. Urol Clin No Am* 14:459-469, 1987.

93. McClure RD: Male Infertility. *Urol Clin No Am* 14:471-488, 1987.

94. Burns PJ and Douglas RH: Reproductive hormone concentrations in stallions with breeding problems: case studies. *J Equine Vet Sci* 5:40-42, 1985.

95. Spratt DI *et al,* in Santen RJ and Swerdloff RS: *Male Reproductive Dysfunction: Diagnosis and Management of Hypogonadism, Infertility and Impotence.* Marcel Dekker, New York, 1986. pp 227-249.

96. Squires EL *et al:* Effect of pulsatile and continuous administration of GnRH on reproductive function of stallions. *Proc Intl Symp Equine Reprod,* 1990. pp 60-61.

97. Boyle MS: The effects of continuous treatment of stallions with high levels of a potent GnRH analogue. *Proc Intl Symp Equine Reprod,* 1990. pp 64-65.

9

Diseases of the Epididymis

Congenital and Familial Diseases

Epididymal Aplasia

Epididymal aplasia is rare in stallions. Segmental aplasia of the epididymis (unilateral aplasia of the cauda epididymis) has been described in horses.[1] Cases of complete epididymal aplasia have been unilateral and associated with testicular agenesis.[2] Other portions of the mesonephric duct, such as the vesicular gland, ampulla or deferent duct, also may be absent, as may the ipsilateral kidney. There is no treatment for epididymal aplasia. Hereditary predisposition is suspected in bulls.[3]

Epididymal Cysts

Cysts can develop in blind vestiges of the extratesticular rete tubules (blind efferent ductules) or mesonephric tubules (aberrant ductules), the blind cranial portion of each mesonephric duct (appendix of the epididymis), or detached segments of the meso nephric tubules (paradidymis).[1] Because the lumina of these channels are lined with secretory epithelium, the potential for cystic dilation exists. Epididymal cysts are uncommon in stallions. Uncomplicated cystic dilations usually do not interfere with epididymal transit of spermatozoa. Large epididymal cysts are clinically detectable as circumscribed fluctuant masses near the caput epididymis, at the craniodorsal aspect of the testicle. These structures can become very large, with the largest reported cyst measuring 7.5 cm in diameter.[4]

Blind efferent ductules, aberrant ductules, and appendices of the epididymis communicate with the lumen of the epididymal duct. Therefore, these remnants can become impacted with spermatozoa, leading to local sperm granuloma formation (see Sperm Granulomas).

Diseases with Physical Causes

Epididymal Lacerations

Though rare, epididymal lacerations can result from severe trauma to the scrotum, even if the insult is nonpenetrating. Epididymal lacerations caused by nonpenetrating scrotal trauma are very difficult to diagnose by noninvasive methods because the attendant scrotal edema and hemorrhage prevent close examination of the scrotal contents by palpation or ultrasound. If the lacerated epididymis is not removed surgically, extravasated spermatozoa probably will produce a granulomatous reaction. This becomes clinically recognizable when scrotal swelling associated with the scrotal injury has subsided. Because the affected epididymis no longer is functional as an organ of sperm transport, the most reasonable treatment is unilateral castration, including removal of the epididymis.

Thermal Injury

Local temperature elevation impairs epididymal spermatozoa as well as spermatogenesis.[5,6] The mechanism of action is unknown. Causes and management of thermally injured scrotal contents are discussed in Chapters 7 and 8.

Torsion of the Spermatic Cord

Protracted torsion of the spermatic cord interferes with the vascular supply to tissues distal to the stricture (including the epididymides and testes), causing ischemic necrosis. Chapter 11 contains a discussion of spermatic-cord torsion.

Inflammatory, Infectious and Immune Diseases

Infectious Epididymitis

Infectious epididymitis of stallions rarely occurs as a primary entity. In men, infectious epididymitis usually is secondary to infections of the urinary tract or accessory genital glands by retrograde dissemination through the deferent ducts. This route of epididymal infection is also possible in the stallion but has not been documented. More commonly, infectious epididymitis is thought to be secondary to, or associated with, concurrent orchitis, either of hematogenous origin or through local invasion via the inguinal canal or scrotal perforation. The tail of the epididymis is most commonly involved, but the head and body may also be affected. The causative agents and mechanisms of dissemination are thought to be similar to those described for bacterial orchitis (Chapter 9). Parasitic migration of *Strongylus edentatus* larvae through the epididymis can also cause epididymitis, occasionally resulting in formation of granulomas.[4,7]

Acute epididymitis results in severe pain with local swelling and edema, usually in conjunction with fever. Acute epididymitis may progress to more chronic forms with abscessation, periorchitis and fibrosis. Sperm granulomas develop if the epididymal basement membrane ruptures, due to extravassation of antigenic spermatozoa. Adhesions may form between the epididymis and its associated tunics.

Diagnosis of epididymitis is based on clinical signs, including pain elicited by palpation of the epididymis(es), change in epididymal shape, texture and size (Figs 1, 2), and detection of adhesions between the epididymis and surrounding tissues. In acute cases, involved portions of the epididymis are painful, soft and fluctuant if abscessation has occurred (Fig 3). Chronicity leads to deposition of connective tissue and hardening of the affected areas. Pain may partially or completely subside. Af-

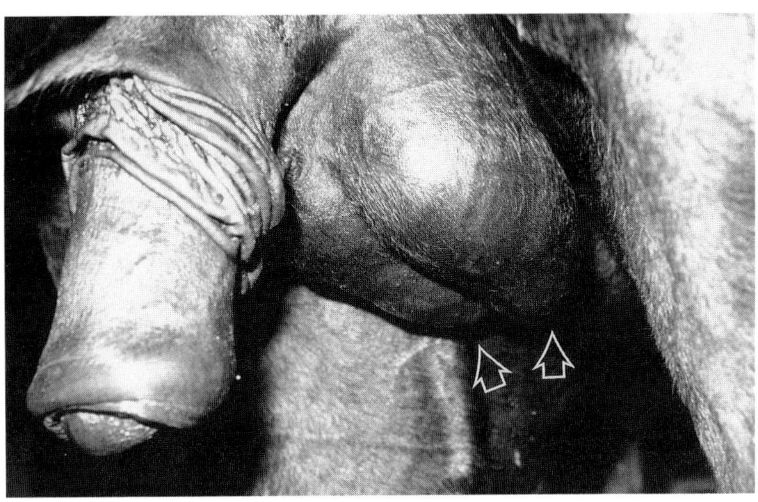

Figure 1. Enlarged cauda epididymides of a stallion with bilateral epididymitis.

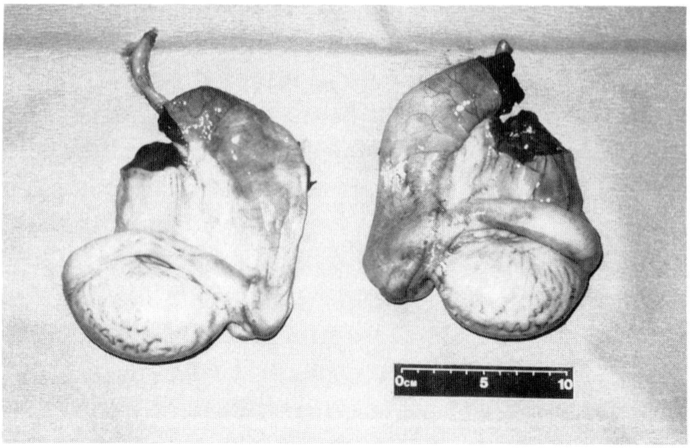

Figure 2. Enlarged and indurated epididymides of a stallion with bilateral epididymitis.

fected stallions may be reluctant to breed and exhibit pain during ejaculation. Inflammatory cells are usually abundant in ejaculates, and spermatozoa are few and morphologically defective (Fig 4). Bacteriologic culture of semen may help identify infectious causes of epididymitis. Obstructions may be present that prevent passage of spermatozoa through the epididymis, thereby precluding collection of semen.

Treatment alternatives are similar to those for infectious orchitis (Chapter 9). In cases of moderate or severe epididymitis, the prognosis for recovery is poor. Obstructions and granulomas usually develop, resulting in sterility. In unilateral cases, removal of the testis, epididymis and spermatic cord on the af-

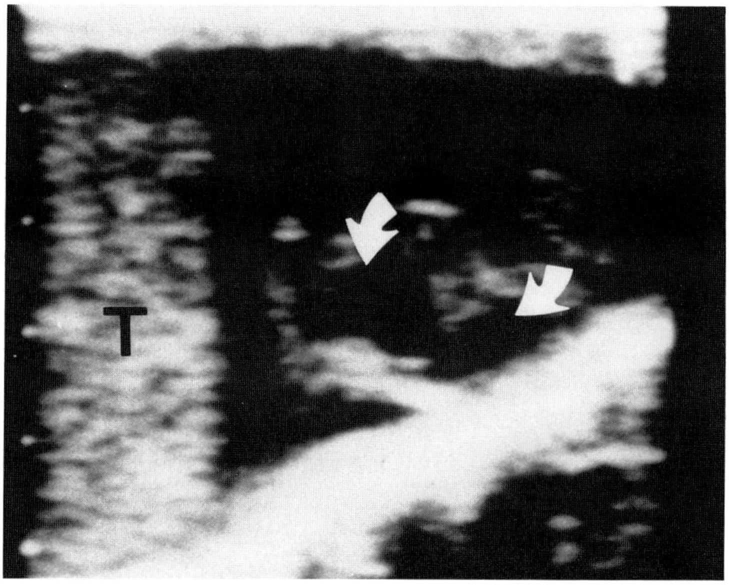

Figure 3. Ultrasonic image of cystic dilatations (arrows) within the cauda epididymidis of a stallion with epididymitis. The cystic areas contained purulent material. Testis (T).

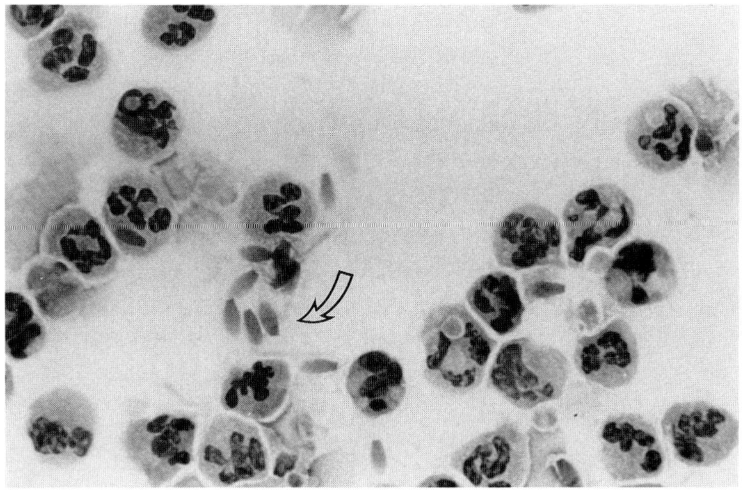

Figure 4. Semen from a stallion with epididymitis, containing numerous neutrophils and scant, defective spermatozoa.

fected side only may salvage a stallion for breeding. Sequential followup examinations and semen cultures are indicated to ensure that spread to remaining reproductive organs has not occurred.

Traumatic Epididymitis

Specific trauma to the epididymis can accompany nonpenetrating scrotal injury. Acute epididymitis is characterized by local pain and swelling. Clinical signs, however, often are masked by the diffuse scrotal edema and discomfort attending scrotal trauma. Sperm granulomas can arise as secondary features of traumatic epididymitis. Modes of treatment are similar to those described for infectious orchitis.

Sperm Granulomas

The antigens of spermatozoa elicit a characteristic granulomatous reaction if spermatozoa escape the seminiferous tubule or excurrent duct luminae and contact the stromal tissue.[1,3,4] Epididymal sperm granulomas are infrequent in stallions, and underlying causes are quite varied. Parasitic migration (*Strongylus edentatus*) is considered a major mediator of sperm granulomas by releasing spermatozoa from the epididymal lumen.[7] Bacterial or traumatic epididymitis also may predispose the basement membrane of the epididymis to violation by spermatozoa. Extravasation of sperm is obvious in cases of epididymal lacerations. Epididymal adenomyosis, an outgrowth of the epithelial lining into the epididymal musculature, has been described in stallions. Sperm granulomas can develop if spermatozoa become embedded within this diverticulum.[4,7] Similarly, impaction of blind efferent ductules, aberrant ductules or the appendix of the epididymis with spermatozoa can lead to formation of sperm granulomas.[1]

In the acute phase, sperm granulomas exist as locally painful swellings but become indurated, painless masses with time. Obliteration of the epididymal lumen can occur subsequent to granuloma formation, obstructing transit of spermatozoa. If sperm blockage has occurred, it probably will be permanent. There is no effective treatment for this condition.

Idiopathic Diseases

Spermiostasis

Spermatozoal transit time through the cauda epididymis varies from 7 to 10 days in stallions, depending on frequency of ejaculation (see Chapter 1).[5,8] Under normal circumstances, spermatozoa probably are not stored in the cauda epididymis for prolonged periods. If they are not removed by ejaculation through mating or masturbation, they are thought to be emitted intermittently from the cauda epididymides (and deferent ducts) into the pelvic urethra and voided during micturition. However, studies involving other species have indicated that spermatozoa may remain viable for several weeks within cauda epididymides. Phagocytosis and resorption are insignificant means of spermatozoal removal from the epididymal lumen.

Some stallions have an impaired ability to emit epididymal and deferent ductal spermatozoa spontaneously, even though they may ejaculate normally. As a result, spermatozoa accumulate abnormally in the epididymis and deferent ducts during sexual rest. Retained spermatozoa undergo degenerative changes, as evidenced by reduction of spermatozoal motility and morphologically normal spermatozoa in ejaculated semen. Typically, a high incidence of spermatozoal head-tail separations (60-80%) is seen in the ejaculates of these stallions. Semen samples have an irregularly high spermatozoal concentration (*eg,* 500-1800 million spermatozoa/ml) and normal volume, resulting in an abnormally high ejaculate sperm number (*eg,* 35-60 billion spermatozoa). Degenerating spermatozoa may be ejaculated in clumps or "casts." Sheets of epithelial cells lining the lumina of the cauda epididymides and deferent ducts also occasionally shed in ejaculates.

Spermatozoa occasionally become impacted within the epididymal/deferent duct lumina to the point that they are not even released by the strong muscular contractions of the ducts at the time of ejaculation. Serial ejaculations usually are required to restore normal semen quality in these stallions. Collection of 10-20 ejaculates over a 1- to 2-week period may be required to correct the problem. Relapse is likely if an affected stallion does not ejaculate regularly (2-3 times weekly). An attempt should be made to determine the frequency of semen collection necessary to maintain maximum semen quality. Semen should then be collected on this schedule, even if mares are not available for breeding. Spermiostasis that results in azoospermia may require an alternative therapeutic approach (see Chapter 16). The underlying cause of spermiostasis is unknown. We are currently investigating the effectiveness of pharmacologic agents (*eg*, beta-adrenergic blockers) in correcting spermiostasis.

Multifactorial Diseases

Generalized Epididymal Dysfunction

The epididymis does not serve simply as a conduit and storage depot for spermatozoa. Spermatozoa leaving the testis are immotile and incapable of fertilizing ova. During epididymal transit, spermatozoa undergo a maturational sequence, characterized by structural, physiologic and biochemical changes, to assume normal progressive motility and fertilizing capacity (see Chapter 1). The specific role the epididymis plays in this maturational process is poorly understood. Unique resorptive and secretory functions of the epididymal epithelium are thought to create a special milieu within the epididymal lumen that is responsible for proper spermatozoal maturation. Apparently these maturational changes occur in the caput and corpus segments of the epididymis. The cauda epididymis is required only for continued spermatozoal transit, storage of spermatozoa, and spermatozoal emission into the attached deferent duct. The biochemical composition of epididymal fluid and epithelial morphology is not constant along the length of the epididymal duct; rather, regional variations exist and are considered critical to normal maturation of spermatozoa.[6,9,10]

Little is known about epididymal function, but it is conceivable that a clinically inapparent disruption in epididymal function could prevent spermatozoa from becoming fully functional. Alterations in the epididymal epithelium might result from a

of the tunica vaginalis commonly produces adhesions between its visceral and parietal layers. Dense fibrous adhesions also may develop between the parietal layer of the tunica vaginalis and surrounding loose scrotal fascia. These sequelae to acute inflammation restrict mobility of the testis within the scrotum. Chronic (fibrous) periorchitis may permanently interfere with spermatogenesis by insulating the encapsulated testis (see Testicular Degeneration in Chapter 8).

Multifactorial Diseases

Hydrocele

Hydrocele refers to an abnormal collection of fluid between the visceral and parietal layers of the tunica vaginalis (within the vaginal cavity or space). Hydrocele can accompany inflammatory and noninflammatory types of scrotal edema. (See Chapter 7 for a discussion of scrotal edema.) Hydrocele also can arise without concurrent scrotal edema.

The vaginal cavity communicates with the peritoneal cavity, thereby permitting abdominal fluid to transfer into the vaginal cavity in some cases of ascites. Local lymphedema has been postulated to contribute to hydrocele also.[1] The fluid character is usually serous (a modified transudate with low cellularity), suggesting it may occur in response to trauma to the visceral or parietal vaginal tunics.[2] Uncomplicated hydroceles also can develop, acutely or insidiously, without an apparent cause.

Affected tunics usually are affected bilaterally, but unilateral hydroceles can occur. The condition may be temporary or permanent. Hydroceles can occur in hot weather, resolving in the fall of the year when the ambient temperature drops. We have observed hydrocele without coexistent scrotal edema in a stallion with suspected equine viral arteritis. Disruptions of the secretory/absorptive functions of the tunica vaginalis are thought to cause noninfectious primary hydrocele.

Initial diagnosis is based on palpation of the scrotal contents. A hydrocele feels like a large compressible fluid-filled bag. The scrotum is enlarged and generally not painful; however, greatly distended vaginal cavities can cause discomfort (Fig 1). The testis and epididymis may not be easily palpable but tend to remain freely movable within the scrotum. Ultrasonic examination reveals fluid of anechoic to semi-echoic character surrounding the involved testes and epididymides (Fig 2). Palpation per rectum rarely reveals the presence of enlarged vaginal rings, which would readily allow transfer of abdominal fluid into the vaginal space(s). Definitive diagnosis is based on aseptic needle aspiration of fluid from the vaginal cavity (Fig 3). The fluid content of each vaginal cavity may range from 10 ml to >1 L. If a surgical tap is performed to identify and drain the fluid

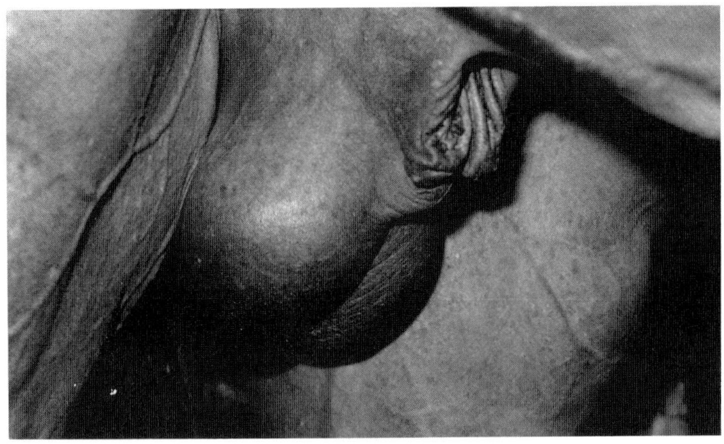

Figure 1. Bilateral hydrocele in a stallion. Note the diffuse enlargement of the exposed (right) scrotal pouch. The cauda epididymis in this pouch was difficult to palpate because of marked fluid accumulation within the vaginal space.

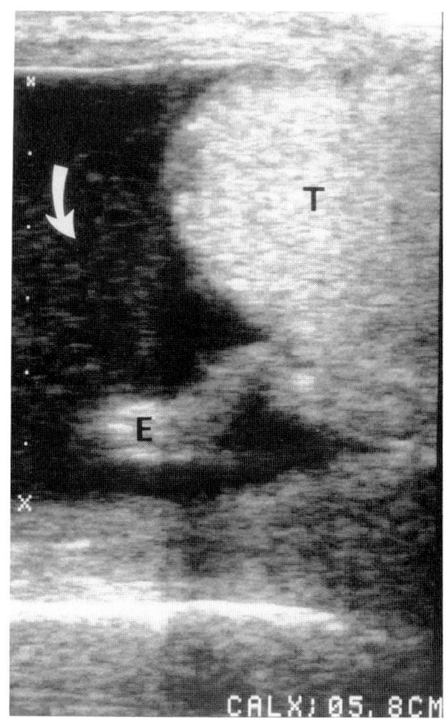

Figure 2. Ultrasonic image of the testis (T), cauda epididymidis (E) and vaginal space (arrow) in a stallion with a pronounced hydrocele.

Figure 3. Removing fluid from the vaginal space of a stallion's scrotum by needle aspiration. The skin overlying the aspiration site was first prepared for aseptic surgery.

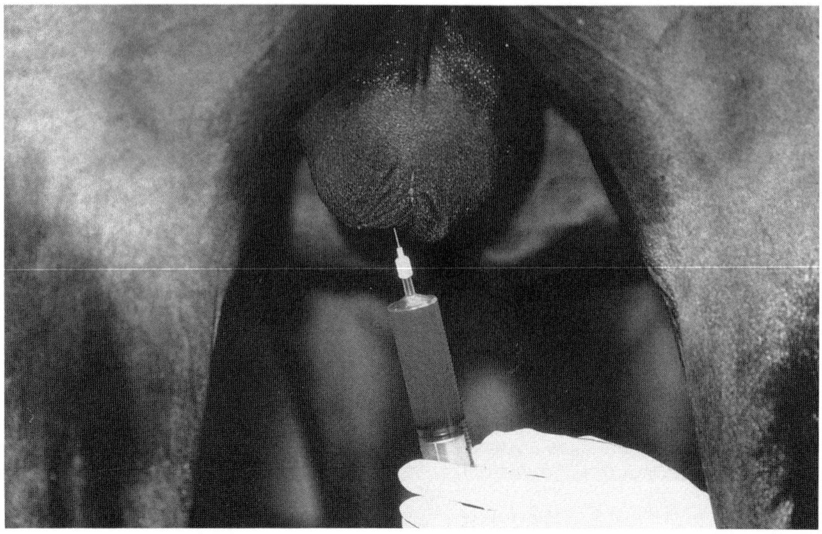

present, great care should be taken to maintain asepsis and to avoid penetration of the testis or epididymis.

Treatment is aimed at removing the underlying cause of the hydrocele, if it can be identified. Hydroceles associated with some underlying conditions (*eg,* infectious conditions or malnutrition) may take some time to resolve. Exercise may help control fluid accumulation is some cases, yet improvement may only be transient. Fluid usually reaccumulates when drained from the vaginal cavity by needle aspiration, unless an inciting factor for the hydrocele is identified and corrected.

While mild cases of hydrocele may not adversely affect fertility, accumulation of a significant volume of fluid causes heat-induced testicular degeneration with a resultant decline in semen quantity and quality.[1,3,4] If a persistent hydrocele is unilateral, surgical removal of the affected testis and surrounding tunics may prevent/correct thermal injury to the contralateral testis.[2]

Inguinal/Scrotal Herniation

An inguinal or scrotal hernia is a protrusion of abdominal viscera, usually small intestines, into the inguinal canal or scrotum. The hernia is inguinal if viscera extend only into the inguinal canal (*ie,* between the vaginal and external inguinal rings) and scrotal if viscera extend beyond the external inguinal ring and enter the scrotum.

The hernia may be direct if the viscera lie external to the vaginal cavity, or indirect if they lie within the vaginal cavity.[5] A direct inguinal or scrotal hernia occurs when the viscera protrude into the inguinal canal through a rent in the peritoneum and transversalis fascia adjacent to the vaginal ring.[6] An indirect inguinal or scrotal hernia occurs when the viscera protrude through the vaginal ring and into the inguinal canal. In domestic animals, the peritoneal and vaginal cavities normally communicate throughout life. In men they communicate only in abnormal instances. Because of this communication, inguinal or scrotal hernias of horses are predominantly indirect. Indirect hernias may rupture through the parietal tunic and lie partially outside the inguinal canal. These hernias are called ruptured inguinal hernias.

Inguinal/scrotal hernias in horses occur almost exclusively in intact males. Most are present at birth or develop soon after as a result of congenitally large vaginal rings.[7] They may be caused by excessive outgrowth of the extraabdominal part of the gubernaculum, which results in a vaginal process with an unusually wide neck.[8] The larger the ring, the greater the predisposition for herniation. The heritability of congenitally large vaginal rings has not been determined.[9] Inguinal or scrotal hernias also may develop following trauma, such as falls, and often are reported following breeding or exercise.[10] Acquired hernias may result from increased intraabdominal pressure and alteration of the architecture of the inguinal canal. In some horses the size of the vaginal ring appears to have no influence on development of the hernia.[11] A genetic predisposition to acquired inguinal or scrotal hernias has not been reported, but Standardbreds have a higher incidence than other breeds.[12]

Congenital hernias usually are of the scrotal type and appear soon after birth as a viscera-filled scrotum (Fig 4). The condition may be unilateral or bilateral. Congenital scrotal hernias can easily be reduced into the abdomen manually, and most show no tendency to incarcerate. The hernias often reduce spontaneously over 3-6 months. Intestines occasionally may become strangulated and require surgical reduction. Congenital inguinal hernias may become apparent only after castration, when the hernial contents eventrate through the scrotal incision. Congenital inguinal and scrotal hernias usually cause no problems; however, if the condition is longstanding, testicular hypoplasia/atrophy or adhesions between the testis, viscera and

Figure 4. Bilateral scrotal hernias of a newborn colt in dorsal recumbency. Note the bowel-filled scrotum.

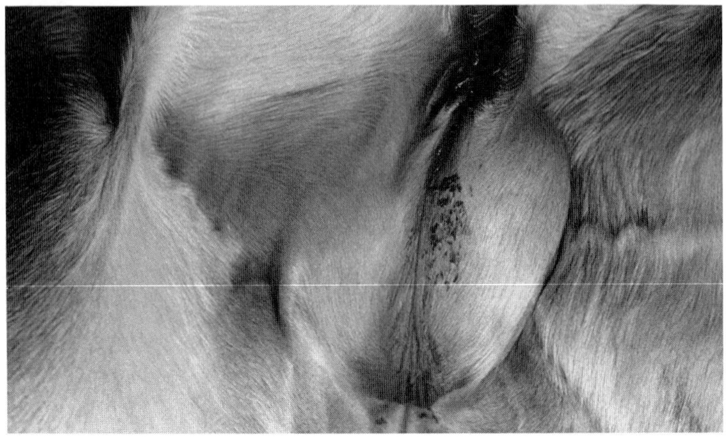

vaginal tunic may occur. In addition, the chance of intestinal incarceration is always present.

Treatment of congenital inguinal/scrotal hernias generally is not required. In the absence of abdominal pain or gross enlargement of the scrotum, only close observation of the colt is necessary. A most conservative form of therapy consists of manually reducing the herniated viscera manually several times daily. This maneuver also permits prompt diagnosis of intestinal incarceration, should it occur. Alternatively, a "foal diaper" can be used to correct persistent hernias. To apply this, the foal is sedated and placed in dorsal recumbency. The hernia is completely reduced, and the external inguinal rings are packed with cotton pledgets, which are covered by an elastic bandage applied in a figure-8 fashion over both inguinal rings (Figs 5, 6). Care should be taken to prevent occlusion of the anus or preputial orifice. Similarly, excessive pressure should not be applied to the penis where it courses ventral to the pelvis. The bandage can be left in place for up to a week. One bandage change may be required before hernia repair is complete. Once the bandage is applied, the external inguinal rings should be palpated intermittently under the bandage each day to ensure that herniation has not recurred.

Surgical intervention is indicated only as a last resort, particularly if a foal has a potential career as a breeding stallion, because castration usually accompanies herniorrhaphy surgery.

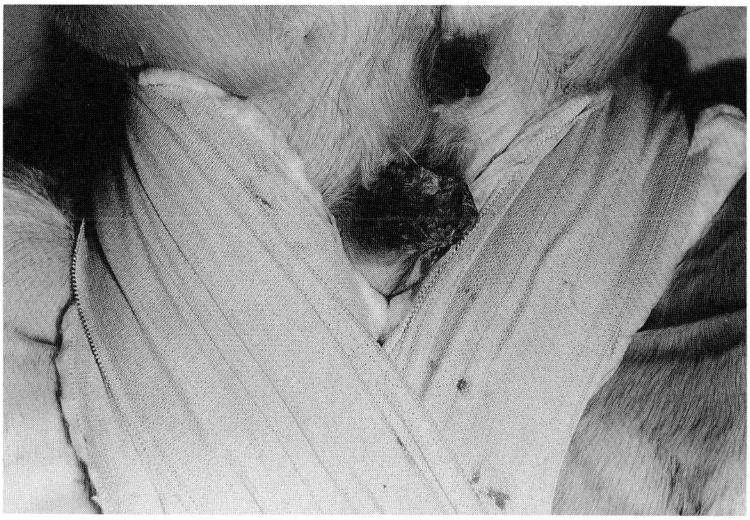

Figure 5. Application of a "diaper" in a foal to correct bilateral inguinal hernias (ventral view).

If an attempt is made to salvage the testes during herniorrhaphy, reherniation, testicular hypoplasia or even necrosis may result from compromised testicular blood supply. Obviously, surgical reduction is indicated if intestinal incarceration occurs. If the colt is to be castrated, a closed or modified-closed technique is used (see Chapter 5). The hernia is reduced, and the testis and attached spermatic cord are twisted to close the lumen of the vaginal cavity. The neck of the vaginal sac is ligated and transfixed to the superficial inguinal ring. The spermatic cord then is transected distal to the ligature with an emasculator. Even though only one inguinal canal may appear to be affected, the other testis should be removed in a similar fashion, as an inapparent hernia may exist in the other canal.

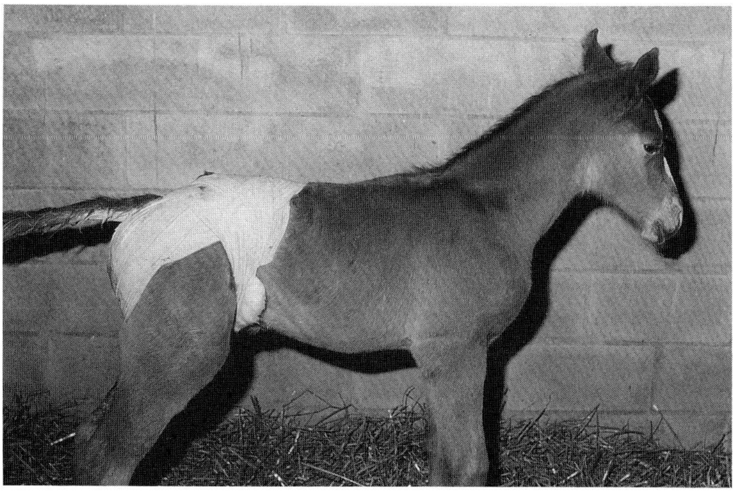

Figure 6. "Diaper" applied to a foal to correct bilateral inguinal hernias.

Acquired inguinal/scrotal hernias occur most commonly in adult horses and usually are attended by signs of acute abdominal pain. The possibility of an acquired inguinal or scrotal hernia always should be considered in stallions exhibiting abdominal pain. In most horses, the scrotum on the affected side is enlarged, and the herniated viscera are incarcerated. If the hernia is inguinal, percutaneous palpation of the herniated viscera may not be possible, but if a rectal examination is performed, viscera are found entering the vaginal ring. Because the internal abdominal oblique muscle extends caudally beyond the vaginal ring, the vaginal process loops around the caudal edge of the muscle and lies in the inguinal canal between the belly of the internal abdominal oblique muscle and the fibrous tendon of the external abdominal oblique muscle. Strangulation of the hernial contents results from constriction of the vaginal ring and because the hernial contents must negotiate the S-shaped inguinal canal.

Most acquired inguinal or scrotal hernias require immediate treatment to avoid irreversible vascular damage to the hernial contents. Reduction of the hernia by external massage may be successful, particularly if the herniation has been diagnosed soon after the onset of clinical signs. To perform this task, the horse is sedated, then the scrotum and spermatic cord are massaged to reduce edema, while moderate downward traction is placed on the testicle with one hand to narrow and tense the vaginal cavity. The distal end of the entrapped viscera is "milked" proximally within the vaginal cavity with the other hand. The other hand prevents the viscera from slipping ventrally again and also provides continued ventral traction on the spermatic cord. The first hand is placed proximal to the second hand, and the process is repeated. The hands are alternated until the hernia is reduced.[10]

If reduction of the hernia by external massage fails, retraction of the entrapped viscera per rectum may be attempted. The horse should be sedated and the rectum relaxed by administration of epidural anesthesia. Alternatively, the stallion can be placed under general anesthesia and in lateral recumbency with the hindquarters raised. Visceral retraction per rectum then may be attempted in conjunction with external massage. Potential complications of this method include damage to the rectum or entrapped viscera. The likelihood of the hernia's recurrence after nonsurgical reduction depends upon the size and integrity of the vaginal ring. Nonsurgical reduction does not permit visual assessment of the hernial contents, so the horse should be observed carefully for several days after hernial reduction for signs of intestinal infarction. Collection and examination of peritoneal fluid may aid assessment of intestinal viability.

Surgical reduction of the hernia is indicated if manual reduction fails, if there is evidence of enlarged or damaged vaginal rings, or if infarction of the entrapped viscera is suspected (Fig 7). The horse is anesthetized and placed in dorsal recumbency, and the inguinal area and ventral midline are prepared for aseptic surgery. Depending on the size of the horse, an 8- to 14-cm skin incision is made over either the scrotum or external inguinal ring on the affected side. The incision is extended through the subcutaneous fascia to isolate the vaginal sac. The parietal tunic is incised longitudinally, using care not to incise the herniated viscera in the process. The incision is extended proximally to the external inguinal ring, exposing the spermatic cord and herniated viscera. If the viscera are viable, they are returned to the abdomen through the vaginal ring. To return the viscera to the abdominal cavity, it may be necessary to enlarge the vaginal ring at its cranial margin with scissors or a bistury. Intestine that has suffered irreversible vascular damage must be resected. Exteriorization of diseased intestine through the superficial inguinal ring may not be possible, especially if the ileum is involved. In this case, resection and anastomosis should be performed through a ventral midline celiotomy in the previously prepared site.

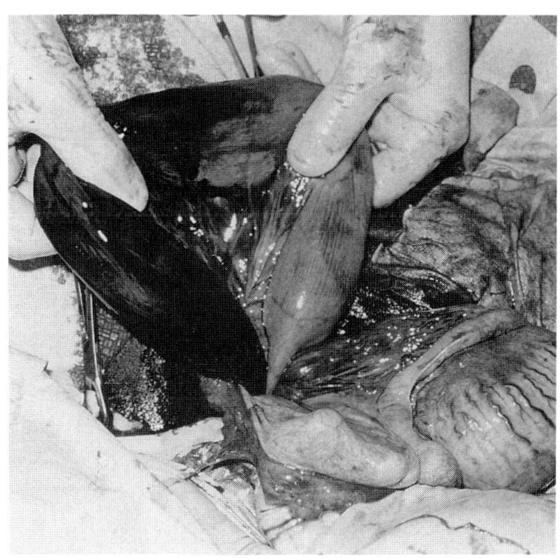

Figure 7. Surgical correction of a unilateral scrotal hernia in a stallion. Note the discoloration of the entrapped intestine. (Courtesy of Dr. T.S. Ford)

Traction on the viscera from inside the abdomen may aid reduction of incarcerated viscera. Twisting the testis and spermatic cord closes the lumen of the vaginal cavity, and the vaginal sac is ligated and transfixed to the external inguinal ring. After the spermatic cord is transected distal to the ligature with an emasculator, the external inguinal ring may be sutured for added assurance against reherniation. If the testis is viable and is to be saved, the caudal 2.5 cm of the superficial inguinal ring must remain unsutured. Usually the testis is removed, as salvage of the testis increases the risk of reherniation.

Most stallions remain fertile with only one testis. The inguinal fascia and skin can be left to heal as an open wound or sutured. The midline celiotomy incision is closed in a routine fashion. The testis on the unaffected side is removed if the horse is not to be used for breeding. Because the heritability of inguinal hernias is unknown, it can be argued that horses with this condition should not be used as sires in breeding programs.

References

1. Ladds PW, in Jubb KVF *et al: Pathology of Domestic Animals.* 3rd ed. Vol 3. Academic Press, New York, 1985. pp 409-459.

2. Hopkins SM *et al:* Unilateral castration as treatment for hydrocele in a bull. *JAVMA* 178:837-838, 1981.

3. McEntee K, in Jubb KVF and Kennedy PC: *Pathology of Domestic Animals*. 2nd ed. Vol 1. Academic Press, New York, 1970. pp 443-485.

4. Roberts SJ: *Veterinary Obstetrics and Genital Diseases.* David & Charles, North Pomfret, VT, 1986. pp 752-893.

5. Ashdown RR: The anatomy of the inguinal canal in the domesticated mammals. *Vet Record* 75:1345-1351, 1963.

6. Schneider RK *et al:* Acquired inguinal hernia in the horse: a review of 27 cases. *JAVMA* 180:317-320, 1982.

7. Wright JG: The surgery of the inguinal canal in animals. *Vet Record* 75:1352-1363, 1963.

8. Wensing CJG, in Hafez ESE: *Descended and Cryptorchid Testes*. Martinus Nijhoff, Boston, 1980. pp 125-137.

9. Hayes HM: Congenital umbilical and inguinal hernias in cattle, horses, swine, dogs, and cats: risk by breed and sex among hospital patients. *Am J Vet Res* 35:839-842, 1974.

10. Goetz TE *et al:* Inguinal and scrotal hernias in colts and stallions. *Compend Cont Ed Pract Vet* 3:S272-S276, 1981.

11. Schneider RK *et al:* Acquired inguinal hernia in the horse: a review of 27 cases. *JAVMA* 180:317-320, 1982.

12. Sembrat RF: The acute abdomen in the horse: epidemiologic considerations. *Vet Surgery* 4:34-38, 1975.

11

Diseases of the Spermatic Cord

Inflammatory, Infectious and Immune Diseases

Funiculitis

Funiculitis, or inflammation of the spermatic cord, generally occurs following castration but can follow trauma, parasite migration (*Strongylus edentatus* larvae), or generalized infections. Scirrhous cord and champignon refer to granulomatous and suppurative spermatic cord lesions, respectively. Funiculitis is discussed in the section entitled Postoperative Complications of Castration in Chapter 5.

Idiopathic Diseases

Torsion of the Spermatic Cord

Torsion of the spermatic cord refers to rotation or twisting of the spermatic cord about its longitudinal axis. Often the condition is inappropriately called testicular torsion. While only observed occasionally in stallions, it occurs more commonly than in males of other domestic species (except dogs), probably because the long axis of the testes is positioned horizontally in the equine scrotum. Torsions usually occur in descended testes, either unilaterally or bilaterally, and can be transient or permanent. Chronic recurring spermatic cord torsions are also possible. Most spermatic cord torsions in horses range from 180 to 360 degrees. Clinical signs depend on the severity of the torsion and the extent of circulatory disturbance.

In most instances, 180-degree torsions are subclinical and found incidentally during examination of the external genital organs (Fig 1). In such cases, the torsion is usually not associated with pain, and semen abnormalities are not present.[1] In some stallions, the torsion may only be transient, *ie,* repeated examinations reveal torsion to be present only occasionally.[2] Infrequently, stallions with a 180-degree torsion of the spermatic cord display mild intermittent scrotal pain that becomes most pronounced during athletic activity, such as racing. The consensus is that spermatic cord torsions up to 180 degrees do not produce local circulatory disturbances and so are considered of minor consequence. It is interesting to note, however, that experimental 180-degree spermatic cord torsion in rats resulted in a 36-44% decrease in arterial blood flow, with the greatest interference noted when the parietal tunic was involved in the torsion.[3] No experimental studies of spermatic cord torsion have been reported in horses. A 270-degree torsion of the spermatic cord was reported to result in preputial/scrotal edema in a stallion, even though scrotal pain was not evident.[4]

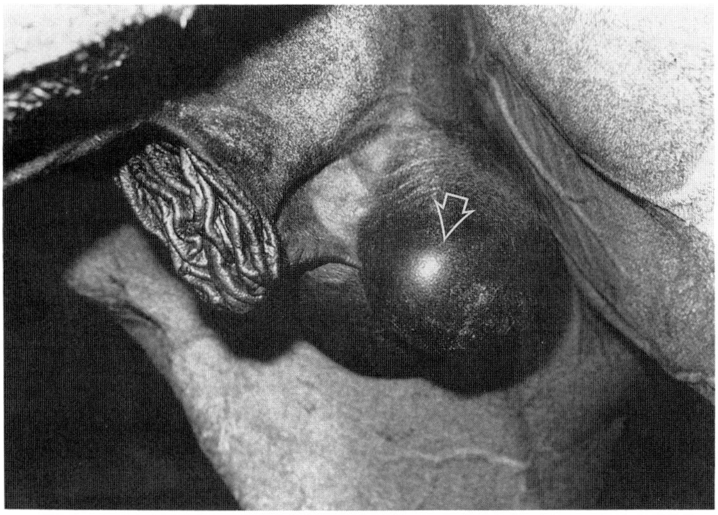

Figure 1. A 180-degree torsion of the left spermatic cord in a stallion. The prominent cauda epididymis of the affected side was directed cranially (arrow) rather than caudally. The condition was not associated with illness.

A 360-degree spermatic cord torsion generally causes acute severe scrotal pain and scrotal enlargement from local edema and hemorrhage. Unrelenting colic and a stilted gait may be evident. Typically this type of torsion is unilateral and permanent; however, temporary torsions are possible and result in recurrent attacks. A 360-degree spermatic cord torsion usually produces severe vascular compromise. Obstruction of the venous circulation (pampiniform plexus) leads to hemorrhagic infarctions and localized edema. Occlusion of the arterial supply results in ischemic necrosis of all ipsilateral scrotal contents distal to the torsion.[4,5]

Factors predisposing to spermatic cord torsion are poorly understood. Elongation of the caudal ligament of the epididymis or proper ligament of the testis and/or an excessively long mesorchium reportedly encourage spermatic cord torsion.[4,6] The relative frequency of intravaginal (excluding the parietal layer of the vaginal tunic) and extravaginal (including the parietal vaginal tunic) spermatic cord torsions has not been reported in horses.

Diagnosis of 180-degree torsion is relatively easy and based on identifying the location of the bulbous cauda epididymis and caudal ligament of the epididymis within the scrotum (Fig 1). The caudal ligament of the epididymis is a remnant of the gubernaculum testis. It typically remains as a small fibrous structure attached to the cauda epididymis, and is generally palpable through the scrotal wall, thereby serving as a landmark for identification of the cauda epididymis. Under normal circumstances, these structures are located at the caudal pole of the testis. Their presence in the cranial scrotum, with no attendant clinical signs, indicates a 180-degree torsion of the testis.

With a 360-degree torsion of the spermatic cord, the cauda epididymis and caudal ligament of the epididymis are palpated in their proper scrotal positions. Other clinical signs and the history suggest spermatic cord torsion.[4,6-8] Acute scrotal pain is detected in conjunction with unilateral scrotal enlargement and edema. The spermatic cord is thickened and firm, and the attached testis may be painful and enlarged. Both structures may be pulled dorsally in the scrotum. Palpation of scrotal contents becomes difficult as scrotal edema and swelling progress. A primary differential diagnosis for torsion of the spermatic cord is inguinal/scrotal herniation. Examination of the suspect vaginal ring by palpation per rectum helps differentiate these conditions, as viscera enter the inguinal canal with the latter condition. An edematous and painful vaginal ring, however, sometimes can be observed with spermatic cord torsion. Other diseases that may mimic spermatic cord torsion include scrotal trauma, orchitis/periorchitis, testicular neoplasia or hematoma, varicocele and thrombosis of spermatic cord vasculature.[4,5,9]

Treatment of 180-degree spermatic cord torsions generally is not necessary, as it rarely interferes with reproductive or athletic performance. If necessary, an orchiopexy can be performed.[4,10] With the horse under general anesthesia, a 3-cm skin incision is made in the scrotum over the intended site of the epididymal tail. The spermatic cord torsion is reduced manually, then a 2-cm incision is made in the parietal tunic. The proper ligament of the testis is exposed through the incision in the parietal tunic, then sutured to the adjacent tunica dartos with nonreactive, nonabsorbable suture material. The vaginal tunic and scrotal skin are closed routinely.[10]

A 360-degree spermatic cord torsion is considered a surgical emergency. Unilateral castration generally is recommended, as affected testes are rarely salvageable. The spermatic cord is ligated and transected proximal to the site of torsion. Removal of the opposite testis is advised if the horse is not to be used for breeding. Early diagnosis and treatment are imperative if the affected testis is to be saved. Studies of affected men indicate that permanent testicular atrophy is likely unless spermatic cord torsion is corrected within 4-10 hours of occurrence.[11,12]

Experimental evidence suggests that unilateral spermatic cord torsion can permanently damage the contralateral testis.[13,14] The supposed mechanism is immunologic, due to antibody formation to spermatozoa liberated from the ischemic testis. Owners of breeding stallions with severe unilateral torsion of the spermatic cord should be made aware of this potential sequela. Interestingly, a stallion was reported to have recurrent bilateral torsion of the spermatic cords. Unilateral castration was performed to correct a severe 360-degree torsion of one spermatic cord. At a later date, orchiopexy was performed to correct a 270-degree spermatic cord torsion on the other side. Season pregnancy rate in mares bred to this stallion the following year was excellent (>90%).[4]

Varicocele

The term varicocele describes abnormally distended and tortuous veins of the pampiniform plexus. This condition is a well-recognized cause of infertility of men and rams. Varicoceles are found infrequently during genital examination but their relationship to fertility has not been critically studied in the stallion. Varicoceles purportedly disturb the local thermoregulatory mechanism, causing increased intrascrotal temperature and subsequent spermatogenic dysfunction. We have detected unilateral varicosities in 2 stallions with normal spermatozoal quality and quantity.

Diagnosis is based on palpation of the characteristic "bag of worms" texture within the spermatic cord, created by the dilated tortuous vessels. In stallions, the condition usually is unilateral and nonpainful on palpation, and does not interfere with breeding performance. However, thrombosis of a varicocele has been reported in a horse.[5] The neck of the scrotum on the affected side may by wider than usual (Fig 2).

Treatment of varicoceles is discouraged in rams because of a possible hereditary predisposition for the disease.[15] Surgical removal of varicoceles (varicocelectomy) has improved semen quality and fertility of some men. Varicocelectomy has not been reported in the stallion. Thrombosis of a varicocele necessitates

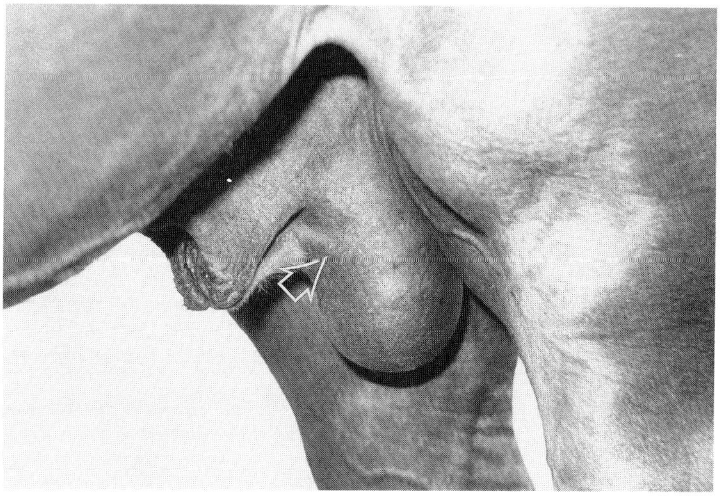

Figure 2. Varicocele of the left pampiniform plexus in a stallion, resulting in abnormal thickening of the scrotal neck (arrow) on the affected side.

unilateral castration, with transection of the spermatic cord proximal to the area of thrombosis.

Thrombosis of Spermatic Cord Vessels

Thrombosis of vessels within the spermatic cord is rare in stallions. Both the pampiniform plexus (venous circulation) and the testicular artery have been affected.[5,9] Only unilateral thrombosis has been reported. The causes of thrombus formation in spermatic cord vessels have not been established. It is possible that verminous migration in the vessel walls could lead to thrombosis. Previous spermatic cord torsion may predispose the vessels to thrombus formation. Clinical signs resemble those described for 360-degree torsion of the spermatic cord, as both conditions result in vascular obstruction. Definitive diagnosis is by surgical exploration. Unilateral castration is the only viable treatment. The spermatic cord should be transected above the site of the lesion.

References

1. Rossdale PD and Ricketts SW: *Equine Stud Farm Medicine.* 2nd ed. Lea & Febiger, Philadelphia, 1980. pp 120-164.

2. Kenney RM: Clinical evaluation of the stallion. *Proc Ann Mtg AAEP,* 1975. pp 336-355.

3. Janetschek G *et al:* Hemodynamic effects of experimental testicular torsion. *Urol Res* 15:303-306, 1987.

4. Threlfall WR *et al:* Recurrent torsion of the spermatic cord and scrotal testis in a stallion. *JAVMA* 196:1641-1643, 1990.

5. Ladds PW, in Jubb KVF *et al: Pathology of Domestic Animals.* 3rd ed. Vol 3. Academic Press, New York, 1985. pp 409-459.

6. Pascoe JR *et al:* Torsion of the spermatic cord in a horse. *JAVMA* 178:242-245, 1981.

7. Horney FD and Barker CAV: Torsion of the testicle in a Standardbred. *Am J Vet Res* 16:272-273, 1975.

8. Pezzoli G *et al:* Plastic operation of the testicular torsion in the horse. *Clin Vet* 102:533-535, 1979.

9. Horney FD and Milne FJ: Thrombosis of the spermatic artery resembling torsion of the spermatic cord in a stallion. *Can Vet J* 5:88-90, 1964.

10. Donawick WJ, Univ Penn: Personal communication, 1987.

11. Wyatt JK and Mundy HB: Torsion of the testicle: a clinical review of 20 cases. *Can Med Assn J* 107:971-973, 1972.

12. Weinerth JL, in Sabiston DC Jr: *Textbook of Surgery.* 13th ed. Saunders, Philadelphia, 1986. pp 1670-1695.

13. Merimsky E *et al:* Assessment of immunological mechanism in infertility of the rat after experimental testicular torsion. *Urol Res* 12:179-182, 1984.

14. Chakraborty J *et al:* Torsion of the spermatic cord - A long term study of the contralateral testis. *Urol Res* 14:257, 1986.

15. Roberts SJ: *Veterinary Obstetrics and Genital Diseases.* David & Charles, North Pomfret, VT, 1986. pp 752-893.

12

Diseases of the Accessory Genital Glands

Congenital and Familial Diseases

Agenesis/Dysgenesis

Developmental anomalies of the accessory genital glands are rare in stallions. Testicular agenesis may be accompanied by agenesis of portions of the ipsilateral mesonephric duct, such as the epididymis, deferent duct, vesicular gland or ampulla. Both cystic dilation of vesicular gland ducts and suspected unilateral ampullar hypoplasia have been described in stallions.[1,2] Anomalous development was suspected in these cases.

Inflammatory, Infectious and Immune Diseases

Bacterial Infections

Bacterial infections of the accessory genital glands are uncommon in stallions. They are noteworthy because of their persistent nature, effect on fertility and proclivity for venereal transmission. The causative bacteria are varied and include *Pseudomonas aeruginosa, Klebsiella pneumoniae, Streptococcus* spp, *Staphylococcus* spp and *Brucella abortus*.[1,3-6] Anaerobic bacteria have not been isolated from diseased accessory genital glands. Possible routes of infection include ascending infectious urethritis, extension of infectious cystitis, ductal spread of infectious epididymitis/orchitis and hematogenous/lymphatic spread of a generalized infection. Bacteria and/or inflammatory lesions have been demonstrated in all 4 accessory genital glands. The vesicular glands seem to be the most frequently involved sites, but bacteria also may invade the other accessory genital glands during the course of an infection.

Clinical manifestations of bacterial infections of accessory genital glands are varied. Acute infections may be manifested as reluctance to breed or ejaculate. Affected stallions may show pain during ejaculation. More often, however, stallions exhibit normal breeding behavior, and signs of accessory genital gland infection are not clinically evident. Examination of the accessory genital glands, via palpation per rectum, is indicated (Fig 1). Infected vesicular glands may be enlarged and firm, occasionally with a lobulated texture and irregular borders. In the acute stages, pain can elicited by palpation. Either unilateral or bi-

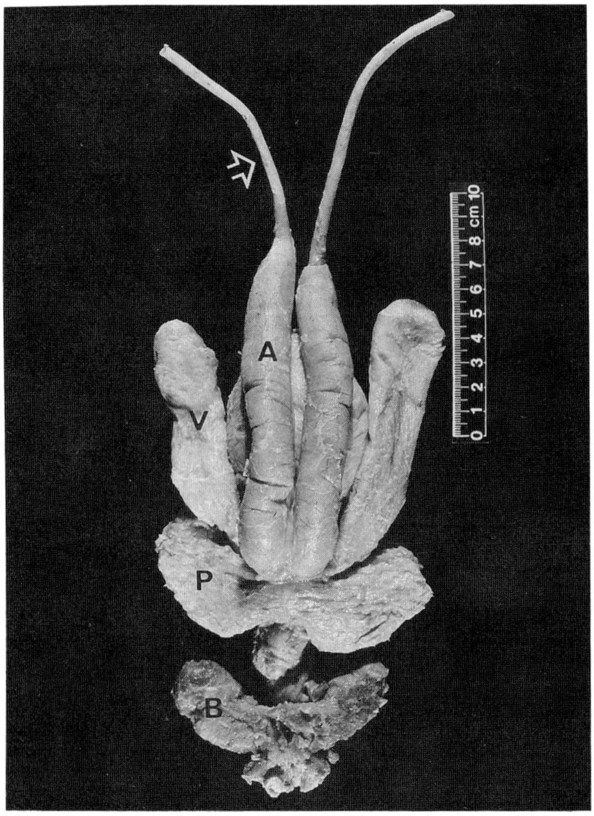

Figure 1. Accessory genital glands of the stallion: Bulbourethral glands (B), bilobed prostate gland (P), vesicular glands (V) and ampullae (A). The deferent ducts are also depicted (arrow).

lateral involvement is possible. Palpable changes in the other accessory genital glands have not been reported, nor has ultrasonographic evaluation of accessory genital gland infections.

Localization of an infection to a specific accessory genital gland often is difficult. Culture and cytologic examination of vesicular gland fluid may aid diagnosis. The stallion is sexually stimulated to promote development of an erection and to distend the vesicular glands. The penis then is washed with a surgical scrub, paying particular attention to the glans penis and fossa glandis, then rinsed and dried. A sterile 100-cm rubber catheter with an inflatable cuff is passed into the urethra until the tip is adjacent to the orifices of the ejaculatory ducts (seminal colliculus).[7] Catheter placement is aided by palpation per rectum. The cuff is inflated and the fluid within the suspect vesicular gland is expressed by manual compression of the gland per rectum. Fluid is collected in a sterile container from the catheter opening at the urethral orifice. Another catheter is similarly placed in the urethra and the procedure repeated if the contents of the opposite gland are to be evaluated. The fluid of the vesicular glands may be contaminated by urethral organisms when using this technique.

Fluid from the bulbourethral glands also can be selectively collected for evaluation. The erect penis of the stallion is prepared as described above. The glans penis is rubbed briskly while the stallion remains in close proximity to a mare exhibiting behavioral estrus. This stimulates release of clear preejaculatory fluid (10-30 ml) from the bulbourethral glands. The fluid is contaminated by contents of the urethral lumen, so bacterial urethritis is difficult to distinguish from infection of the bulbourethral glands when using this technique. Bacterial contamination is difficult to avoid when passing a balloon-tipped catheter to the origin of the bulbourethral gland ducts to collect the fluid.

Selective fluid collection from the prostate gland or ampullae alone is not possible; however, semen collection with an open-ended (Krakow model) artificial vagina may allow detection infection involving the prostate gland, ampullae, deferent ducts or epididymides.[8,9] The stallion's penis in inserted into an open-ended artificial vagina sufficiently to expose the glans penis. After the preejaculatory fluid is completely expelled, the first 2-3 sperm-rich fraction jets of the ejaculate are collected using a sterilized funnel or a sterile plastic bag attached to a urethral prosthetic device (see Chapter 4).[9,10] The sperm-rich fraction contains fluid predominantly from the prostate gland, ampullae, deferent ducts and epididymides. The remainder of the ejaculate can be collected in a separate container. This sperm-poor fraction originates principally from the vesicular glands.[11]

Ejaculates obtained from stallions with infections of the accessory genital glands contain numerous neutrophils and bacteria, and usually red blood cells. Leukocytes in the semen should be distinguished from round immature germ cells, *ie,* spermatogonia, spermatocytes or round spermatids. Air-dried semen smears can be stained with Giemsa's, Wright's or hematoxylin-eosin stains to differentiate inflammatory cells from round germ cells prematurely released from the seminiferous epithelium. A Gram's stain aids identification of the causative organism(s). Ejaculates sometimes contain gross clots of pus and frank blood.

Bacterial infections of the accessory genital glands usually cause infertility. Transmission of the bacteria to the mare during natural mating is unavoidable. Mares that develop genital infections after being bred by stallions with infected accessory genital glands may develop a vulvar discharge, have short interestrus intervals, or simply fail to conceive or maintain a pregnancy.[12-14]

Treatment of bacterial infections involving accessory genital glands often is unsuccessful. Except during an acute inflammatory state, most antibiotics given systemically diffuse poorly into the accessory genital glands. This is because they have an unfavorable pH or pK_a, poor lipid solubility and/or low protein-binding qualities. Trimethoprim-sulfamethoxazole may be the best antibacterial for systemic treatment if the causative organism is susceptible to it. Studies of affected men indicate this drug combination achieves high levels in prostatic fluid when administered systemically.[15,16]

Antibacterial drugs ineffective by systemic administration can be instilled into lumina of the vesicular glands, using a small-diameter (2-mm) catheter placed through the urethral opening of each vesicular gland at the seminal colliculus (Fig 2). Catheter placement is guided endoscopically, and the catheter is passed into the urethral lumen via the biopsy channel of the endoscope. Surprisingly, even a small-bore (7-mm diameter) endoscope can be passed into vesicular gland lumina via the seminal colliculus. This allows vigorous irrigation of each gland lumen before antibacterial drugs are instilled. Preliminary re-

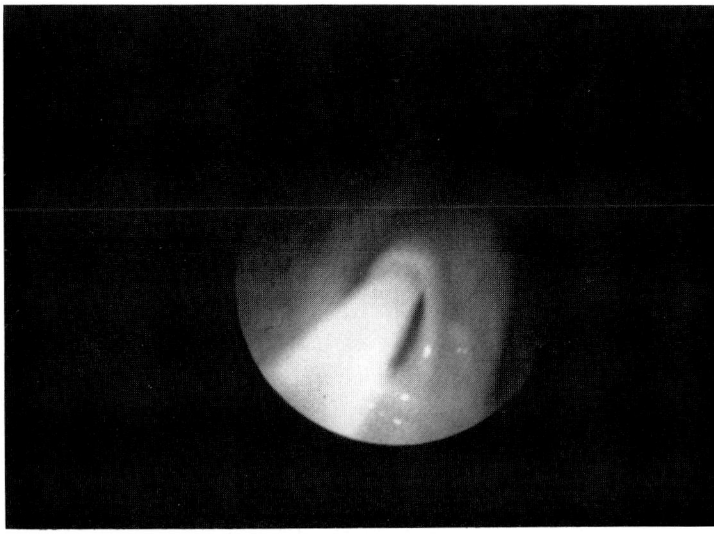

Figure 2. Upon viewing the seminal colliculus with a flexible endoscope, a 2-mm catheter is passed via the biopsy channel of the endoscope into the common opening of the right vesicular-gland duct and ampulla. The catheter is then blindly passed into the lumen of the right vesicular gland. A small-diameter (7 mm) endoscope can be passed directly into either vesicular gland. (The seminal colliculus is located on the dorsal surface of the urethra but appears as shown here through the endoscope because the instrument is directed upside down as it bends around the pelvic ischium en route to the proximal urethra.)

sults in our clinic with this therapeutic approach for infection of the vesicular glands have been encouraging.

Selection of antibacterial drugs always should be based on *in vitro* determination of sensitivity tests. Seminal vesiculectomy is possible, but the technique has not yet been perfected for routine use. Successful elimination of local infection by excision of infected vesicular glands is questionable, as concomitant infection of other accessory genital glands may exist. The effect of seminal vesiculectomy on fertility of stallions also warrants investigation.

If treatment of infected accessory genital glands is unsuccessful in a breeding stallion, fertility of the stallion may be extended, and venereal transmission of the bacterial disease to mares avoided, by using a minimum contamination breeding technique.[14] Semen from the stallion is collected using an artificial vagina, then placed semen extender containing appropriate antibacterial drugs before artificial insemination. The effect of antibacterial drugs on bacterial growth and spermatozoal motility in semen extender should be tested before use. Maintaining the extended semen in a light-protected container at 20-25 C for 15-30 minutes before insemination is usually sufficient for controlling bacterial growth.

If the stallion is to breed by natural service, 100-150 ml of semen extender containing appropriate antibacterials are infused into the mare's uterus immediately before breeding. Uterine lavage with 1-3 L of physiologic saline at 4 hours postbreeding or for 1-3 consecutive days postovulation may also improve pregnancy rate in these mares.[17,18] Antibacterial drugs can be instilled into the uterus following each uterine irrigation. Only drugs to which the bacteria are sensitive should be used.

Viral Infection

Equine arteritis virus can become sequestered in the genital tract of stallions after the acute phase of the disease. The result is a long-term asymptomatic carrier, with virus shed in the semen at the time of mating.[19] Thus, venereal transmission of equine arteritis virus by chronically infected stallions is a primary mode of dissemination. The specific areas of virus sequestration in the genital tract remain unknown. It is possible that the virus persists in the accessory genital glands. Attempts to isolate equine arteritis virus from all internal genital organs of chronically infected stallions should help in identifying specific sites of sequestration.

References

1. Neely DP, in Morrow DA: *Current Therapy in Theriogenology.* Saunders, Philadelphia, 1980. pp 694-706.

2. Ladds PW, in Jubb KVF *et al: Pathology of Domestic Animals.* 3rd ed. Vol 3. Academic Press, New York, 1985. pp 409-459.

3. Klug E *et al:* The effect of vesiculectomy on seminal characteristics in the stallion. *J Reprod Fertil* (Suppl) 27:61-66, 1979.

4. Roberts SJ: *Veterinary Obstetrics and Genital Diseases.* David & Charles, North Pomfret, VT, 1986. pp 752-893.

5. Blanchard TL *et al:* Bilateral seminal vesicu litis and ampullitis in a stallion. *JAVMA* 192:525-526, 1988.

6. Sojka JE and Carter GK: Hemospermia and seminal vesicle enlargement in a stallion. *Compend Cont Ed Pract Vet* 7:S587-S590, 1985.

7. Cooper WC: Methods of determining the site of bacterial infections in the stallion reproductive tract. *Proc Ann Mtg Soc Theriogenol,* 1979. pp 1-4.

8. Sojka JE and Carter GK: Hemospermia and seminal vesicle enlargement in a stallion. *Compend Cont Ed Pract Vet* 7:S587-S590, 1985.

9. Tischner M *et al:* Analysis of the pattern of ejaculation in stallions. *J Reprod Fertil* 41:329-335, 1974.

10. McCarthy PF *et al:* A modified "open" artificial vagina and a urethral prosthetic device for the collection of gel-free semen. *Proc Ann Mtg Soc Theriogenol,* 1979. pp 5-9.

11. Mann T and Lutwak-Mann C: *Male Reproductive Function and Semen.* Springer-Verlag, New York, 1981. pp 1-37, 171-193.

12. Hughes JP *et al:* The occurrence of *Pseudomonas* in the reproductive tract of mares and its effect on fertility. *Cornell Vet* 56:595-610, 1966.

13. Hughes JP and Loy RG: Investigations on the effect of intrauterine inoculations of *Streptococcus zooepidemicus* in the mare. *Proc Ann Mtg AAEP,* 1969. pp 288-292.

14. Blanchard TL *et al:* Use of a semen extender containing antibiotic to improve the fertility of a stallion with seminal vesiculitis due to *Pseudomonas aeruginosa. Theriogenology* 28:541-546, 1987.

15. Stamey TA *et al:* The concentration of trimethoprim in prostate fluid; nonionic diffusion or active transport? *J Infect Dis* 128:S686-S690, 1973.

16. Walsh PC, in Wyngaarden JB and Smith LH Jr: *Cecil's Textbook of Medicine.* 17th ed. Saunders, Philadelphia, 1985. pp 1375-1376.

17. LeBlanc MM and Asbury AC: Rationale for uterine lavage after breeding in mares. *Proc Ann Mtg AAEP,* 1988. pp 623-628.

18. Brinsko SP *et al:* The effect of uterine lavage four hours post-insemination on pregnancy rate in mares. *Proc Ann Conf Res Workers Anim Dis,* 1989. p 42.

19. Timoney PJ *et al:* The carrier state in equine arteritis virus infection in the stallion with specific emphasis on the venereal mode of virus transmission. *J Reprod Fertil* 35:95-102, 1987.

13

Diseases of the Urethra

Diseases with Physical Causes

Trauma

Physical damage to the urethra can take several forms. Penetrating or blunt trauma to the penis can result in urethral bruising, hemorrhage, lacerations or rupture. Ischial injuries can produce similar urethral lesions. The urethral process becomes engorged with blood and protrudes cranially when penile erection occurs. It can therefore be easily lacerated by tail hairs of the mare during the act of breeding, or changed by the breeding dummy during semen collection. Prolonged application of improperly sized plastic "stallion rings" or similar constricting devices around the shaft the penis in an attempt to control masturbation can result in circumferential pressure necrosis of the underlying penile tissues (Fig 1). Indirect damage to the urethra may occur with focal cicatrization. Surgical removal of the distal portion of the urethral process to treat cutaneous habronemiasis may result in proliferation of scar tissue at the excision site. The inelastic scar tissue may tear repeatedly at the time of breeding, as it can no longer dilate in response to engorgement of the corpus spongiosum penis with blood. The consequence is recurrent hemorrhage.

Iatrogenic urethral injury occurs due to incorrect or repeated urethral catheterization or improper endoscope passage, causing diffuse urethritis or isolated areas of mucosal trauma. Use of topical silver nitrate to stimulate mucosal healing can lead to marked necrosis and cicatrization of surrounding tissues. Calculi large enough to become lodged within the urethral lumen during transit can produce necrosis and subsequent scarring of the mucosa. Inversion of the urethral process is an interesting but rare disorder noted during maximal penile tumescence. The underlying cause is unknown, but the malady has been associated with ejaculatory failure, suggesting that it may produce pain.

Diagnosis of external trauma to the urethra begins with close inspection of the penile/perineal integument. Sedation aids exteriorization of the penis, permitting better examination. The presence and location of any contusions or lacerations should be noted. The tracts of penetrating wounds should be explored thoroughly. The penile shaft should be examined for a circumferential depression from an improperly used stallion ring. Close scrutiny of the urethral orifice reveals any lesions of cutaneous habronemiasis. Scar tissue from corrective surgery for cutaneous habronemiasis can be identified readily. Excoriations or lacerations of the urethral process may become infected from bacterial contaminants, thus delaying the healing process. Such lesions may ulcerate, causing profuse hemorrhage when stretched during ejaculation, similar to that seen with *Habronema* granulomas.

Urethral endoscopy allows definitive diagnosis of urethral lesions (Fig 2). Mural lesions, such as ulcerations, lacerations (Fig 3), prolapsed urethral vessels, cicatrices (Fig 4) and luminal

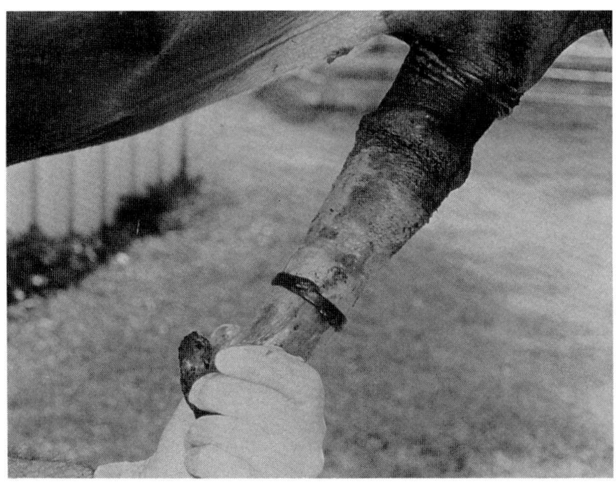

Figure 1. Nonexpandable plastic ring enveloping the free portion of the penile body to discourage masturbation in a breeding stallion. Excessive pressure may result in damage to underlying tissues, including the urethra. (Courtesy of Dr. L.H. Kloppe)

Figure 2. A flexible endoscope can be used to visualize the urethral lumen of the stallion along its entire length.

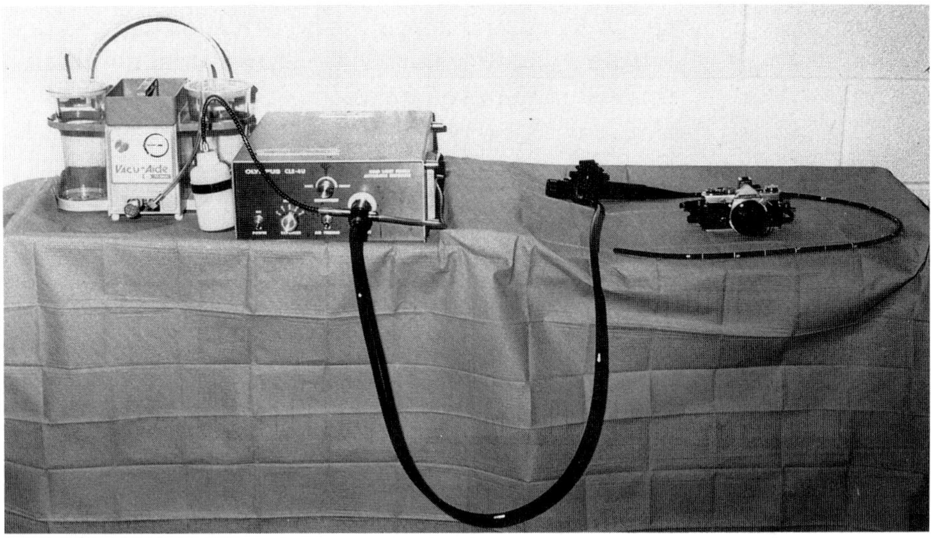

obstructions caused by lodged calculi, are readily identified, as is inflammation.[1] Inflammation should not be confused with the normally vascular urethral wall (Fig 5). A sterilized flexible endoscope, at least 100 cm long, should be used. The instrument is introduced into the urethra at the external urethral orifice and guided along the entire length of the urethral lumen, providing uninterrupted examination of the entire urethra. Perineal urethrotomy is not required.

The patency of the penile urethra and integrity of the wall can be assessed by retrograde urethrograms.[1,2] Both positive-

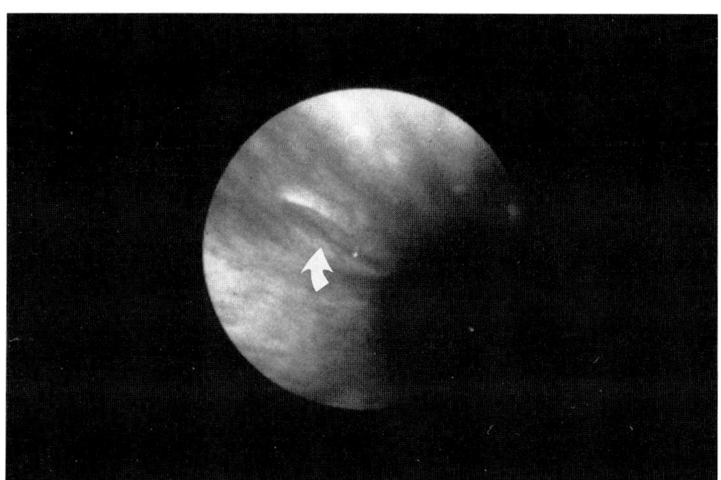

Figure 3. Endoscopic view of a rent in the wall of the pelvic urethra that results in communication between the urethral lumen and the corpus spongiosum penis.

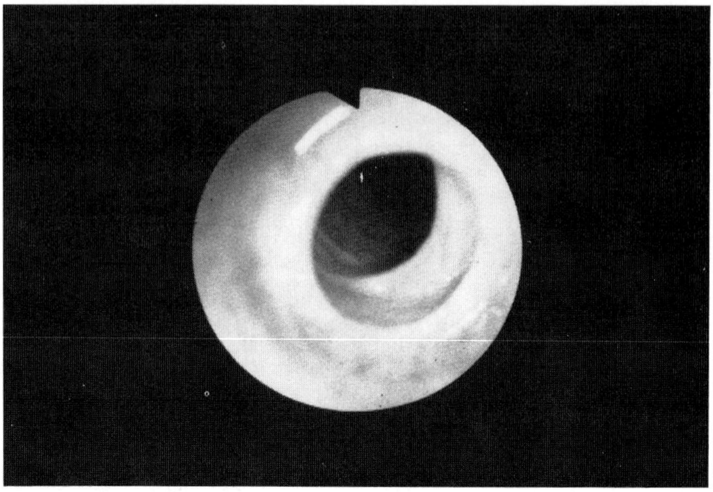

Figure 4. Endoscopic appearance of cicatrices within the lumen of the urethra.

contrast and double-contrast radiographic studies can be performed. Using this diagnostic approach, one can detect space-occupying lesions, such as urethral strictures, prolapsed subepithelial urethral vessels, and proliferation of granulation tissue, as well as pseudomembranes created by urethritis, lacerations, and ulcerations and fistulas of the urethra. Ultrasonographic examination is a useful adjunct to endoscopy and radiography to examine the urethra. This technique is especially useful for locating lodged urethral calculi (either penile or pelvic) before their removal via urethrotomy, and in detecting bladder calculi.

Urolithiasis most commonly involves the bladder, though renal and urethral calculi occur as well. The size of urinary

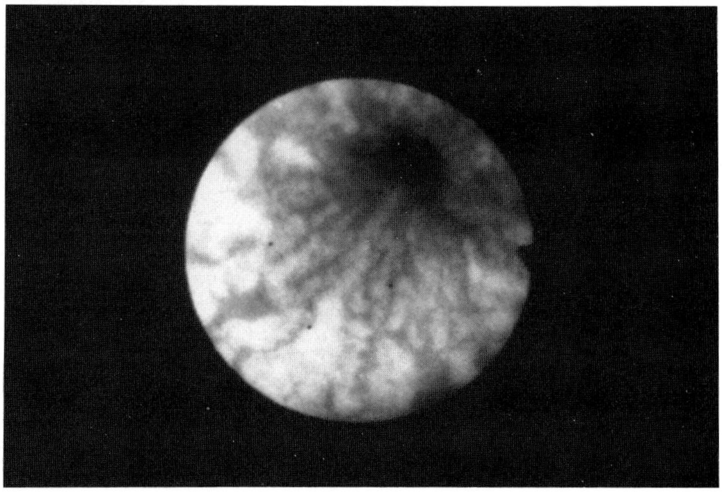

Figure 5. The walls of a stallion's urethra typically have prominent vascular patterns. Such vascularity should not be considered an inflammatory change.

calculi varies, and they may be quiet large (Fig 6). Calcium phosphate uroliths are more common in horses on high-grain diets, while calcium carbonate uroliths are more common in horses fed grass and hay. Clinical signs include dribbling of urine with chronic cystitis, dysuria or stranguria, recurrent colic and a stilted painful gait. Penile protrusion from the preputial orifice is frequent or constant in cases with chronic involuntary dribbling of urine.

Therapeutic measures depend on the form of urethral injury. Curettage, in conjunction with local urethral dilation, can be used to treat strictures, prolapsed urethral vessels, and proliferative granulation tissue that encroach upon the urethral lumen and disrupt its patency.[3]

Recurrent tearing of the urethral process after partial amputation is difficult to control. Gradual stretching of the circumferential cicatrix of the urethral orifice with urethral dilators, local application of emollients, and sexual rest may allow permanent healing of the operative site. In some cases, prolonged sexual abstinence (at least 2 months) is curative.

Iatrogenic injury to the urethral wall following improper instrumentation generally resolves without complication or special therapeutic measures. Sexual rest is indicated.

Calculi lodged within the lumen of the pelvic urethra can be removed via perineal urethrotomy.[2] The operation usually is

Figure 6. Urolith recovered from the bladder of a stallion.

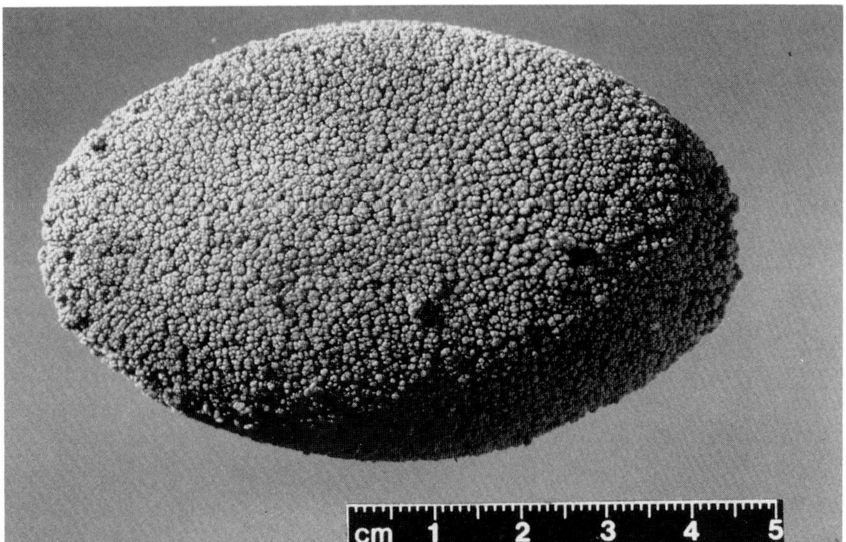

performed on the standing horse using sedation and epidural anesthesia. Infiltration of local anesthetic supplements epidural anesthesia, if needed. A 6- to 8-cm vertical skin incision is made on the perineal midline, beginning 2-3 cm ventral to the anus. Sharp dissection between the retractor penis muscles and through the bulbospongiosus muscle is continued until the urethra is encountered. Catheterization facilitates identification of the urethra. The urethral wall and its enveloping cavernous tissue (corpus spongiosum penis) are incised longitudinally. The indwelling catheter is removed and a lithotrite (or similar forceps) is introduced to retrieve the calculus. Palpation per rectum aids manipulation of the lithotrite within the urethral lumen. Though some small smooth calculi can be removed intact through the urethrotomy site, most calculi must be crushed before removal. This is done *in situ* (if they are impacted) or by repelling them into the bladder lumen. After removal of the calculus, the ischial urethrotomy site generally is allowed to heal as an open wound. Postoperative complications are rare.

Rents or lacerations of the urethral wall that communicate with the adjacent corpus spongiosum penis are refractory to healing (see Hemospermia in Chapter 16). Sexual rest and local medications do not restore the integrity of the urethral wall. One reason for the persistent nature of these lesions may be the increased blood pressure within the corpus spongiosum penis during erection and micturition, and the subsequent oozing from the rent in the urethra. This pathologic entity becomes evident during ejaculation or, occasionally urination as arterial bleeding into the urethral lumen. The bleeding ceases as blood within the corpus spongiosum penis is expelled. Ischial urethrotomy, described above, in conjunction with prolonged sexual rest (at least 2 months) may facilitate urethral healing. Incising the corpus spongiosum penis temporarily converts this semi-closed cavernous space into an open one, encouraging drainage of blood through the urethotomy site rather than the site of the original laceration. This surgical technique may circumvent intraurethral bleeding long enough to permit adequate healing of the urethral wound. Workers at Texas A&M University are investigating a surgical technique for primary closure of lacerations within the pelvic urethra that are refractory to healing.

No treatment has been described for inversion of the urethral process.

Inflammatory, Infectious and Immune Diseases

Bacterial Urethritis

Bacterial urethritis of horses is relatively uncommon. It occurs as a primary disease or as a sequel to infectious cystitis or local injury, and may be associated with hemospermia (see Hemospermia in Chapter 16). Lesions can occur throughout the urethra, including the pelvic urethra in the area of the ejaculatory ducts. The relationship of urethritis in this area to infections of the internal accessory genital glands has not been determined.

Diagnosis of bacterial urethritis is based on isolation of the causative organism from urethral swabs. Urethral endoscopy permits direct visual examination of the mucosal lining for evidence of inflammatory changes. Pseudomembranes may develop in pronounced cases of bacterial urethritis. These membranous structures are detectable by endoscopic examination and occasionally by double-contrast radiographic studies.[1,2] Examination of the accessory genital glands by palpation and ultrasound examination per rectum, and transurethral endoscopy may help determine involvement of these structures in the inflammatory process. Ejaculated semen should also be evaluated for inflammatory cells.

Bacterial urethritis usually responds to systemic antimicrobial therapy in conjunction with instillation of nonirritating antimicrobial drugs into the urethral lumen. Bacterial urethritis involving the proximal urethra may be treated most effectively via instillation of antimicrobial drugs through an ischial urethrotomy site for several consecutive days.[1] After resolution of the urethritis, the urethrostomy is allowed to heal by granulation. Selection of antimicrobial drugs is based on the antimicrobial susceptibility of the causative organism. Medications used should be nonirritating to the urethral mucosa. Sexual rest (at least 2-4 weeks) is a mandatory part of therapy. Underlying conditions, such as cystitis or penetrating wounds, also must be managed properly. Posttreatment cultures of the urethra, urine and semen are required to ensure elimination of the inciting bacteria.

Cutaneous Habronemiasis (Summer Sores)

This parasitic disease commonly affects the urethral process of the penis. Chapter 14 contains a discussion of cutaneous habronemiasis.

Chlamydial Urethritis

Chlamydia spp have been isolated from the urethra of stallions, but their relationship to urethral disease is unclear. Chlamydial urethritis of men is fairly common.

Protozoal Urethritis

Dourine, a disease caused by *Trypanosoma equiperdum*, may be clinically manifested as urethritis with a mucopurulent urethral discharge early in the disease. Generalized signs become evident as the disease progresses (see Chapter 2). Tentative diagnosis is based on clinical signs. Confirmation requires demonstration of the organism or serologic testing. Euthanasia of affected stallions is recommended. Dourine is presently eradicated from the United States.

Toxic Disease

Cantharidin Intoxication

Cantharidin, a hemolymph component in the blister beetle, is a potent irritant/vesicant that primarily affects the gastrointestinal and urinary tracts, and possibly the heart of horses that consume the toxin.[4] Cystitis and urethritis are common manifestations of the disease in horses that survive the initial phase of the intoxication. Frequent urination, dysuria and hematuria may be present.

References

1. Voss JL and Pickett BW: Diagnosis and treatment of haemospermia in the stallion. *J Reprod Fertil* 23:151-154, 1975.

2. Walker DF and Vaughan JT: *Bovine and Equine Urogenital Surgery*. Lea & Febiger, Philadelphia, 1980. pp 105-182.

3. Voss JL and Wotowey, JL: Hemospermia. *Proc Ann Mtg AAEP*, 1972. pp 103-112.

4. Schmitz DG and Reagor JC, in Robinson NE: *Current Therapy in Equine Medicine 2*. Saunders, Philadelphia, 1987. pp 120-122.

14

Diseases of the Penis

Diagnostic and Therapeutic Considerations

Exteriorization of the Penis

Critical examination of the penis requires its exteriorization from the preputial cavity. This prerequisite is met in patients with paraphimosis, penile paralysis or priapism. Under usual circumstances, however, when the stallion is not sexually stimulated, the penis is detumescent and within the prepuce. Therefore, psychic manipulation, drugs, manual procedures or a combination of these must be employed to exteriorize the penis. Exposure to an estrous mare usually elicits an erection; however, penile tumescence may be lost before the genital examination is completed if the stallion is not accustomed to examination. Alternatives in uncooperative stallions and geldings include tranquilization and/or manual retrieval.

For cooperative stallions, the penis can be extracted by passing a hand through the preputial orifice, grasping the penis behind the glans and manually removing it from the preputial cavity. With this technique, deliberate and continuous ventral force must be exerted to override the resistance of the retractor penis muscles. Because most horses actively oppose this method, light tranquilization often is used. Intravenous xylazine or acepromazine maleate produces spontaneous protrusion of the penis. The effect usually is more pronounced following tranquilization with acepromazine maleate. The examiner should be aware of the possible deleterious consequences of tranquilization. By a mechanism that is not fully understood, tranquilization, especially with phenothiazine tranquilizers, such as acepromazine maleate, can lead to irreversible penile prolapse and its attendant problems.[1-7]

Phimosis

Phimosis is the inability of the penis to protrude from the prepuce as a sequel to preputial injury or disease (Fig 1). Preputial edema, as occurs following castration or blunt genital trauma, chronic posthitis and neoplastic/granulomatous lesions of the prepuce, is a common cause of phimosis. Involuntary containment of the penis within the prepuce causes preputial urine accumulation, leading to inflammation of the penis and preputial laminae (balanoposthitis), and secondary bacterial infection. For a more thorough discussion of phimosis, see Chapter 15.

Paraphimosis

Paraphimosis refers to inability to retract the penis into the prepuce as a result of preputial injury or disease (Fig 2). Paraphimosis often follows acute preputial trauma but may develop as an aftermath of protracted penile prolapse, *eg,* with penile paralysis associated with debility, or penile paralysis/priapism following use of some tranquilizers.[1,8]

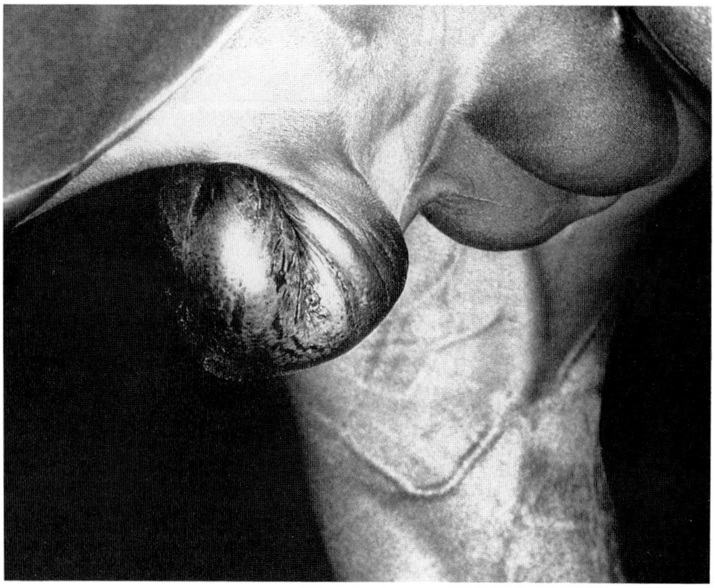

Figure 1. Phimosis caused by excessive swelling at the preputial orifice.

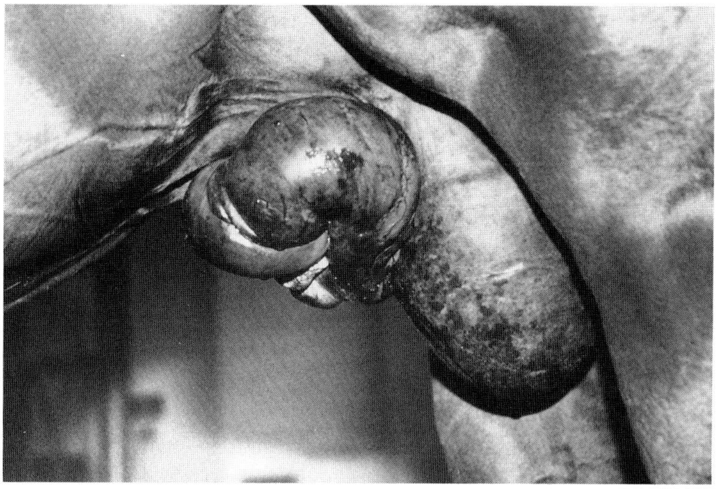

Figure 2. Paraphimosis associated with acute swelling of the prepuce.

Inflammatory edema of the prepuce is a predictable response to direct preputial trauma. Gravitational edema also may result from scrotal/inguinal trauma, as occurs following castration. If the penis extrudes from the prepuce during this inflammatory episode, the preputial swelling presents a mechanical impediment to penile retraction. Once penile prolapse occurs, the edema preventing penile retraction becomes even more pronounced, compounding the problem.

Protracted penile prolapse, no matter what the origin, causes impaired venous and lymphatic drainage and, within hours, edematous swelling of the penis and prepuce. Initially a large "collar" of edema tneds to form near the preputial ring. Constriction caused by this edematous collar often leads to further penile swelling. If treatment is not instituted, the process becomes self-perpetuating because of worsening vascular compromise and the pendulous nature of the organ. Edematous fluid eventually oozes through the penile and preputial integuments, which become increasingly friable. Cellulitis develops and the integument becomes thickened, inelastic, desiccated, necrotic and irreversibly damaged. Gangrenous changes of the penile tissue can occur unless the condition is reversed (Fig 3).

The first consideration in treatment of paraphimosis is to support the penis and reduce secondary gravitational edema. If

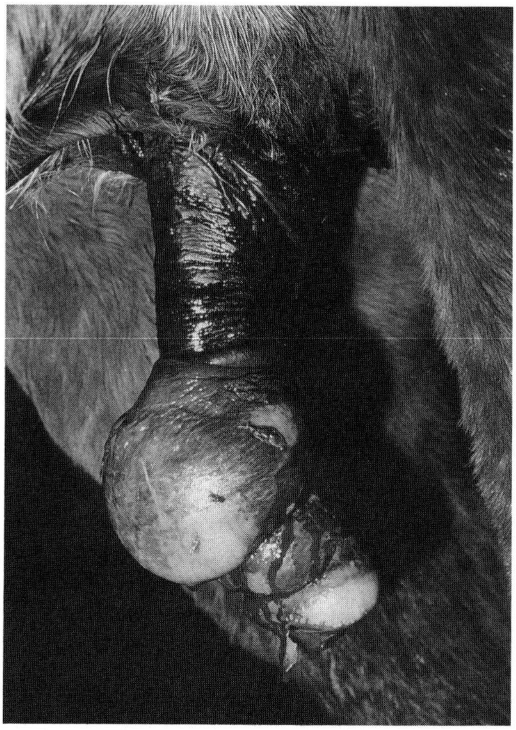

Figure 3. Necrotic changes in a prolapsed penis of long-standing duration.

possible, the penis should be replaced within the preputial cavity. It can be retained there with towel clamps or a purse-string retention suture placed near the preputial ring or preputial orifice (Fig 4). Better yet, the penis can be kept within the preputial cavity with a retention device fabricated from a 500-ml narrow neck plastic bottle (Fig 5).[9] The bottom (base) of the bottle is removed and the edges padded with several layers of tape. Two 5-ft lengths of rubber tubing or rolled gauze are secured to the bottle neck at their midpoints. The penis is inserted into the plastic bottle until the urethral process abuts the opening at the bottle neck. The penis then is replaced within the preputial cavity, along with the overlying plastic bottle. The bottle is held in position with the tubing (or gauze) secured to the bottle neck. One length of tubing is passed laterally and dorsally around both flanks and tied over the horse's back. The other length of tubing passes caudally along each side of the scrotum and between the hind legs, and then is fastened to the tubing over the horse's back. If the penis is positioned properly within the plastic bottle, urine can escape through the opening in the bottle neck. A loose-mesh suspensory harness (Fig 6) may be applied in a similar fashion to maintain the position of the

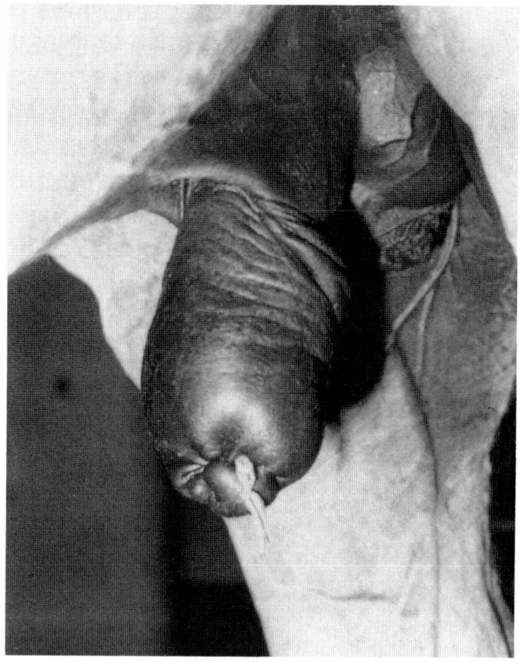

Figure 4. Pursestring suture inserted in the internal prepuce to prevent penile prolapse.

plastic bottle. In some instances, the suspensory harness alone may prevent prolapse of the penis. The penis should be removed from the preputial cavity at least twice daily for examination and application of emollients. Use of the apparatus can be discontinued when the horse voluntarily retains the penis within the preputial cavity.

Figure 5. Device fabricated for retaining the penis within the preputial cavity of stallions with penile prolapse.

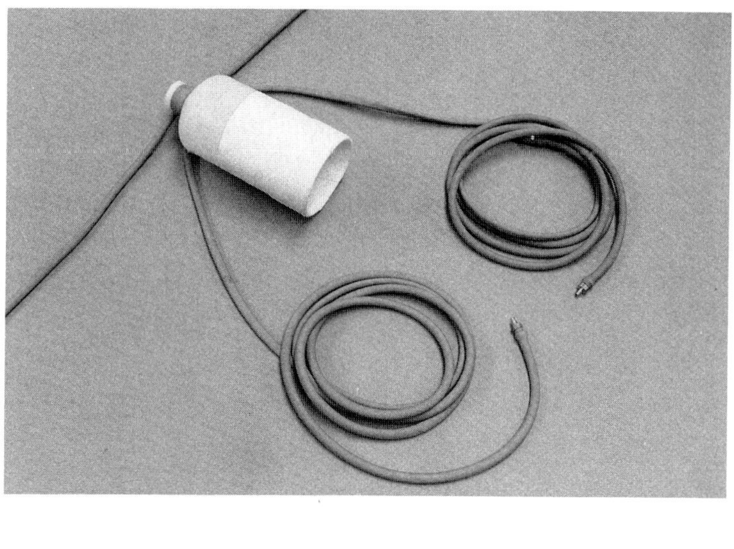

In acute cases, penile/preputial edema usually can be relieved by gentle massage with emollients, cold pack applications (see discussion of cryotherapy in Chapter 7), and the supportive measures described above. Temporarily wrapping rubber or pneumatic bandages around the penis hastens reduction of edema in pronounced or refractory cases. If the edema cannot be reduced sufficiently to permit replacement of the penis within the preputial cavity, the penis should be supported against the ventral abdominal wall with abdominal wraps. Once the penis is supported, either against the body wall (Fig 7) or within the preputial cavity (Fig 6), the horse should be exercised regularly to promote local venous and lymphatic drainage.

Emollients should be applied to the penis periodically to prevent drying and cracking of the integument. If the integument has been damaged, local and systemic antimicrobial therapy is indicated, as well as judicious use of diuretics and nonsteroidal antiinflammatory agents.

Recovery can be expected if irreversible damage to the integument has not occurred and if protracted penile paralysis or priapism does not accompany paraphimosis (see Penile Paralysis and Priapism below). Extensive fibrosis of the integument may result in preputial dysfunction, necessitating scar revision by elliptic incision or circumcision (discussed under Preputial Resection in Chapter 15). If unresponsive penile paralysis or

Figure 6. Nylon mesh, with attached tubing, fitted over the preputial orifice of a stallion to aid retention of the device shown in Figure 5 within the preputial cavity.

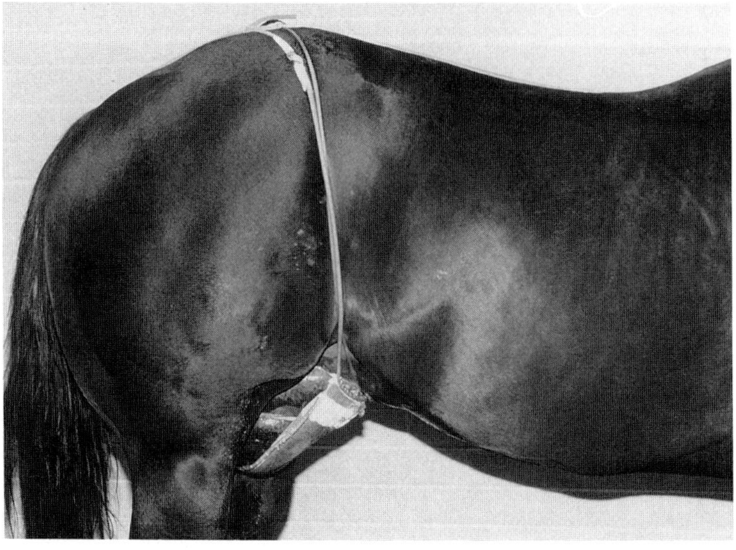

priapism is associated with the paraphimosis, surgical retraction of the penis (see Phallopexy) or amputation of the penis (see Phallectomy) may be required. Extensive damage to the penile cavernous tissue or nervous supply may impair sexual function in breeding stallions.

Penile Paralysis and Priapism

Reports of penile paralysis and priapism sometimes do not differentiate between these distinctly different conditions. Penile paralysis occurs secondary to reduced retractor penis muscle tone.[10] It has occurred in exhausted or debilitated horses, with myelitis or spinal injury, and following use of phenothiazine-derivative drugs.[1,4-6,8,10,11] Motor innervation of the retractor penis muscles of the stallion is thought to be solely supplied by alpha-adrenergic nerve fibers; therefore, paralysis of this muscle and penile prolapse occur when alpha-adrenergic blocking drugs, such as the phenothiazine derivatives, are administered.[12]

The prolapsed penis is flaccid and cannot be maintained in a retracted position within the preputial cavity, culminating in extensive penile swelling and trauma. Venous and lymphatic drainage are impaired and, if unrelieved, fluid continues to accumulate as the disorder progresses to a chronic ulcerative

Figure 7. Prolapsed penis held close to the body wall with an abdominal wrap to reduce dependent edema.

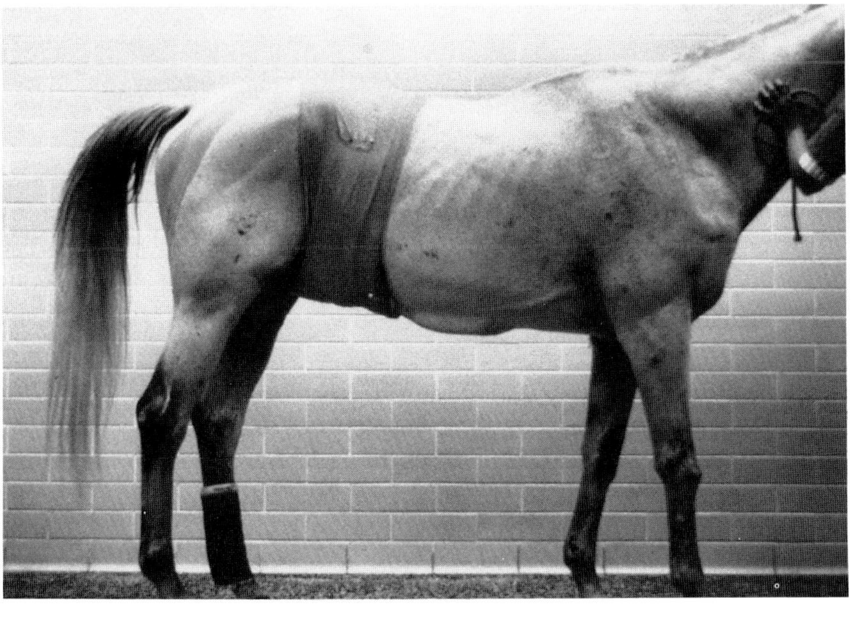

balanoposthitis (Fig 3). The epithelial surfaces of the exposed penis become dried, thickened and inelastic.[1,10] The protracted gravitational pull associated with prolonged penile prolapse has been postulated to cause damage to the pudendal nerves and smooth muscle cells of erectile tissue in the corpus cavernosum penis and the retractor penis muscles.[1,10] The pudendal and caudal rectal nerves, both of which are derived from the third and fourth sacral nerves, supply both sensory and motor innervation to muscles and skin of the genitalia, including the erectile bodies of the penis and the retractor penis muscles.[13,14] Local anesthesia of the pudendal nerves, alone or in conjunction with the caudal rectal nerves, results in prolapse of the penis from the preputial cavity. [14,15] Therefore, damage to these nerves would explain long-term penile paralysis and diminution or loss of cutaneous sensation of the penis noted in some affected stallions.

Priapism is a persistent erection without sexual arousal, and is initially unassociated with penile paralysis. It occurs from protracted engorgement of the corpus cavernosum penis with blood. The corpus spongiosum penis and corpus spongiosum glandis remain relatively empty (see Chapter 1 for a discussion of the cavernous tissue of the penis). While full erection may not be achieved, the penis is not flaccid as in cases involving only penile paralysis (Fig 8).[5-7] Failure of the corpus cavernosum penis to detumesce as a result of disturbances of blood flow,

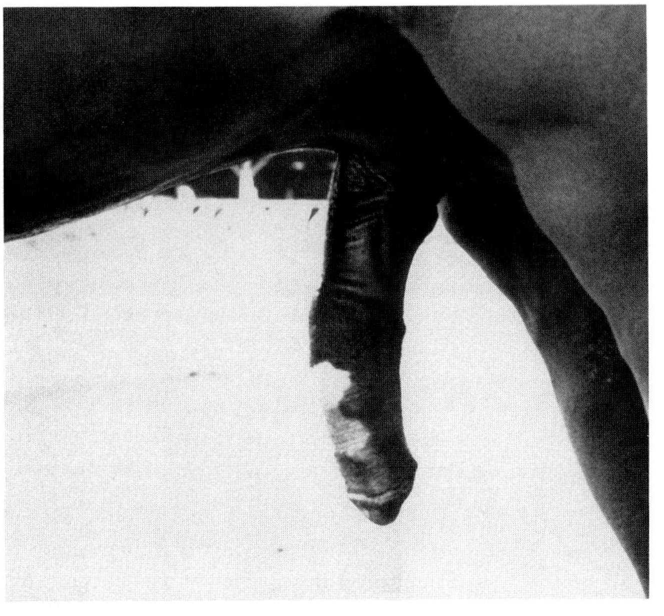

Figure 8. Firm, partially erect penis of a stallion with priapism.

either arterial or venous, has been incriminated as the cause of priapism in men, though the precise causes of these hemodynamic disturbances are unknown.[16,17] Priapism in men is often idiopathic, but hematologic disorders that increase sludging of erythrocytes can induce priapism by retarding venous outflow from the corpus cavernosum penis.[18] When the penis fails to detumesce, CO_2 tension in the corpus cavernosum penis rises, increasing the viscosity of blood, and venous occlusion occurs where collecting veins join the cavernous spaces. Edematous swelling of corporeal septae further reduces chances of venous outflow and favors irreversible venous obstruction. Fibrosis of the cavernous trabeculae and arteriolar occlusion follow (Figs 9-11). Disruption of the arteriovenous supply and fibrosis of the corpus cavernosum penis lead to permanent mechanical interference with erection.

Priapism in horses occurs primarily following administration of phenothiazine tranquilizers.[5-7] The condition has been reported in geldings, but is more common in stallions.[5,19] Androgens may maintain activity of smooth muscle cells in the cavernous erectile tissue and thereby play a key role in maintaining the size of the cavernous spaces. In the absence of androgens, these smooth muscle cells are thought to atrophy, leading to decreased size of the cavernous blood spaces. Vascular filling of the corpus cavernosum penis following tranquilization would

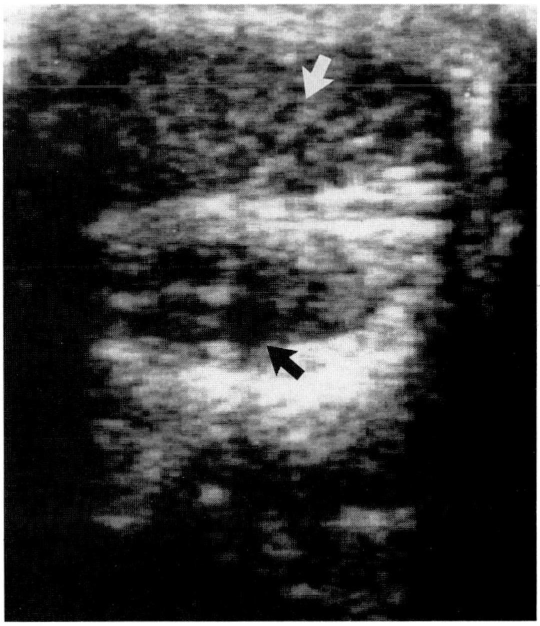

Figure 9. Ultrasonic image of the normal penile body of a stallion, revealing the trabecular spaces of the corpus cavernosum penis (white arrow) and the urethral lumen, surrounded by the corpus spongiosum penis (black arrow).

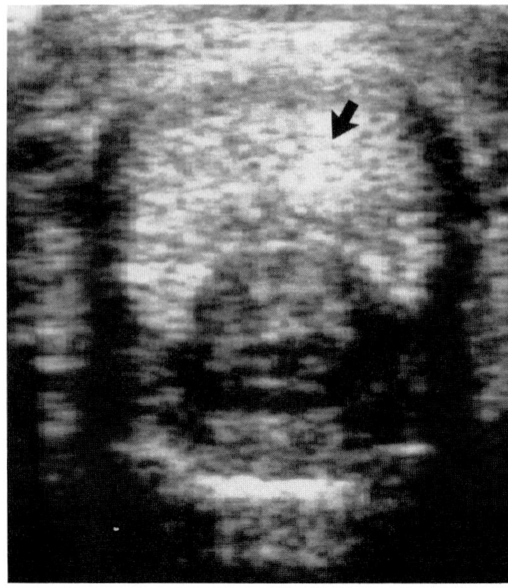

Figure 10. Ultrasonic image of the penile body of a stallion with long-standing priapism.[51] Note the uniform, highly echogenic pattern of the corpus cavernosum penis (arrow), a finding consistent with thrombosis.

likewise be reduced in geldings.[10] This hypothetical mechanism would explain initial tumescence of the corpus cavernosum. However, in men, failure of the detumescence mechanism is considered necessary for priapism to persist.[16] Phenothiazine tranquilizers may cause priapism by blockade of the alpha sympathetic impulses that mediate detumescence.[18]

If the erection does not subside in a few hours, penile and preputial swelling ensue, and the penis undergoes progressive necrotic changes similar to that described above for penile paralysis and paraphimosis (Fig 12).

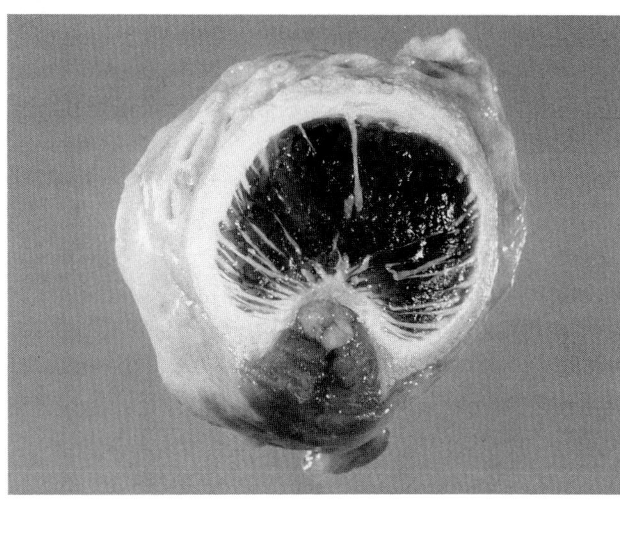

Figure 11. Cross-section of the penile body of a stallion with protracted priapism, revealing marked thrombosis of the corpus cavernosum penis.

Penile paralysis or priapism should be differentiated from paraphimosis. In paraphimosis, the penis cannot be retracted because of preputial injury or disease.

Medical treatment of horses with penile paralysis consists of penile massage, application of slings, administration of diuretics, and replacement of the penis into the preputial cavity. The section on Paraphimosis contains a detailed discussion of therapy.

Medical treatment of horses with priapism has generally been unsuccessful but has included penile massage, application of emollient dressings and slings, and administration of corticosteroids and diuretics systemically to reduce dependent edema. Manual compression of the penis with the horse anesthetized has been unsuccessful.[7] Administration of the ganglionic blocker, benztropine mesylate (8 mg IV), brought about detumescence in one gelding treated within 2 hours after onset of priapism but was unsuccessful in treatment of a stallion when administered 4 days after the onset of priapism.[19,20]

In the early stages of priapism in men, alpha-adrenergic agents are injected into the corpus cavernosum penis to promote stimulate contractility of cavernous and arterial smooth muscle and promote penile detumescence.[17,21] This technique has not been described in horses.

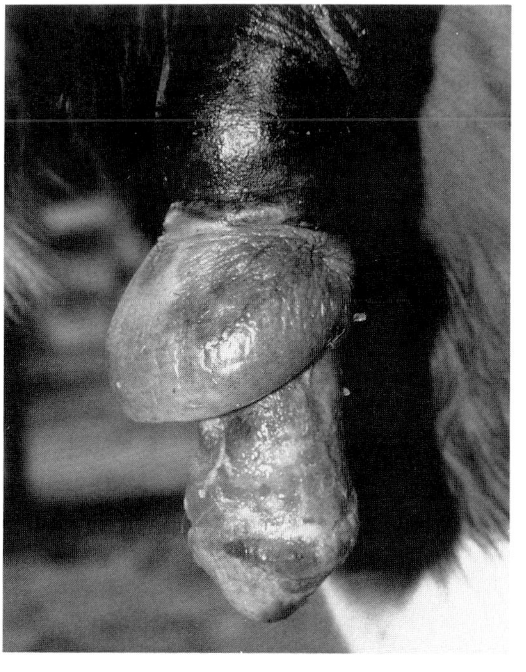

Figure 12. Balanoposthitis in a stallion with long-standing priapism.

In men, further treatment for priapism includes removal of congealed acidotic blood from the corpus cavernosum penis, and creation of shunts to establish venous drainage from the corpus cavernosum penis into the corpus spongiosum penis.[17] Both of these procedures have been performed in stallions.[17] To flush the corpus cavernosum penis to remove sludged blood, the horse is anesthetized and positioned in dorsal recumbency, and the penis, prepuce and inguinal region are prepared for aseptic surgery. Heparinized saline solution is flushed, under pressure, into the corpus cavernosum penis through a 12-ga needle inserted into cavernosal tissue proximal to the glans penis. The sludged blood and saline solution are drained through 1 or 2 12-ga needles inserted into the corpus cavernosum penis 10-15 cm caudal to the base of the scrotum. The cavernous spaces are irrigated until fresh blood is seen in the efflux. Evacuation of cavernosal blood may be of no benefit by itself if venous outflow is occluded because continued arteriolar inflow maintains turgidity of the erectile body. If fresh blood is not seen, arteriolar damage has also probably occurred.

Surgical management is indicated if conservative therapy does not restore venous outflow. The point at which venous occlusion becomes irreversible is not clear, but creation of a venous shunt is indicated in men that fail to respond to medical therapy or cavernosal lavage, regardless of the duration of the priapism.[22] The effect of the shunting procedure on the erectile mechanism in stallions is not known.

To create a shunt, the corpus cavernosum penis is exposed caudal to the scrotum and a side-to-side anastomosis is created between the corpus cavernosum penis and the corpus spongiosum penis (Fig 13).[20] Because the corpus spongiosum penis is not involved in initial development of an erection, its patent cavernous spaces and collecting veins provide an exit route for the blood within the corpus cavernosum penis. Postoperatively, inability to develop an erection may be due either to damaged erectile tissue or to the shunt itself. Low-pressure and low-flow shunts may collapse and thrombose when venous outflow resumes, but it is not known if closure of these shunts is required for return to normal sexual function.

The prognosis for return to normal reproductive function is quite bleak. However, some stallions can impregnate mares successfully even though the penis does not become rigid when fully engorged. These stallions require assistance with intromis-

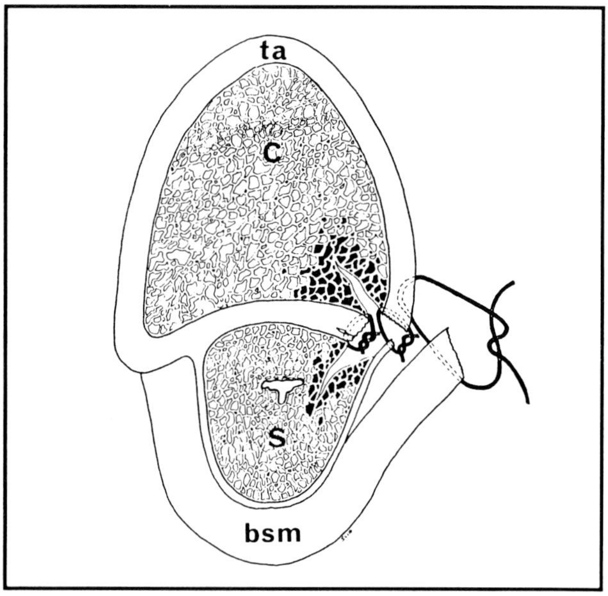

Figure 13. Creation of a vascular shunt between the corpus cavernosum penis (C) and the corpus spongiosum penis (S) as a surgical treatment for priapism in stallions. After incising the corpus cavernosum penis and corpus spongiosum penis, the incised tunica albuginea of the corpus spongiosum penis is sutured to the incised tunica albuginea overlying the lateral aspect of the corpus cavernosum penis. The incised bulbospongiosus muscle (bsm) is then resutured to the tunica albuginea of the corpus cavernosum penis.

sion. Repeated breeding attempts may encourage recanalization of damaged cavernous tissue.[23] Intracavernosal injection of vasoactive drugs, such as papaverine, phenoxybenzamine and phentolamine, has improved erectile function of men with damaged cavernosal tissue.[17] Similarly affected horses may also benefit from intracavernosal administration of these drugs.

Refractory cases of penile paralysis or priapism require phallopexy or partial phallectomy.

Phallopexy

(Bolz Operation)

Penile prolapse unresponsive to exhaustive nonsurgical corrective measures generally requires phallopexy (penile retraction surgery) or partial phallectomy (penile amputation). Phallopexy is the more conservative of the 2 penile surgeries, but candidates must meet certain prerequisites before this procedure can be recommended over phallectomy. First, castration should be performed at or near the time of phallopexy, and the horse should not be allowed exposure to mares in the postoperative period. Erection or coital attempts can damage the operative site. Second, the penis must be capable of being retracted fully into the preputial cavity, and inflammation/infection of the penis and prepuce must be controlled before phallopexy is performed.

The Bolz operation is performed under general anesthesia with the horse in dorsal recumbency. The urethra is catheterized, and the inguinal region, scrotum and penis are prepared for aseptic surgery. A 10-cm skin incision is made on the perineal raphe just caudal to the base of the scrotum, or 5 cm caudal to the residual castration scars.[24] The penis is isolated, then carefully freed from its surrounding fascia by digital dissection. Injury to the vascular network on the dorsum of the penis should be avoided. The shaft of the penis is retracted through the skin incision until the annular ring, formed by the reflection of the inner lamina of the internal prepuce onto the penis, is visible at the cranial end of the skin incision. This preputial attachment is freed of loose fascia, and a heavy, nonabsorbable suture is passed deeply through the lateral surface of the penis in a dorsoventral direction. An assistant should palpate the fornix of the preputial cavity to ensure that the suture has not entered the preputial cavity accidentally. Entering the fornix with the suture could lead to abscessation. The suture must be placed through the lateral surface of the penis to avoid perforation of the urethra, which could result in urethral fistula formation. The indwelling urethral catheter facilitates identification of the urethra and protects against inadvertent injury.

Using eyed needles, both ends of the secured suture material are passed caudally through the skin, exiting 2 cm apart near the center of the skin incision. The suture material exits the skin 4-5 cm lateral to the midline. The same suture pattern is repeated on the opposite side of the penis. The ends of each suture are tied over a roll of gauze, button or rubber tubing to minimize skin necrosis from suture tension (Fig 14). If adequate suture tension is applied, the penis is contained within the preputial cavity, with the tip of the glans penis just inside the preputial orifice. Inadequate retraction results in protrusion of the glans penis from the preputial orifice, while excessive traction results in urination within the preputial cavity and associated balanoposthitis. Both sutures should be tied in a bow knot so that suture tension can be adjusted after the horse is standing. An alternative method of penile retraction and fixation is to anchor the preputial reflection to the subcutaneous fascia near the center of the perineal incision with heavy absorbable suture.[25] This approach prevents necrosis of the skin underlying the

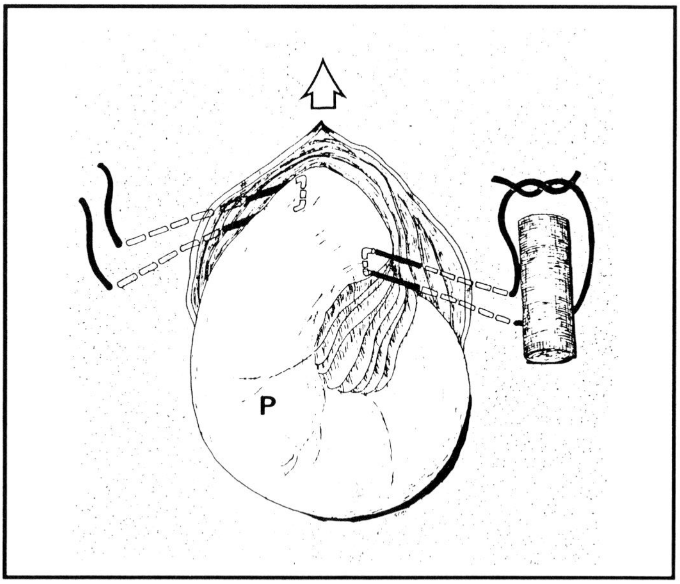

Figure 14. The Bolz procedure, showing the method for anchoring the penis (P), in a retracted position, to the subcutaneous tissue behind the scrotum. Arrow is pointing cranially.

tension sutures but precludes adjustment of suture tension postoperatively.

Phallopexy produces a sigmoid curvature in the penis, but blood supply and urine flow remain unimpeded. The fascia and skin are closed separately in a routine manner. Placement of a Penrose drain in the surgical site is optional. If a drain is used, the horse should be kept in cross-ties until the drain is removed, 6-7 days postoperatively, to prevent contamination of the wound. Tetanus pro phylaxis and systemic antibiotic therapy are indicated. Use of diuretics to control local edema is advised. The horse should be exercised twice daily to reduce postoperative swelling. If percutaneous retention sutures are used, they can be removed along with the sutures in the skin incision 12-14 days postoperatively. By this time, the retention sutures probably will be loose due to some skin necrosis beneath the tension bolsters. The horse usually can resume work 3-4 weeks after surgery.

If a stallion has not been castrated before phallopexy, this should be done after the phallopexy has healed. Castration should not be performed at the same time as the phallopexy if the castration site is to heal as an open wound, as the open scrotal wound may interfere with healing of the closed perineal wound. Both procedures can be performed simultaneously if the castration site is sutured. Alternatively, the stallion can be castrated before phallopexy, but the formidable task of caring for the prolapsed penis is prolonged while the castration wounds heal.

Phallectomy

(Amputation of the Penis)

Phallectomy (or more properly, partial phallectomy) is a radical surgical procedure reserved for horses with intractable paraphimosis, extensive penile injury or a serious penile disease, such as squamous-cell carcinoma. The operation is performed with the horse under general anesthesia and in lateral or dorsal recumbency. The penile urethra is catheterized to facilitate its identification, and the genital area is prepared for aseptic surgery. The penis is maintained in extension by manual traction on a length of sterile gauze looped around the collum glandis. A tourniquet of rubber tubing is secured around the penis proximal to the intended site of amputation to control hemorrhage. If amputation is performed because of persistent penile prolapse, the penis is transected at the preputial orifice (Fig 15). The penile remnant should not protrude from the preputial orifice; but, to avoid urine scalding, the sutured end of the penis should also not be located high within the preputial cavity.[1]

Various techniques of penile amputation have been devised to minimize local hemorrhage and urethral strictures, both of

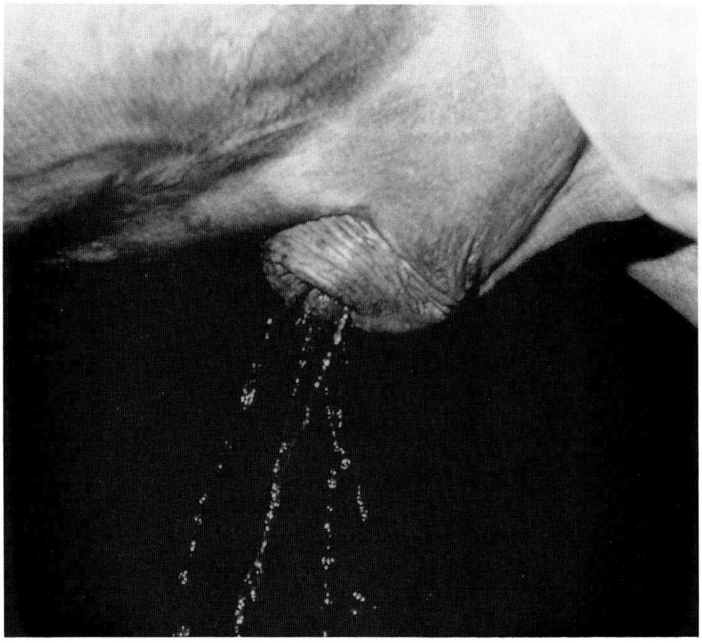

Figure 15. Urination following partial penile amputation, showing proper site for penile transection to avoid urine scalding of the preputial cavity.

which are common postoperative complications. We prefer a technique described by Scott, with some minor modifications.[26] At the intended point of penile transection, a circumferential incision is made through the skin and underlying loose connective tissue until the vessels on the dorsum of the tunica albuginea are encountered. These vessels are ligated individually with absorbable suture and severed. Sharp dissection is continued through the corpus cavernosum penis (CCP). These corporeal bodies are severed in a slightly oblique, craniodorsal to caudoventral plane. The corpus spongiosum penis (CSP) encircling the urethra also is transected without entering the urethra. The urethra is identified easily by the indwelling catheter previously placed in the lumen. A 4- to 5-cm section of the urethra is carefully dissected free from the distal segment of the penis. Following removal of the urethral catheter, the urethra is transected, saving the 5-cm segment dissected from the distal penis. When the penile amputation is complete, a portion of the urethra, freed of its enveloping CSP, should project beyond the remaining penis.

Hemorrhage from the incised CCP is controlled by suturing the dorsal and lateral tunica albuginea to the ventral portion bordering the urethral groove with 0 absorbable suture material in an interrupted suture pattern (Fig 16). Proper alignment of the larger (outer) perimeter of the tunica albuginea to the smaller (inner) perimeter is achieved by preplacing the first 3 sutures. Hemorrhage from the sinusoidal spaces of the CSP is controlled by suturing its thin tunica albuginea to the urethral stump. The urethral stump is flared in a fan-like fashion over the sutured end of the CCP, and sutured to the skin with simple-interrupted 2-0 absorbable or nonabsorbable suture material (Fig 16). The urethra is easily stretched to cover a large area. To prevent retraction of urethral tissue, each suture should include a bite in the underlying tunica albuginea of the CCP. Nonabsorbable sutures are removed in 10-14 days.

An alternative method of securing the urethral stump to the skin has been described.[26] The urethral stump is incised into 3 triangular segments, with the apex of each triangle located distally. These segments then are intermeshed in a dove-tailed fashion and sutured to similarly prepared segments of penile or preputial skin.

Another commonly used technique of penile amputation uses a triangular incision, 4 cm long and 3 cm wide, on the ventrum of the penis proximal to the site of amputation.[27] The apex of the incision points proximally, and the base marks the intended site of penile transection. The incisions extend through the skin, retractor penis muscles, bulbospongiosus muscles and CSP but do not enter the urethral lumen. This triangle of tissue is dissected off the catheterized urethra and discarded. A longitudinal incision is made through the exposed triangle of urethra on a line from the apex to the middle of the base of the triangle. The urethral wall is sutured to the penile skin in a simple-interrupted pattern with 2-0 absorbable or nonabsorbable suture material. The catheter is withdrawn, and the penis is obliquely transected from the base of the triangle dorsodistally. The vessels on the dorsum of the penis, overlying the tunica albuginea of the CCP, are ligated individually. Nonabsorbable noncapillary 0 sutures are placed in an interrupted pattern through the urethral wall and tunica albuginea of the urethral groove across (not through) the sinusoidal tissue of the CCP and through the tunica albuginea and skin on the dorsal and lateral penile surfaces. This creates a 4-bite suture pattern. The first 3 sutures are preplaced at equal intervals before being tied to ensure even closure. When the sutures are tightened, the urethral mucosa

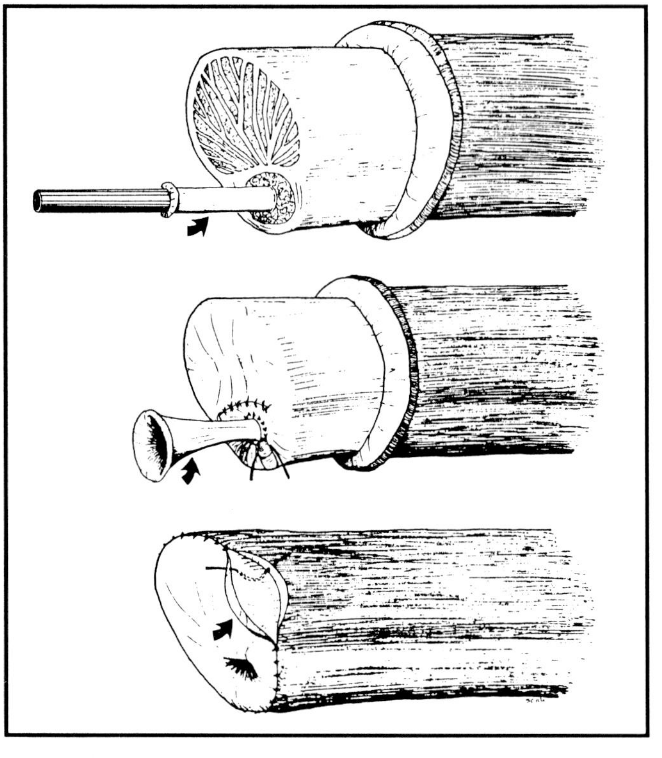

Figure 16. Amputation of the equine penis, with separate closures of the corpus cavernosum penis and corpus spongiosum penis, followed by fixation of the flared urethral mucosa (arrows) to the skin of the penis.

and skin are apposed and the cavernous spaces are compressed. Sutures are removed 10-14 days postoperatively.

Minor hemorrhage through the suture lines can be expected for several days, especially when the horse extends its penis to urinate. Minor dehiscence of the suture line is expected and causes little problem. Excessive dehiscence can result in urethral stenosis and may necessitate further reconstructive surgery.

En-bloc resection and penile retroversion have been described for treatment of extensive involvement of the penis, prepuce and/or superficial inguinal lymph nodes.[28] The horse is anesthetized and positioned in dorsal recumbency. The bladder is catheterized and the inguinal area prepared for aseptic surgery.

A skin incision is created 6 cm cranial to the prepuce and continued 10 cm caudally around each side of the prepuce. The subcutaneous tissue is incised to expose the abdominal tunic, and the plane of dissection is extended to the superficial inguinal rings. The external pudendal vessels are ligated, and the superficial inguinal lymph nodes are removed. The penis is amputated 6-8 cm caudal to the prepuce. Four centimeters of urethra and CSP are left beyond the penile stump. The CCP is closed with preplaced interrupted absorbable sutures.

A 6-cm incision is created on the perineal raphe 20 cm ventral to the anus, and penile fascia is separated by blunt dissection to free the distal tip of the penis from the penile fascia. Six centimeters of the penile stump are retracted through the perineal incision. The tunica albuginea of the retroverted penis is sutured to the subcutaneous tissue of the ventral aspect of the perineal incision, and the penile fascia is sutured to the subcutaneous tissue of the lateral and dorsal aspects of the subischial incision. The dorsum of the exposed urethra is longitudinally incised, and the urethral incision is sutured to the skin of the perineal incision with nonabsorbable suture. Penrose drains are placed in the subcutaneous space of the site of *en-bloc* resection, and the subcutaneous tissue and skin are closed.

Congenital and Familial Diseases

Agenesis, Dysgenesis

Congenital absence or abnormal formation of the penis and prepuce has been associated with various forms of intersexuality (see Chapter 7). The most common form of intersexuality is male pseudohermaphroditism. Retroversion of the penis has also been observed in genotypic, gonadal and phenotypic males.[10] Affected horses have undescended testes and malformed prepuce. Plastic and reconstructive surgery has been performed on some malformed external genital organs to provide a more cosmetic appearance.[196] Penile hypoplasia also has been described.[76] Affected horses have a normal external genital organ configuration, but the penis is smaller than normal. The cause has not been studied, so transmissibility of the defect to offspring is unknown. Inadequate contact of the hypoplastic penis with the vaginal wall during intravaginal thrusting may impede ejaculation.

Diseases with Physical Causes

Lacerations and Abrasions

Lacerations, contusions and abrasions of the penis generally occur when the penis is erect, as it is well protected within the confines of the preputial cavity when detumescent. Breeding makes the penis very vulnerable to kicks from a nonreceptive mare. Tail hairs of the mare or an improperly placed "breeding stitch" in the mare's vulva are common sources of injury to the penis at the time of intromission. Improperly constructed or poorly maintained artificial vaginas or breeding phantoms also can produce penile injuries during semen collection. Paraphimosis, penile paralysis and priapism expose the penis to the environment for long periods. In addition to the rapidly progressive congestion and edema that accompany such penile disorders, the prolapsed penis is quite susceptible to secondary injury. Less commonly, the penis is involved in inguinal lacerations (Fig 17) or ischial trauma.

Prompt appropriate therapy is the key to successful treatment of penile injuries. Initial treatment of a traumatized penis is directed at controlling acute inflammation and edema. When begun immediately, gentle but persistent penile massage using demulcents and cold packs works remarkably well to curb local swelling. The section entitled Scrotal Trauma, Chapter 7, contains a discussion of specific therapeutic principles; these principles are also applicable to the penis. Delayed treatment can lead to massive penile/preputial/scrotal edema and increases the likelihood of irreversible damage to the external genitalia. Systemic antiinflammatory and diuretic medications are useful adjuncts to local therapy. Prophylactic antimicrobial therapy also should be instituted to control cellulitis. A tetanus toxoid booster is recommended if the horse has not been vaccinated against tetanus within the past year.

A serious sequela of penile trauma is penile paralysis and/or paraphimosis, both of which have potentially devastating consequences. Returning a prolapsed penis to its normal detumescent position within the preputial cavity is critical to prevention of both complications. Extensive trauma to the exposed penis may occasionally lead to cutaneous desensitization that, upon penile healing, interferes with the stallion's ability to copulate and ejaculate. Specific guidelines for reducing a prolapsed penis are discussed above in the sections on Paraphimosis and Penile Paralysis.

Superficial penile lacerations heal remarkably well as open wounds if local infection and edema are controlled and sexual rest is enforced until healing is complete. Debridement and suturing are recommended for deep lacerations of the penis. In a horse treated by suturing, measures to prevent tissue infection and inflammatory edema also should be instituted. Prolonged sexual abstinence is essential to healing. If lacerations have penetrated cavernous tissue, the overlying tunica albuginea is sutured to prevent hemorrhage when the cavernous spaces become engorged. Penetration of the urethral wall can occur with penile lacerations, especially those on the ventrum of the penis. Surgical repair is indicated in these instances to prevent

Figure 17. Inguinal laceration in a yearling colt, with exposure and penetration of the underlying penis. (Courtesy of Dr. J.P. Watkins)

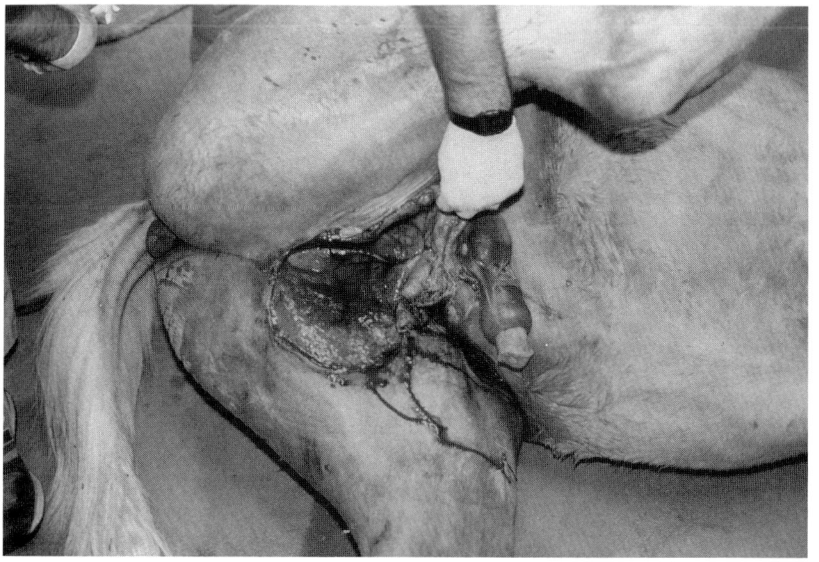

fistula formation. Severe penile injury may necessitate amputation. The section entitled Phallectomy contains a description of the surgical procedures for penile amputation.

Stallion Ring-Induced Ischemic Necrosis

Stallion rings are nonexpansive bands, generally plastic, placed immediately proximal to the glans penis to discourage masturbation in breeding stallions (Fig 18). Ribbon has been tied around the penis in this location to provide the same effect. These encircling devices are thought to restrict penile tumescence by causing pain when the penis becomes erect. The efficacy of these appliances has not been critically tested. Nevertheless, many stallion managers use these devices routinely to control masturbation by stallions during the breeding season.

If used, stallion rings (or ribbons) must be properly fitted, and inspected, cleaned and changed at least weekly to prevent penile/urethral damage. Tightly fitting rings or prolonged applications compress the underlying penile and urethral tissue, leading to ischemic necrosis and constricting fibrosis. Such injury often results in urethral strictures or failure of erection, primarily involving the corpus spongiosum glandis (interference with belling of the glans penis). Nerve damage also may develop, causing hypoesthesia or anesthesia of the penis distal to the constricting lesion. Pinching the penile integument does not elicit a reaction from stallions with desensitization.

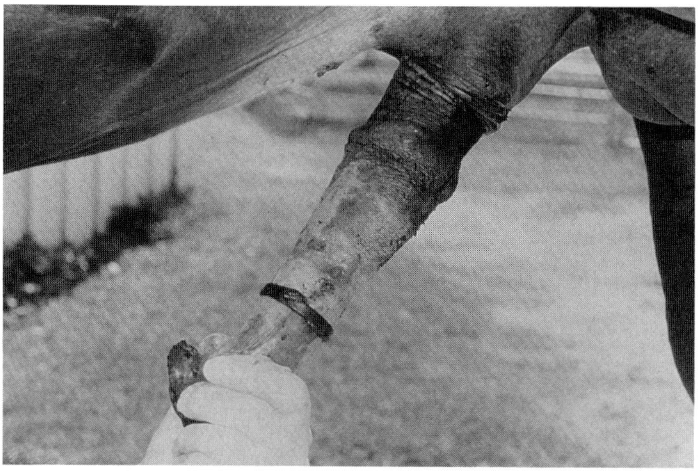

Figure 18. Nonexpandable plastic ring enveloping the free portion of the penile body to discourage masturbation in a breeding stallion. (Courtesy of Dr. L.H. Kloppe)

Endoscopic examination of the urethral lumen provides information about the extent of urethral involvement, as may contrast radiography.[29] Treatment of urethral strictures usually consists of local curettage combined with luminal dilation. Because the affected area is distal on the penis, it is usually accessible for surgical correction via the urethral orifice, thus avoiding the need for urethrotomy. In most instances, the regenerative capacity of the urethra is remarkably good. Repair of damaged erectile tissue is difficult. Persistent erectile dysfunction often results, usually because of inability of the corpus spongiosum glandis to fill properly with blood during sexual stimulation. Repeated stimulation encourages erection and reestablishes patency of the constricted sinusoidal spaces. Specific treatment for damaged innervation has not been determined.

Rupture of the Penile Suspensory Ligaments

The paired suspensory ligaments of the penis support the proximal shaft of this organ through attachments to the ventral pelvis. Rupture of this suspensory apparatus is very rare.[10] The affected penis develops a characteristic ventral bow proximal to the prepuce; phimosis with secondary preputial dermatitis from urine scalding may occur. Treatment consists of reapposition of the torn edges of the suspensory ligament.[30] The effect of this disorder on stallion reproductive performance is not known due to its infrequent occurrence.

Penile Hematoma

Penile hematomas usually result from blunt trauma to the erect penis during breeding. Usually this occurs from a kick by an unreceptive mare or inadvertent bending of the penis during intromission. Delayed deflection of a stallion's penis away from a breeding phantom during semen collection can cause penile trauma. Improper use of an artificial vagina also may produce a penile hematoma, by acute penile bending, particularly in vigorous-breeding stallions.

Penile hematomas in stallions rarely result from rupture of the tunica albuginea that envelops the corpus cavernosum penis, as occurs in bulls. Rather, hemorrhage generally emanates from ruptured vessels of the rich venous plexus lying on the dorsum of the penis superficial to the cavernous tissue. Hemorrhage from these vessels causes rapid swelling at various locations along the length of the penis, often beginning beneath the internal laminae of the prepuce (Figs 19, 20). In many instances, the swelling becomes so pronounced that the penis no longer can be retracted. Extravasation of blood is attended by venous congestion, lymphatic obstruction and inflammation, exacerbating swelling. Progressive preputial and scrotal edema also develop. For this reason, paraphimosis is a common sequel to untreated penile hematomas.

Treatment is directed at countering hemorrhage, penile swelling and paraphimosis. Initially, compression bandages are applied to the penis to reduce hemorrhage. Local application of cold packs also is indicated, as described in the section entitled Scrotal Trauma, Chapter 7. If the hematoma continues to expand despite treatment, rupture of the tunica albuginea should be suspected, and the site of the hematoma should be surgically

Figure 19. Penile hematoma, with extravasation of blood into the subcutaneous tissue of the prepuce and penis (arrows).

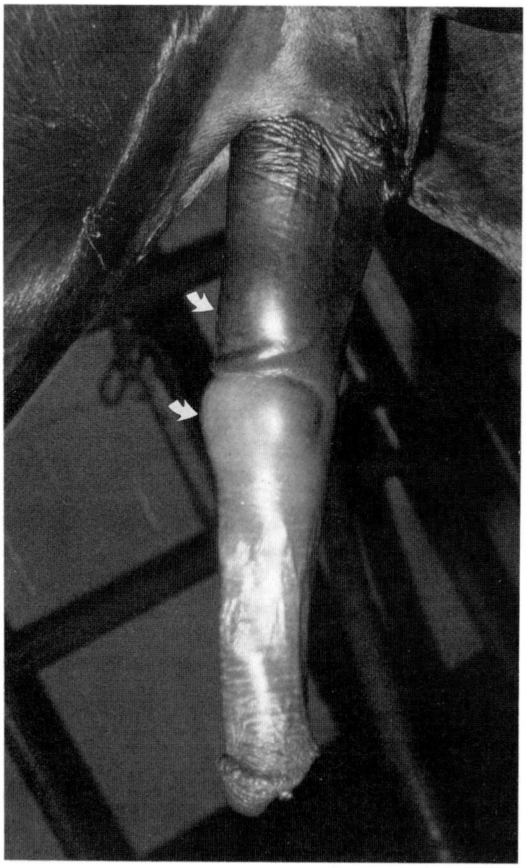

Figure 20. Penile hematoma, with extravasation of blood into the subcutis of the proximal prepuce (arrow).

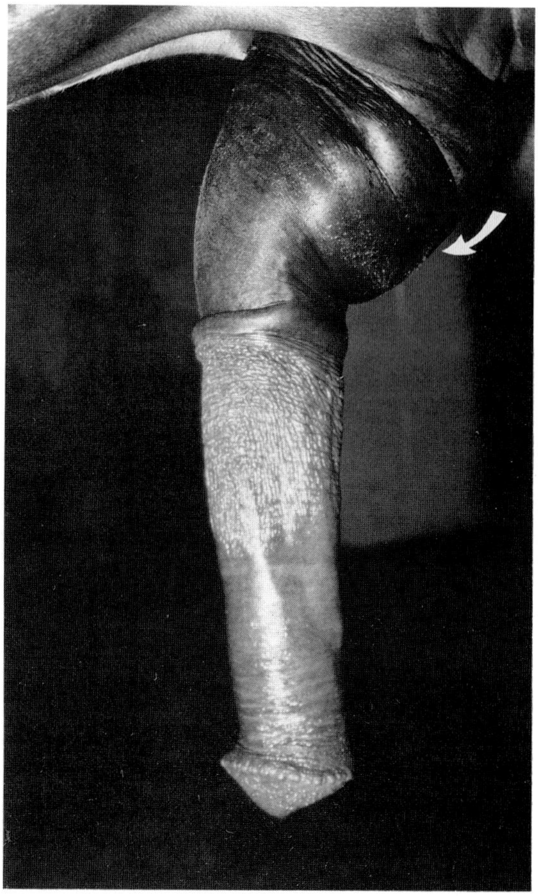

explored. Failure to repair ruptures of the tunica albuginea could result in shunts between erectile tissue and dorsal veins of the penis, producing dysfunction of the erectile mechanism.

Systemic antiinflammatory and diuretic medications are given to help control inflammation and edema. Efforts are made to reduce the swelling sufficiently so the penis can be replaced within the preputial cavity. Specific treatment methods for managing the prolapsed penis are discussed in the section above on Paraphimosis.

Once the acute phase of the injury has subsided and the penis can be retracted voluntarily, efforts should be made to minimize formation of subcutaneous fibrous tissue that can invade areas of hemorrhage and inflammatory edema. Daily penile massage with emollients is recommended to maintain tissue pliability. Three weeks after initial injury, the stallion should be exposed to a mare to evaluate the integrity of the penis during erection. Residual fibrous tissue often creates adhesions that, in turn, produce directional deviation of the penis during erection (Fig 21). Penile deviations should be treated by daily manipulation of the erect penis, which involves gentle pulling of the penis back into its normal position to override the restricted extension caused by scar tissue. The penile hematoma also can produce local nerve damage, causing hypoesthesia or anesthesia of the penis distal to the injury. There is no treatment for this complication. Nerve damage obviously interferes with sexual function in breeding stallions.

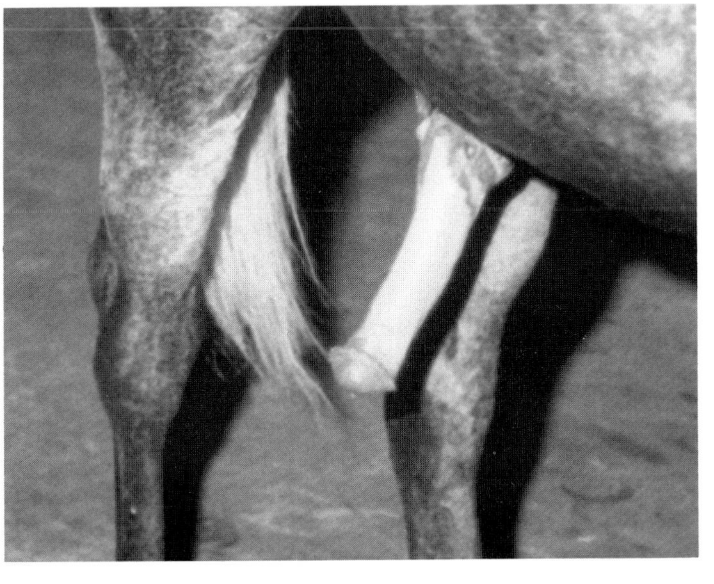

Figure 21. Lateral deviation of the penis resulting from fibrous tissue reaction to previous penile trauma (from a kick by the mare during breeding).

Swelling and edema from penile and preputial trauma may be sufficient to interfere with testis thermoregulation. Stallions may be oligospermic or azoospermic after penile healing is complete, with spermatozoal output not returning to normal for up to several months following the onset of the injury.

Smegma Accumulation

Secretions of the preputial sebaceous and sweat glands combine with dirt and desquamated epithelial cells to form a gray to black caseous, foul-smelling and often putty-like substance termed smegma. Smegma accumulates on the surface of the prepuce and penis (Fig 22). If penile hygiene is ignored, excessive amounts of smegma collect on the prepuce and penis, occasionally becoming impacted within the 3 recesses of the fossa glandis on the distal end of the penis (Fig 23). Irritation caused by retained smegma can produce low-grade balanoposthitis. In fact, it has been postulated that smegma is carcinogenic and may predispose stallions to squamous-cell carcinomas of the prepuce and penis.[11] Abnormally large accumulations of smegma within the recesses of the fossa glandis may evoke some discomfort during urination or possibly ejaculation.

The penis and prepuce of geldings and stallions should occasionally be cleansed with warm water. Generally, use of soaps is discouraged. The sudsing action of various soaps aids removal of smegma, but it may remove the normal bacterial flora of the

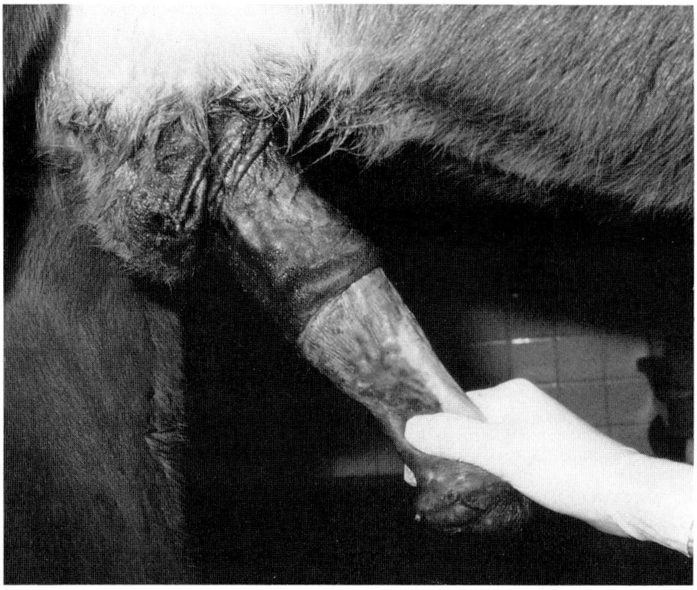

Figure 22. Excessive smegma accumulation on the surface of the proximal prepuce of a middle-aged gelding.

Figure 23. Formed masses of smegma recovered from the diverticula within the fossa glandis of a stallion's penis.

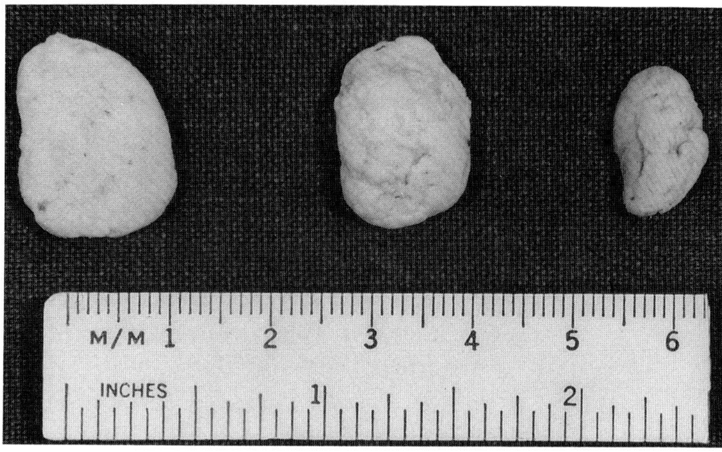

penis, causing overgrowth of potentially pathogenic organisms, such as *Pseudomonas aeruginosa* or *Klebsiella pneumoniae*.[58] Because of its emulsifying properties, dioctyl sodium sulfosuccinate has been used infrequently to remove smegma from the penis and prepuce. The effects of this product on the skin's integrity and bacterial flora have not been studied. It is generally considered innocuous when used once or twice a year.

Inflammatory, Infectious and Immune Diseases

Coital Exanthema

Coital exanthema is a viral venereal disease of horses. The causative agent, equine herpesvirus-3 (EHV-3), is antigenically distinct from the other equine herpesviruses, EHV-1 (rhinopneumonitis virus) and EHV-2 (cytomegalovirus). Lesions generally are confined to the external genitalia of stallions and mares. The penis and prepuce are the most commonly affected areas of stallions. The course of the disease follows a predictable pattern. Lesions begin as small (5-15 mm), white to gray, discrete circumscribed vesicles or pustules that often become confluent (Fig 24). Within a few days, the vesicles and pustules rupture to form superficial ulcers. Edematous genital swelling is uncommon but sometimes follows.

The clinical disease typically is self-limiting, with complete resolution within 3-5 weeks. Focal areas of depigmentation may remain. Similar lesions occur on the surface of the vulva and vestibule of infected mares. Though an uncommon feature, coincident extragenital lesions have been observed in a mare with lesions around the mouth and nostrils.[32] Infected horses infrequently develop transient fever and lethargy. Infection of horses with EHV-3 has not been documented to cause infertility or abortion under natural circumstances;[33] however, some investigators believe that susceptible mares bred to stallions infected with EHV-3 may have a lowered conception rate for that cycle.[34]

Clinical disease usually is observed during the breeding season, as virus transmission occurs through genital contact. Though coitus is the major pathway of disease transmission for stallions, mares may become infected following artificial insemination or possibly by examination per rectum using contaminated rectal sleeves. Flies have been proposed as mechanical vectors of the virus, but this mode of transmission has not been confirmed.[35]

Treatment consists of sexual rest and daily applications of protective emollients, as the lesions are quite painful during the acute phase of the disease. Secondary bacterial infection is a rare

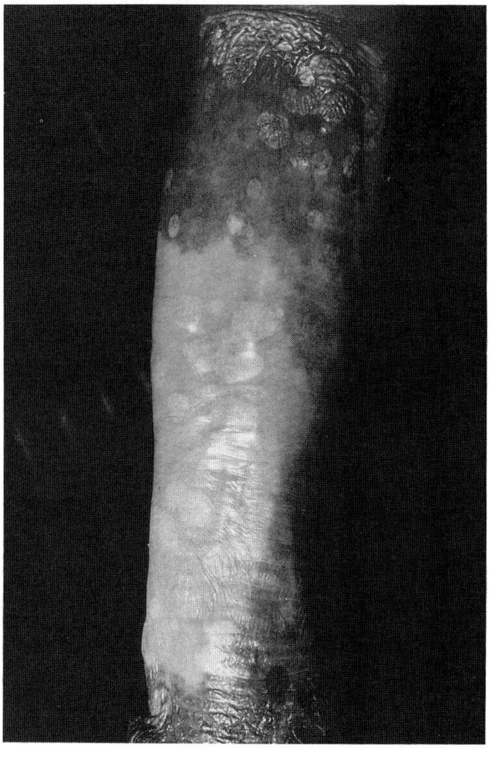

Figure 24. Lesions of coital exanthema on the penile body of a breeding stallion.

complicating factor. The antiviral compound, acyclovir, used to treat *herpes simplex* and *varicella/zoster* infections in people, has not been adapted for use against EHV-3, primarily because of its expense and the transient nature of this disease in horses. Sexual rest should be observed until genital lesions are healed completely to minimize the likelihood of disease transmission. To keep a stallion from breeding for such a long time puts considerable pressure on stallion managers. Alternatively, semen can be collected in an artificial vagina, preferably using an open-ended model (see Chapter 4), after the acute (painful) phase of the disease has subsided.

Mares are inseminated artificially in an attempt to lessen the chance for disease transmission; however, breed regulations regarding breeding policy must be acknowledged.

Recurrence of equine coital exanthema in previously infected stallions has not been critically studied. It has been postulated that disease propagation can result from coitus with clinically normal carrier mares. The virus possibly remains in the latent form in infected horses, with occasional recrudescence occurring spontaneously or in immunocompromised horses.[35] Complement fixation and serum neutralization antibodies peak 2-3 weeks following infection. Complement-fixation antibodies decrease rapidly thereafter, but serum-neutralization antibodies persist for at least a year, providing sustained serologic evidence of infection.[35]

Contagious Equine Metritis

Taylorella equigenitalis, the causative agent of contagious equine metritis (CEM), is the only bacterium known to consistently produce venereal disease in horses. This microaerophilic Gram-negative coccobacillus was unrecognized before its isolation during a disease outbreak in European Thoroughbreds in 1977.[36] It since has been recovered from a large number of infected horses, primarily Thoroughbreds, in several countries, including the United States. The global distribution of CEM has not been mapped thoroughly because the methods of culture are somewhat complex and are not available in all countries. *Taylorella equigenitalis* is very fastidious, requiring a selective medium and special incubation conditions for successful *in-vitro* cultivation.

Contagious equine metritis is highly contagious, with horizontal transmission occurring primarily via coitus. The disease has been spread inadvertently by unhygienic reproductive management practices, such as handling mare and stallion genitalia without disposable gloves or using contaminated veterinary instruments. *Taylorella equigenitalis* has been isolated from placentas and newborn foals, indicating a vertical mode of disease transmission.[37,38]

The disease causes temporary infertility of mares. These mares typically develop a copious vulvar discharge a few days following coitus (or other means of disease contraction). Outward signs of endometritis/cervicitis/vaginitis occasionally are not evident, but the diestrous period is reduced, suggesting endometrial irritation. The clinical signs of disease tend to dissipate within 2 weeks of infection, but the organism can persist in the reproductive tract for prolonged periods, especially in the clitoral sinuses, clitoral fossa, oviducts and ovarian surface.[36,39] Such mares become inapparent carriers of the disease. In marked contrast to mares, stallions never become clinically infected upon genital exposure to *Taylorella equigenitalis*. Rather, they serve as asymptomatic carriers of the organism. If untreated, *Taylorella equigenitalis* can persist on the surface of the penis and prepuce indefinitely, but migration of the organism to the internal genital organs has not been reported.

Diagnosis of CEM is especially difficult in stallions because lesions and clinical signs associated with the disease are absent. In addition, serologic methods of diagnosis are unsuccessful in stallions because superficial contamination of the external genitalia does not stimulate a humoral response. Confirmation of the disease in stallions usually is based on bacterial isolation from the external genitalia. Culture swabs are obtained from the urethral sinus (within the fossa glandis), urethra, penile skin and preputial folds. Preejaculatory fluid also should be collected for bacteriologic culture, if possible. All swabs must be placed in Amies' transport medium separately, then shipped to an appropriate diagnostic laboratory within 24 hours. Samples should be cooled (4 C), but not frozen, during shipment to the laboratory.

The environmental and commensal bacteria that flourish on the external genitalia of stallions tend to inhibit growth of *Taylorella equigenitalis* on culture plates, making isolation of the organism difficult. To overcome the problems of bacterial isolation, suspect stallions also should be bred to properly screened test mares. These mares are examined bacteriologically and serologically postbreeding to detect disease transmission.

Some "positive" stallions may not transmit the disease to all test mares, probably because of the site of bacterial seclusion within the deep recesses of the fossa glandis. An additional diagnostic approach, which follows, has been proposed to reduce the likelihood of false-negative results.[40] Smegma, collected from the urethral fossa of suspect stallions, is mixed with 30 ml sterile saline and inoculated into the uterus of selected test mares, using an insemination pipette. The test mares are examined bacteriologically and serologically for disease transmission.

Treatment of infected stallions has been quite successful. The extruded penis and prepuce are washed thoroughly for 5 minutes daily with chlorhexidine solution (Nolvasan: Fort Dodge, at least a 2% solution) for 5 consecutive days. Particular attention is given to cleansing the 3 recesses of the fossa glandis, as they are primary sites of infection. Following each cleansing session, the penis and prepuce are dried and coated liberally with an ointment containing nitrofurazone (Bactofur: Whitney). This treatment did not impair semen quality of stallions, even though penile washing with chlorhexidine in a separate study was associated with decreased motility and an increased incidence of morphologic aberrations in stallion spermatozoa.[41,42] Large doses of nitrofurantoin have also been found to be gonadotoxic in men.[43]

Constant surveillance programs are required to prevent dissemination of CEM, both domestically and internationally. Isolation and prompt treatment of infected horses are mandatory to containment of the disease, and must be directed by appropriate federal authorities. If the disease is suspected, federal veterinarians must be contacted immediately.

Bacterial Colonization

The surface of the stallion's penis and prepuce normally is inhabited by a variety of commensal bacteria that cause unavoidable contamination of the mare's reproductive tract at the time of coitus. These bacteria constitute the normal microflora of the stallion's external genitalia and rarely produce genital infection in immunologically competent mares. Occasionally the normal bacterial flora is disrupted, and potentially pathogenic bacteria colonize the penis and prepuce. Though these organisms rarely produce clinical disease in stallions, they can be transmitted to the mare's genital tract at the time of breeding, causing infectious endometritis and associated infertility. *Pseu-*

domonas aeruginosa and *Klebsiella pneumoniae* are the most common venereal pathogens. Both are common environmental organisms and, as such, easily can gain access to the external genitalia of the stallion.

Factors that precipitate accumulation of opportunistic pathogens on the surface of the external genitalia have not been determined. Some investigators contend that the normal bacterial microflora of the stallion's external genitalia combats proliferation of pathogens and that frequent washing of the penis, especially with soap, removes these nonpathogenic resident organisms, increasing the susceptibility of the penis and prepuce to colonization by potentially pathogenic organisms.[44,45] Other workers dispute this philosophy, asserting that repeated washing of the external genitalia alone does not contribute to overgrowth of potential pathogens.[46] The environment in which a stallion is housed possibly can influence the type of organisms harbored on the external genitalia. The organisms also can be acquired at the time of coitus with a mare with a genital infection.

Bacterial colonization of a stallion's external genitalia by pathogens usually is suspected if postcoital endometritis and infertility are noted in a high percentage of mares bred. Bacteriologic culture of the fossa glandis, free portion of the penile body, and folds of the external lamina of the prepuce provides an overall perspective of the microbial population.[47] However, interpretation of the bacteriologic findings can be quite difficult. For instance, *Pseudomonas aeruginosa* and/or *Klebsiella pneumoniae,* though usually not in pure culture, often are isolated from the external genitalia of stallions with normal fertility. Most often they represent a small proportion of a mixed bacterial population. It also is important to recognize that the virulence of the various serotypes of *Pseudomonas aeruginosa* and *Klebsiella pneumoniae* apparently differ.[48,49] *Klebsiella pneumoniae* capsular types 1 and 5 are considered the most virulent of this species. Similar information is not available for *Pseudomonas aeruginosa.*

If a stallion harbors suspected bacterial pathogens on the external genital organs, the most reliable approach to determining their pathogenicity is to test breed the stallion to suitable maiden mares. These mares subsequently are examined for pregnancy 12-15 days postovulation using transrectal ultrasonography. If they are confirmed nonpregnant or display an abnormal vulvar discharge in the early postbreeding period, their bacteriologic status should be examined. Mares infected at breeding occasionally display shortened interestrus intervals;[50] however, mares with normal immunologic uterine resistance mechanisms often eliminate the infection from the reproductive tract soon after breeding, so bacteriologic cultures may be uninformative.[50-53]

If a stallion is a confirmed carrier of bacteria that cause genital disease in mares, managerial adjustments must be made to maintain the stallion in the breeding program. The best corrective measure is artificial insemination (AI). Semen, collected with an artificial vagina, is mixed with a semen extender containing antibiotics selected by bacterial susceptibility before mare insemination.[54] The penis and prepuce of the stallion are washed thoroughly, then rinsed and dried before semen collection to minimize contamination of the ejaculate with the pathogenic bacteria. Semen collection using an open-ended artificial vagina yields a more bacteria-free ejaculate, if the bacteria are limited to the external genitalia.[55,56] Of course, these procedures can be used only in breeds whose registries approve breeding by AI.

In breeds that do not permit AI, control of disease transmission becomes more difficult because bacterial contamination of the mare's reproductive tract is inevitable at the time of coitus. Before breeding, the stallion's penis and prepuce are washed thoroughly with a povidone-iodine scrub, then rinsed and dried to minimize bacterial inoculation of the mare's reproductive tract during coitus. In addition, immediately before breeding, the uterus of the mare is infused with 100-125 ml of semen extender containing appropriate antibiotics.[50] At 4-6 hours after breeding and/or 1-3 days postovulation, uterine lavage may be indicated to control bacterial endometritis. [57,58] Uterine lavage before 4 hours postbreeding may reduce pregnancy rates in mares.[59]

Once a stallion's penis becomes colonized with pathogenic bacteria, it is very difficult to reestablish the normal bacterial microflora. Use of systemic antibiotics to control the problem almost always is unsuccessful. Daily cleansing of the penis and prepuce (as described above), followed by local application of antibacterial ointments or creams, helps control bacterial growth. Use of emollients also protects the integument against chafing and cracking induced by frequent cleansing. Local ap-

process. Granulomatous lesions may become friable and bleed when handled. Stretching of the urethral process during penile engorgement and ejaculation may result in hemospermia. Small yellow caseous masses, composed primarily of eosinophils and nematode larvae, are present throughout the granulation tissue. These masses help differentiate this disease from other vegetative lesions, such as squamous-cell carcinoma, sarcoids and exuberant granulomas.[68-70]

Definitive diagnosis is by identifying the larvae or their tracts microscopically. Impression smears of crust-free lesions occasionally confirm the presence of larvae when prepared with Wright's stain; larvae are difficult to identify, however, in smear preparations.[67,68] Biopsies taken from both caseous and granulomatous areas of lesions are usually required to confirm the diagnosis. Histologic sections of infested tissue generally reveal numerous dead eosinophils surrounding cross sections of larvae and multiple caseous granules throughout the granulomatous tissue. Biopsies are required to differentiate cutaneous habronemiasis from sarcoids and squamous-cell carcinoma because ulcerating neoplasms attract flies and may become secondarily infected with parasitic larvae.[68-70]

Treatment is directed at reducing hypersensitivity to the larvae and eliminating larvae from the wound. Antiinflammatory drugs, such as diethylcarbamazine or corticosteroids, usually alleviate the foreign-body reaction against the larvae.[64] Organophosphate insecticides are often administered intrale-

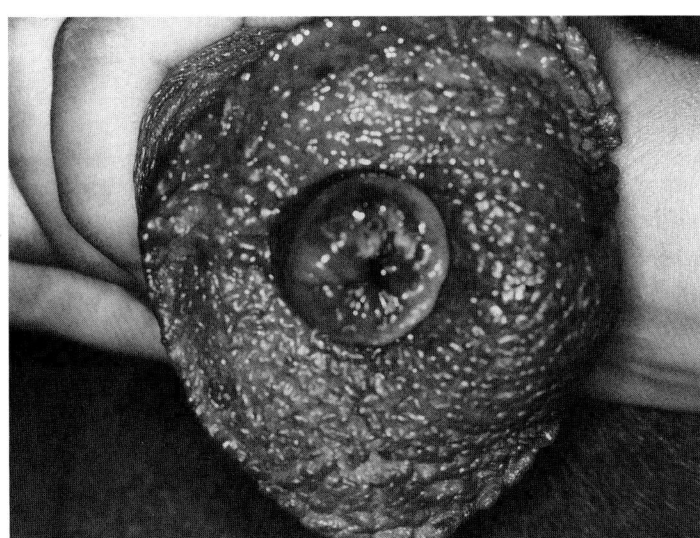

Figure 26. Caseous masses associated with cutaneous habronemiasis at the mucocutaneous junction of the distal urethra.

sionally, PO, IV or topically to kill the parasitic larvae.[64] Topical organophosphate therapy of large lesions is often futile. Systemic treatment with organophosphate insecticide, when combined with local therapy, has yielded good results when administered at 2- to 4-week intervals until lesions are healed.[64,66,67] Systemic treatment with organophosphates is not without risk, and horses should be monitored for signs of organophosphate toxicity or other adverse reactions.[64,71]

Ivermectin is reported to prevent and cure cutaneous habronemiasis, due to its larvicidal activity. Intramuscular administration of ivermectin (0.2 mg/kg) kills most larvae and leads to rapid clinical improvement (within 1 week) and resolution (within 1-5 weeks) of most *Habronema* lesions.[72] Some horses (about 16%) fail to respond to a single dose of ivermectin and require a second treatment to remove larvae and resolve lesions. Oral administration of ivermectin (0.2 mg/kg) once monthly is reported to result in a similar rate of improvement.[73] Early *Habronema* lesions can be expected to respond to a single treatment, while 3 treatments at 10-day intervals are more appropriate for more severe lesions.[74] Large or secondarily infected lesions may require additional therapy, such as cryotherapy or surgical ablation, for complete resolution.[65]

Horses affected concurrently with ventral or scrotal onchocerciasis may develop edematous reactions in affected skin as the *Onchocerca* microfilariae die.[75] Midventral pruritus and edema were reported in 10% of 3616 horses treated with ivermectin in Louisiana.[76] Concurrent administration of corticosteroids may reduce this reaction;[77] however, swelling is reported to regress in 2-3 days even without administration of corticosteroids.[74] If onchocerciasis is suspected, delaying systemic treatment until conclusion of the breeding season may be advisable to avoid the transient adverse effect of scrotal edema on spermatogenesis.

Cryotherapy or surgical removal may be necessary to resolve large or nonresponding *Habronema* granulomas in locations other than on the urethral process. A double freeze-thaw cycle, consisting of a quick freeze and unaided thaw followed by a second quick freeze and unaided thaw, has been successful with such lesions.[78] A controlled spray of liquid nitrogen is directed over the lesion until the freeze line extends about 1 cm beyond the perimeter of the lesion, taking care to not freeze too deeply. Extremely large lesions can be frozen in segments. Fly repellent is applied locally until healing is complete to prevent reinfestation. Affected horses are examined one week following treatment to ensure that all portions of the lesion are inactive.

Chronic infestation of the urethral process causes marked periurethral fibrosis, necessitating amputation. Amputation of the urethral process can be performed in the standing horse after infiltration of the base of the urethral process with local anesthetic, or with the horse under general anesthesia.[79] The penis is prepared for aseptic surgery, and the urethra is catheterized to facilitate dissection. Retention needles can be inserted through the urethral process and catheter just caudal to the granuloma to facilitate surgery. A circumferential incision, extending through all the tissue layers, is made around the base of the urethral process, proximal to the lesion. The incision should be beveled so that the epithelium of the urethral process is slightly larger than the mucosa. The urethral mucosa is sutured to the skin of the stump of the urethral process, using 2-0 absorbable material in a simple-interrupted pattern. By beveling, the circumferential incision in the outer epithelial surface of the urethral process is rolled inward to prevent mucosal eversion, which predisposes to injury of the urethral mucosa after healing. On followup examinations, remaining hemorrhagic or ulcerative lesions can be lightly cauterized with silver nitrate sticks. Sexual rest is indicated until lesions have healed sufficiently to avoid interference with breeding or fertility. Cicatrization associated with the surgery can result in bleeding during ejaculation because the scar tissue may tear during maximal erection.

To prevent reinfestation, fly control with baits or spray insecticides is necessary. Manure must be disposed of properly. Wounds or abrasions are protected with bandages and protective ointments that contain insecticides or repellents.[80] Regular cleansing of the prepuce and sheath may prevent development of lesions.[65] Regular deworming with products that control the parasite is indicated. An additional benefit of including ivermectin in the deworming program is that reactions to *Onchocerca* microfilariae seldom occur after the first treatment.[74]

Squamous Papilloma

(Warts)

Squamous papillomas may occur on the penis or prepuce of horses, though their incidence is very low. Papovaviruses are thought to incite their development. See Neoplasia below for further discussion of squamous papillomas.

Neoplasia

Squamous-Cell Carcinoma

Squamous-cell carcinoma, derived from statified squamous epithelium, is the most common neoplasm of the external genitalia, and originates primarily on the glans penis or internal lamina of the prepuce.[1,81,82] Penile and preputial squamous-cell carcinoma occurs most commonly in aged horses and is most prevalent in breds with nonpigmented genitalia, such as American Paint Horses and Appaloosas. Lack of pigmentation may predispose to carcinoma of the external genitalia, even though these tissues are rarely exposed to direct sunlight.[83]

Smegma has been suggested to be a factor in development of the neoplasm.[84] It may provoke malignant change by causing chronic irritation, or it may actually contain carcinogens.[85] Bacteria in smegma may convert the cholesterol in smegma into a carcinogen. Smegma applied to the skin, vagina and cervix of mice has induced neoplasia;[84,85] yet, a carcinogenic effect of smegma on equine epithelium has not been demonstrated. Because smegma may cause squamous-cell carcinoma, geldings and older horses may be predisposed to the disease because they tend to accumulate more smegma than do stallions and young horses.

The neoplasms may initially appear as a small, keratinized plaques on the genitalia. Being invasive, they generally develop into a shallow, crested, ulcerative lesions that become necrotic and foul smelling.[62] Papillary growths of varying sizes may also develop, some of which have a cauliflower-like appearance (Figs 27-29).[62] Penile or preputial lesions with these characteristics should be considered a squamous-cell carcinoma until proven otherwise. Extensive proliferative growths associated with squamous-cell carcinoma may mechanically interfere with copulation. Advanced lesions may result in protrusion of the penis from, or retention within, the preputial cavity. Impingement of the urethra by the neoplasm may cause dysuria. Squamous-cell carcinomas involving the penis or prepuce tend to grow slowly and remain localized until late in the course of the disease, then invade other sites of the preputial cavity. Metastasis may eventually occur, primarily to the superficial and deep inguinal lymph nodes. Metastasis to distant systemic sites (lung or liver) is rare.[82,86]

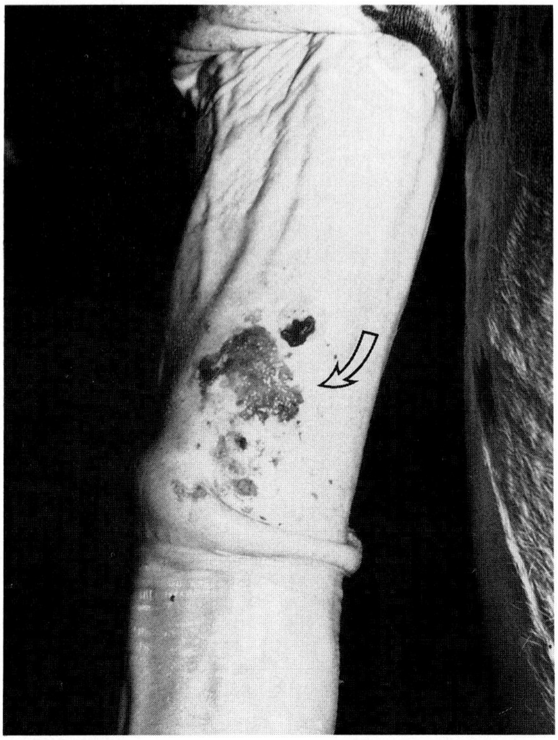

Figure 27. Squamous-cell carcinoma involving the prepuce of a stallion (arrow).

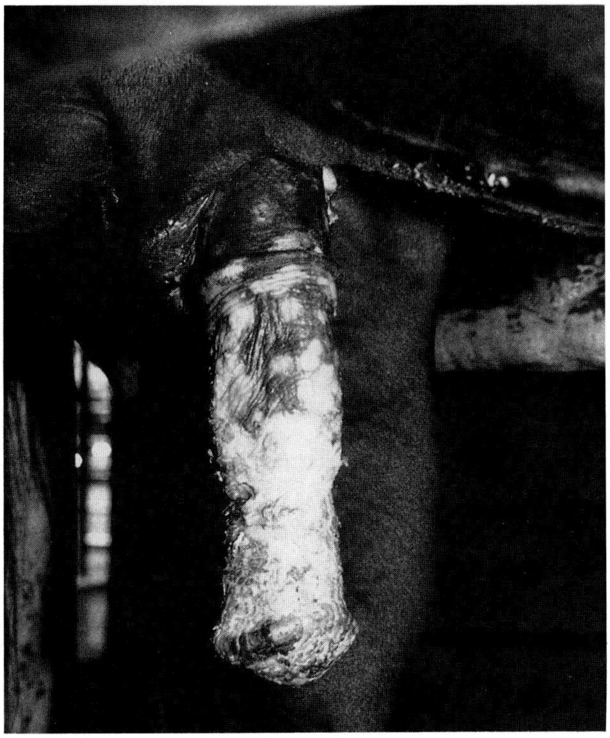

Figure 28. Diffuse involvement of a gelding's penis with lesions of squamous-cell carcinoma. (Courtesy of Dr. J.R. Joyce)

Definitive diagnosis of squamous-cell carcinoma is based on histologic examination of a biospy. The neoplasm is usually well differentiated and characterized by irregular cords (rete pegs) consisting of large epithelial cells, with intercellular bridges, that penetrate the dermis (Fig 30), and formation of keratin "pearls" (Fig 31).[86,87] The neoplasm is often surrounded by inflammatory cells, and may contain areas of calcification or necrosis. Secondary invasion by *Habronema* larvae is also possible.

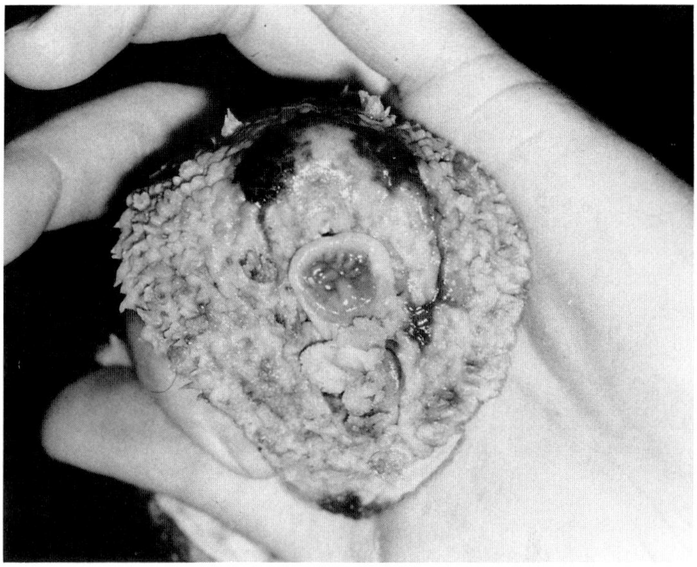

Figure 29. Papillary growths of squamous-cell carcinoma involving the distal penis.

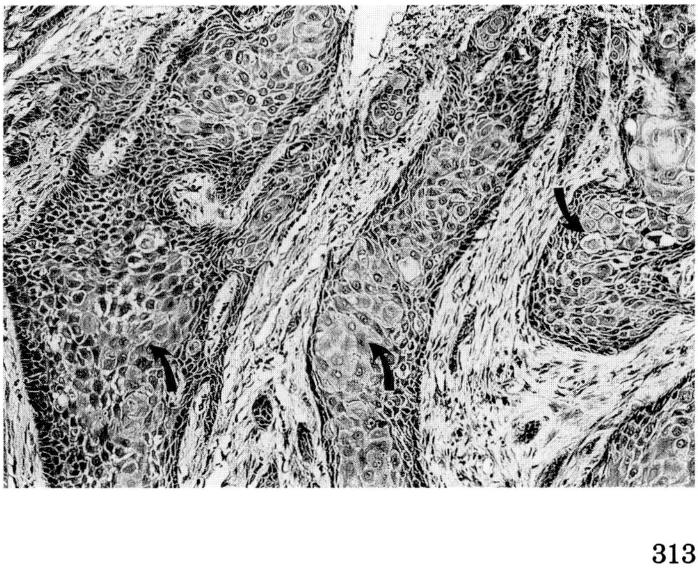

Figure 30. Histologic section of a squamous-cell carcinoma involving the skin of a horse's penis. Note the prominent rete pegs containing neoplastic epithelial cells (arrows). (hematoxylin & eosin, 10X magnification) (Courtesy of Dr. J.F. Edwards)

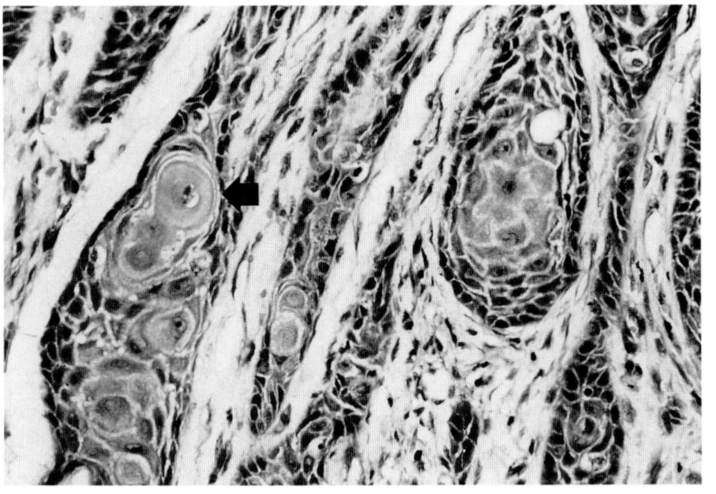

Figure 31. Histologic section of a squamous-cell carcinoma involving the skin of a horse's penis. Note the keratin pearls (arrow), a distinguishing characteristic of this type of tumor. (hematoxylin & eosin, 25X magnification) (Courtesy of Dr. J.F. Edwards)

Treatment may involve cryosurgery, hyperthermia, local excision, reefing operation, and phallectomy. Cryotherapy is generally recommended for early neoplastic lesions.[88,89] Lesions are frozen to -20 to -30 C with liquid nitrogen, either as a spray or cryoprobe. Both depth and degree of freezing should be monitored with a thermocouple. Several (2-3) freeze-thaw cycles are recommended. Fast freezes and slow thaws are thought to be most effective for elimination of the neoplastic tissue. Cryonecrosis of the tumor is caused by direct damage from the cryogen, and from anoxia caused by thrombosis of the microvasculature.

Radiofrequency-induced hyperthermia has been recommended for ocular squamous cell carcinomas, but its use for similar tumors involving the external genitalia has not been reported.[90]

Use of a localized current field radiofrequency (LCF RF) capable of heating the neoplasms to 50 C for 30 seconds caused complete regression of ocular squamous-cell carcinoma in 6 of 8 horses.[90]

In addition to cryotherapy or hyperthermia, small neoplastic lesions can be excised or treated with applications of 5-fluorouracil (an antimetabolite). Usually such lesions go unnoticed, and help is sought only after the lesions become more extensive.

A reefing operation can be performed to excise larger neoplasms involving the internal lamina of the prepuce, if simple excision of the lesions is impossible (see Chapter 15). The amount of internal preputial lamina that can be removed while still preserving copulatory function of the penis has not been determined.

Phallectomy is indicated in horses with lesions too large or numerous to treat using the above approaches. This surgical approach would, of course, be performed to salvage a horse for purposes other than breeding. Reportedly, amputation of only the glans penis may not always interfere with copulation. Methods for performing penile amputation have been discussed above (See Phallectomy).

Horses with extensive neoplastic involvement of the external genitalia may require *en-bloc* resection of the penis, prepuce and superficial inguinal lymph nodes, combined with perineal urethrostomy (See Phallectomy above). The preputial cavity and penis should be meticulously examined for small metastases, and other sites of predilection, such as the nictitating membranes, should be examined for involvement. The superficial and deep inguinal lymph nodes should be palpated for enlargement but it should be kept in mind that lymphadenitis may be due to secondary infection rather than metastasis.

Squamous Papilloma

(Warts)

Squamous papillomas, or warts, are relatively common in horses. They develop only rarely on the penis or prepuce of horses. The neoplasm is generally thought to be caused a papovavirus.[91] Squamous papilloma has been described as a benign form of squamous-cell carcinoma;[92] however, the structural antigens of papovavirus have not been detected in squamous-cell carcinomas.[91,93,94]

Squamous papillomas appear as multiple proliferative cutaneous growths (Figs 32, 33). Histologically they are characterized by benign hyperplasia of epithelium, occasionally with lymphoplasmacytic infiltration.[92] The virus multiplies within the nucleus of epidermal cells, sometimes invading the cytoplasm through the nuclear pores.[62]

Treatment of nongenital squamous papillomas is generally not required because actively acquired immunity results in their spontaneous regression within 1-6 months. A variety of topical agents have been used for treatment of nongenital squamous papillomas, including podophyllin cream, DMSO, retinoic acid

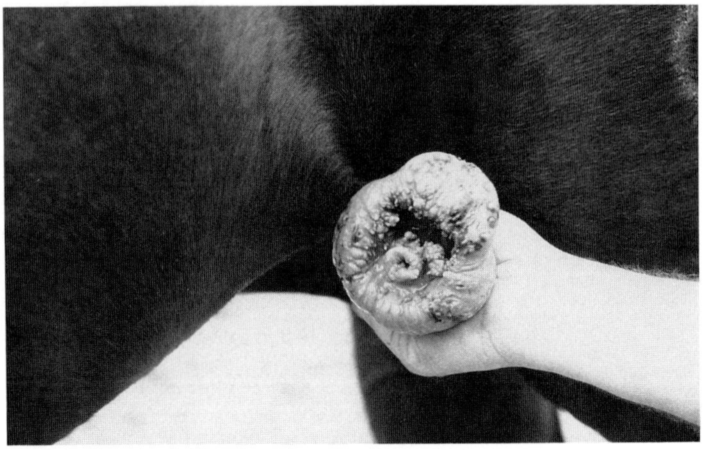

Figure 32. Fibrous papillomas involving the distal penis.

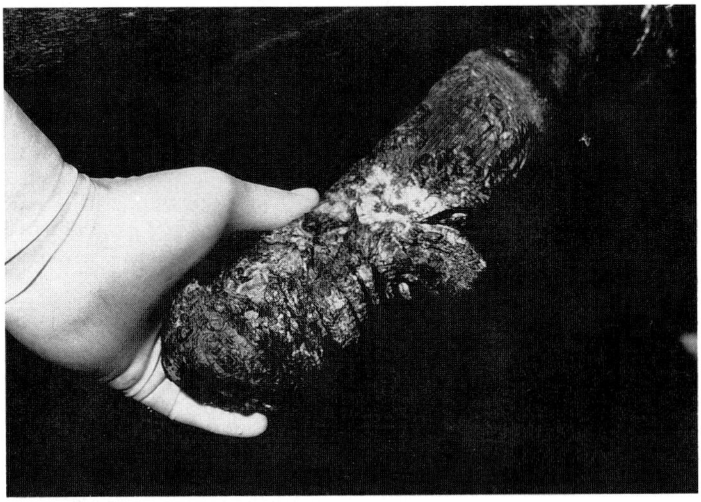

Figure 33. Diffuse involvement of a stallion's penis with fibrous papillomas.

cream, castor oil and glacial acetic acid.[62,91] Excision and cryotherapy are also reported to be successful for removal of isolated papillomas.[91] Use of autogenous vaccines for treatment of squamous papillomas has not been critically investigated. In contrast to nongenital squamous papillomas, genital forms generally are quite refractory to treatment. These tumors are found on the external genitalia of horses only rarely.

References

1. Walker DF and Vaughan JT: *Bovine and Equine Urogenital Surgery*. Lea & Febiger, Philadelphia, 1980. pp 105-182.

2. Memon MA *et al:* Penile paralysis and paraphimosis associated with reserpine administration in a stallion. *Theriogenology* 28: In press, 1990.

3. Whittle BA and Crooks JL: Penile prolapse with immobilon. *Vet Record* 101:312, 1977.

4. Wheat JD: Penile paralysis in stallions given propiopromazine. *JAVMA* 148:405-406, 1966.

5. Lucke JN and Sansom J: Penile erection in the horse after acepromazine.*Vet Record* 105:21-22, 1979.

6. Gerring EL: Priapism and ACP in the horse. *Vet Record* 109:64, 1981.

7. Pearson H and Weaver BMQ: Priapism after sedation, neuroleptanalgesia and anaesthesia in the horse. *Equine Vet J* 10:85-90, 1978.

8. Simmons HA *et al:* Paraphimosis in seven debilitated horses. *Vet Record* 116:126-127, 1985.

9. Taylor TS and Bowen JM: Personal communication, 1986.

10. Bolz W: The prophylaxis and therapy of prolapse and paralysis of the penis occuring in the horse after administration of neuroleptics. *Vet Med Rev* (Leverkusen) 4:255-263, 1970.

11. Roberts SJ: *Veterinary Obstetrics and Genital Diseases.* David & Charles, North Pomfret, VT, 1986. pp 752-893.

12. Ambache N and Killick SW: Species differences in postganglionic motor transmission to the retractor penis muscle. *Brit J Pharm* 63:25-34, 1978.

13. Nickel R *et al: The Viscera of Domestic Animals.* Springer-Verlag, New York, 1973. pp 303-349.

14. Schumacher J *et al:* Pudendal and caudal rectal nerve blocks in the horse-an anesthetic procedure for reproductive surgery. *Theriogenology* 24:457-464, 1985.

15. Magda II: Local anesthesia in operations on the male perineum in horses. *JAVMA* 113:559, 1948.

16. Hinman F: Priapism: reasons for failure of therapy. *J Urol* 83:420-428, 1960.

17. Pohl J *et al:* Priapism: a three-phase concept of management according to aetiology and prognosis. *Brit J Urol* 58:113-118, 1986.

18. Dorman BW and Schmidt JD: Association of priapism in phenothiazine therapy. *J Urol* 116:51-53, 1976.

19. Sharrock AG: Reversal of drug-induced priapismin a gelding by medication. *Aust Vet J* 58:39-40.

20. Schumacher J and Hardin DK: Surgical treatment of priapism in a stallion. *Vet Surgery* 16:193-196, 1987.

21. Lue TF *et al:* Priapism: a refined approach to diagnosis and treatment. *J Urol* 136:104-108, 1986.

22. Falk D and Loos DC: Spongiocavernosum shunt in the surgical treatment of idiopathic persistent priapism. *J Urol* 108:101-103, 1972.

23. Hurtgen JP, in Robinson NE: *Current Therapy in Equine Medicine 2.* Saunders, Philadelphia, 1987. pp 558-563.

24. Berge E and Westhues M: *Veterinary Operative Surgery.* Williams & Wilkins, Baltimore, 1966. pp 273-277.

25. Kersjes AW *et al: Atlas of Large Animal Surgery.* Williams & Wilkins, Baltimore, 1985. pp 51-82.

26. Scott EA: A technique for amputation of the equine penis. *JAVMA* 168:1047-1051, 1976.

27. Williams WL: *Diseases of the Genital Organs of Domestic Animals.* 3rd ed. Ethel William Plimpton, Worcester, MA, 1950. pp 218-221,436-437.

28. Markel MD *et al:* Genital neoplasms treated by en bloc resection and penile retroversion in horses: 10 cases (1977-1986). *JAVMA* 192:396-400, 1988.

29. Voss JL and Pickett BW: Diagnosis and treatment of haemospermia in the stallion. *J Reprod Fertil* 23:151-154, 1975.

30. Swanstrom OG and Krahwinkel DJ: Preputial hernia in a horse. *VM/SAC* 69:870-871, 1974.

31. Bowen JM *et al:* Effects of washing on the bacterial flora of the stallion's penis. *J Reprod Fertil* 32:41-45, 1982.

32. Krogsrud J and Onstad O: Equine coital exanthema: isolation of a virus and transmission experiments. *Acta Vet Scand* 12:1-14, 1971.

33. Pascoe RR: The effect of equine coital exanthema on the fertility of mares covered by stallions exhibiting the clinical disease. *Aust Vet J* 57:111-114, 1981.

34. Bitsch V: Cases of equine coital exanthema in Denmark. *Acta Vet Scand* 13:281-283, 1972.

35. Pascoe RR and Bagust TJ: Coital exanthema in stallions. *J Reprod Fertil* 23:147-150, 1975.

36. Powell DG, in Morrow DA: *Current Therapy in Theriogenology 2.* Saunders, Philadelphia, 1986. pp 786-792.

37. Powell DG and Whitwell K: The epidemiology of contagious equine metritis (CEM) in England 1977-1978. *J Reprod Fertil* 27:331-335, 1979.

38. Timoney PJ: Isolation of the contagious equine metritis organism from colts and fillies in the United Kingdom and Ireland. *Vet Record* 111:478-482, 1982.

39. Acland HM *et al:* Contagious equine metritis: distribution of organisms in experimental infection of mares. *Am J Vet Res* 44:1197-1202, 1983.

40. Swerczek TW: Contagious equine metritis: test for suspect carriers.*Vet Record* 108:420-421, 1981.

41. Cahill C: Contagious equine metritis in the stallion. *Proc Ann Mtg AAEP,* 1978. pp 279-282.

42. Rath D *et al:* Influence of chlorhexidine on seminal patterns in stallions. *J Reprod Fertil* (Suppl) 35:109-112, 1987.

43. Herlihy R *et al*, in Pryor JP and Lipshulz LI: *Andrology*. Butterworths, Boston, 1987. pp 242-260.

44. Bowen JM *et al:* Effects of washing on the bacterial flora of the stallion's penis. *J Reprod Fertil* 32:41-45, 1982.

45. Swerczek TW: Aggravation of strangles, equine clostridial typhlocolitis (colitis X) and bacterial venereal diseases in the horse by antibacterial drugs. *Proc Ann Mtg AAEP*, 1979. pp 305-311.

46. Jones RL *et al:* The effect of washing on the aerobic bacterial flora of the stallion's penis. *Proc Ann Mtg AAEP,* 1984. pp 9-16.

47. Cooper WC: Methods of determining the site of bacterial infections in the stallion reproductive tract. *Proc Ann Mtg Soc Theriogenol,* 1979. pp 1-4.

48. Bowen JM, in Robinson NE: *Current Therapy in Equine Medicine 2.* Saunders, Philadelphia, 1987. pp 567-570.

49. Simpson DJ, in Robinson NE: *Current Therapy in Equine Medicine 2.* Saunders, Philadelphia, 1987. pp 513-516.

50. Blanchard TL *et al:* Use of a semen extender containing antibiotic to improve the fertility of a stallion with seminal vesiculitis due to *Pseudomonas aeruginosa. Theriogenology* 28:541-546, 1987.

51. Hughes PJ and Loy RG: Investigations on the effect of intrauterine inoculations of *Streptococcus zooepidemicus* in the mare. *Proc Ann Mtg AAEP*, 1969. pp 289-292.

52. Peterson FB *et al:* Studies on the pathogenesis of endometritis in the mare. *Proc Ann Mtg AAEP*, 1969. pp 279-287.

53. Varner DD and Blanchard TL: An update on uterine defense mechanisms in the mare. *J Equine Vet Sci* 10:169-175, 1990.

54. Kenney RM *et al:* Minimal contamination techniques for breeding mares: technique and preliminary findings. *Proc Ann Mtg AAEP,* 1975. pp 327-336.

55. Tischner M *et al:* Analysis of the pattern of ejaculation in stallions. *J Reprod Fertil* 41:329-335, 1974.

56. McCarthy PF *et al:* A modified "open" artificial vagina and a urethral prosthetic device for the collection of gel-free semen. *Proc Ann Mtg Soc Theriogenol,* 1979. pp 5-9.

57. LeBlanc MM and Asbury AC: Rationale for uterine lavage after breeding in mares. *Proc Ann Mtg AAEP*, 1988. pp 623-628.

58. Brinsko SP *et al:* The effect of uterine lavage four hours post-insemination on pregnancy rate in mares. *Proc Ann Conf Res Workers Anim Dis*, 1989. p 42.

59. Brinsko SP *et al:* The effect of postbreeding uterine lavage on pregnancy rate in mares. *Theriogenology* 33:465-475, 1990.

60. Johnson TL *et al: Pseudomonas* infection in a stallion: a case report. *Proc Ann Mtg AAEP,* 1980. pp 111-116.

61. Kenney RM and Cummings MR: Potential control of stallion penile shedding of *Pseudomonas aeruginosa* and *Klebsiella pneumoniae*. *Proc Symp Voortplanting Paard,* 1990.

62. Montes LF and Vaughan JT: *Atlas of Skin Diseases of the Horse.* Saunders, Philadelphia, 1983. pp 104-111, 132-147.

63. Soulsby EJL: *Helminths, Arthropods and Protozoa of Domesticated Animals.* 7th ed. Bailliere Tindall, London, 1982. pp 285-287.

64. McMullan WC, in Mansmann RA and McAllister ES: *Equine Medicine and Surgery.* 3rd ed. American Veterinary Publications, Goleta, CA, 1982. pp 789-883.

65. Foil L and Foil C: Parasitic skin diseases. *Vet Clin No Am* (Equine Pract) 2: 403-437, 1986.

66. Wheat JD: Treatment of equine summer sores with a systemic insecticide. *Vet Med* 56:477-478, 1961.

67. Scott B and Allen K: Cutaneous habronemiasis. *Missouri Vet* 28:5-7, 1978.

68. Fadock VA and Mullowney PC: Dermatologic diseases of horses Part 1. Parasitic dermatoses of the horse. *Compend Cont Ed Pract Vet* 5:S615-S622, 1983.

69. Miller RI and Campbell RSF: A survey of granulomatous and neoplastic diseases of equine skin in north Queensland. *Aust Vet J* 59:33-37, 1982.

70. Murray DR *et al:* Granulomatous and neoplastic diseases of the skin of horses. *Aust Vet J* 54:338-341, 1978.

71. Steckel RR *et al:* Equine pulmonary habronemiasis with acute hemolytic anemia resulting from organophosphate treatment. *Equine Pract* 5(2):35-39, 1983.

72. Herd RP and Donham JC: Efficacy of ivermectin against cutaneous *Draschia* and *Habronema* infection (summer sores) in horses. *Am J Vet Res* 42:1953-1955, 1981.

73. Bridges ER: The use of ivermectin to treat genital cutaneous habronemiasis in a stallion. *Compend Cont Ed Pract Vet* 7:S94-S97, 1985.

74. Anderson RR: The use of ivermectin in horses: Research and clinical observations. *Compend Cont Ed Pract Vet* 6:S516-S520, 1984.

75. Herd RP and Donham JC: Efficacy of ivermectin against *Onchocerca cervicalis* microfilarial dermatitis in horses. *Am J Vet Res* 44:1102-1105, 1983.

76. Karns PA and Luther DG: A survey of adverse effects associated with ivermectin use in Louisiana horses. *JAVMA* 185:782-783, 1984.

77. Bello TR: Ivermectin from a researcher-clinician viewpoint. *Proc Ann Mtg AAEP,* 1983. pp 328-331.

78. Migiola S *et al:* Cryosurgical treatment of equine cutaneous habronemiasis. *VM/SAC* 73:1073-1076, 1978.

79. Stick JA: Amputation of the equine urethral process affected with habronemiasis. *VM/SAC* 74:1453-1457, 1979.

80. Boyd CL and Bullard TL: Organophosphate treatment of cutaneous habronemiasis in horses. *JAVMA* 153:324, 1968.

81. Baker JR: Histological survey of tumours of the horse, with particular reference to those of the skin. *Vet Record* 96:419-422, 1975.

82. Jubb KVF and Kennedy PC: *Pathology of Domestic Animals.* 2nd ed. Vol 1. Academic Press, New York, 1970. pp 443-485.

83. Akerejola OO *et al:* Equine squamous-cell carcinoma in Northern Nigeria. *Vet Record* 103:336-337, 1978.

84. Plaut A and Kohn-Speyer AC: The carcinogenic action of smegma. *Science* 105: 391-392, 1947.

85. Pratt-Thomas HR *et al:* The carcinogenic effect of human smegma: An experimental study. *Cancer* 9:671-680, 1956.

86. Hall WC *et al:* Tumours of the prostate and penis. *Bull World Health Org* 53: 247-256, 1976.

87. Stannard AA and Pulley LT, in Moulton J: *Tumors of Domestic Animals.* 2nd ed. Univ California Press, Berkeley, 1978. pp 16-74.

88. Stick JA and Hoffer RE: Results of cryosurgical treatment of equine penile neoplasms. *J Reprod Med Surg* 2:505-507, 1978.

89. Joyce JR: Cryosurgical treatment of tumors of horses and cattle. *JAVMA* 177: 226-229, 1976.

90. Grier RL *et al:* Treatment of bovine and equine ocular squamous cell carcinoma by radiofrequency hyperthermia. *JAVMA* 177:56-61, 1980.

91. Scott DW: *Large Animal Dermatology*. Saunders, Philadelphia, 1988. pp 419-467.

92. Ladds PW, in Jubb KVF *et al: Pathology of Domestic Animals*. 3rd ed. Vol 3. Academic Press, New York, 1985. pp 409-459.

93. Junge RE *et al:* Papillomas and squamous cell carcinomas of horses. *JAVMA* 185: 656-659, 1984.

94. Sundberg JP *et al:* Immunoperoxidase localization of papilloma viruses in hyperplastic and neoplastic epithelial lesions of animals. *Am J Vet Res* 45:1441-1446, 1984.

15

Diseases of the Prepuce

Diagnostic and Therapeutic Considerations

Phimosis

Phimosis refers to inability to exteriorize the penis as a result of a congenital or acquired constriction of the preputial orifice/preputial ring, or other local lesion that causes compression/fixation of the penis within the preputial cavity. The free portion of the penis in a newborn colt *normally* is adhered to the internal lamina of the internal prepuce during the first few weeks of postnatal life, resulting in a form of congenital phimosis. During this period, the internal prepuce can be exteriorized voluntarily, but the penis is fixed within the cavity of the internal prepuce. The epithelia of the apposed penile and preputial integuments gradually separate. Complete separation usually occurs 4-6 weeks after birth.[1]

Acquired phimosis usually is secondary to acute or chronic posthitis (preputial inflammation) or space-occupying lesions of the prepuce (abscesses, neoplasia or granulomas).

Acute posthitis often accompanies injury to the prepuce, as well as infections, such as equine coital exanthema and dourine. Inflammatory edema is a common component of acute posthitis and is especially prominent following trauma (Fig 1). Gravitational effects can worsen preputial edema. Excessive preputial edema can induce prolapse of the external prepuce while trapping the penis in the swollen internal prepuce with a constricting preputial ring. If the penis extrudes from the prepuce during an acute inflammatory episode, paraphimosis is likely (see Paraphimosis in Chapter 14).

Preputial edema can be relieved by administration of diuretics, vigorous exercise, cold pack application, and local massage with demulcents. Specific therapeutic principles for edema of the external genitalia have been discussed previously (see Scrotal Trauma in Chapter 7 and Paraphimosis in Chapter 14). Suturing scrotal incisions after castration or premature closure of scrotal incisions that are healing as open wounds can sometimes lead to marked accumulation of serum and blood within the scrotum, especially if the area becomes septic. The attendant scrotal edema often extends to the preputial tissues. If this occurs, drainage should be established in the ventral scrotum, and the therapeutic regimen described for preputial/scrotal edema should be initiated. System antimicrobial therapy and tetanus prophylaxis also are indicated.

The preputial skin can become sclerotic and nonpliable following chronic posthitis, sometimes to the extent that the normal telescoping ability of the prepuce is impaired, affecting protrusion of the penis. Affected horses urinate within the preputial cavity, heightening inflammation. Cicatricial constriction of the preputial orifice and phimosis eventually occur.[2]

Cicatricial constriction of the preputial orifice can be relieved surgically by preputiotomy.[3] A triangular portion of skin is removed from the ventral surface of the sheath (external lamina

Figure 1. Acute posthitis in a stallion from a kick at the time of breeding.

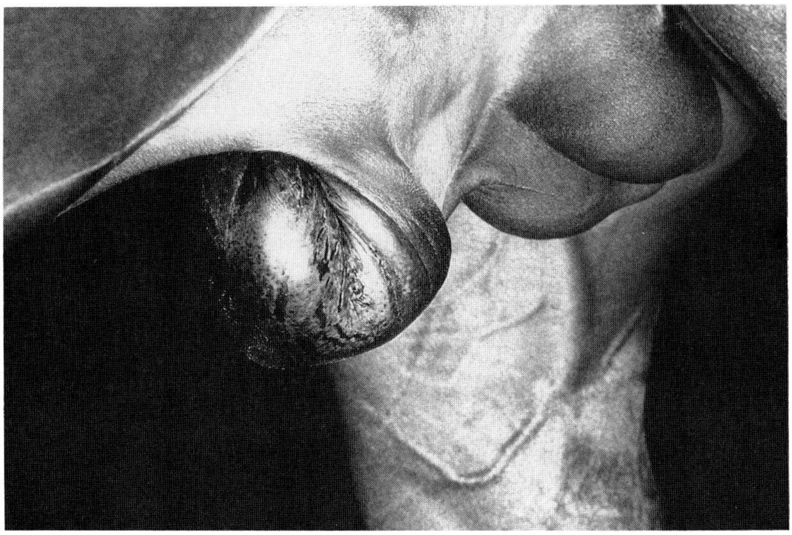

of the external prepuce). The base of the triangular incision is situated at the preputial orifice. The incision is extended down to, but not through, the internal lamina of the external prepuce. This wedge of skin is dissected free from the underlying skin of the internal lamina and discarded. The skin of the internal lamina of the external prepuce is incised on the midline, from the middle of its base to the apex of the formed triangle. The skin of the internal lamina is apposed to the adjacent skin of the external lamina with 2-0 absorbable suture material.

Large neoplastic and granulomatous lesions of the prepuce may compress the contained penis or occlude the preputial orifice sufficiently to prevent penile extrusion. Nonsurgical management of these conditions is a viable option under certain circumstances, but surgical correction often is required.

Preputial Resection

(Reefing Operation, Circumcision, Posthioplasty)

This operative procedure is indicated when diseased preputial skin must be removed circumferentially *en bloc* to restore normal preputial function. The horse is anesthetized and positioned in dorsal or lateral recumbency, and the penis/prepuce are prepared for aseptic surgery. The penis is maintained in extension by traction applied to a length of sterile gauze looped proximal to the glans penis. To facilitate the surgery, a rubber tourniquet is placed tightly around the penis proximal to the surgical site, and the urethra is catheterized. Two circumferential skin incisions are made in the prepuce, marking the proximal and distal borders of the preputial area to be resected. These incisions are connected by a longitudinal skin incision. A plane of tissue dissection is established, parallel to the skin surface, in the loose subcutaneous connective tissue underlying the preputial skin to be removed (Fig 2). The elevated cuff of skin is freed from the underlying tissue and discarded. The tourniquet is loosened to detect vessels requiring ligation. The large branches of the external pudendal artery and vein lying dorsal and lateral to the tunica albuginea of the corpus cavernosum penis are preserved. To establish complete hemostasis, meticulous identification and ligation of bleeding vessels are necessary.

The loose connective tissue underlying the proximal and distal skin incisions is apposed with 2-0 or 0 absorbable suture material in a simple-interrupted pattern. Proper tissue alignment is ensured by initial placement of sutures at four equidis-

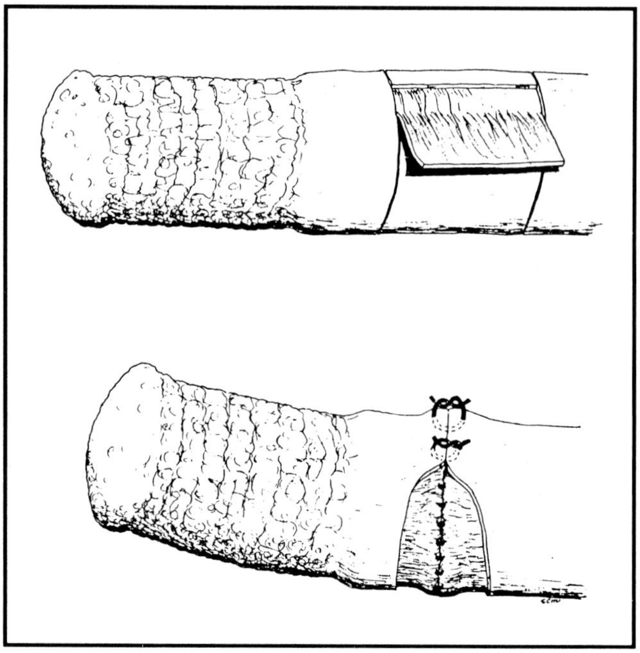

Figure 2. Reefing operation, or circumferential excision of a length of prepuce, with subsequent closure of the preputial defect.

tant points around the penis. The skin is apposed with a simple-interrupted or interrupted horizontal mattress pattern of 2-0 suture material. Either absorbable or nonabsorbable suture material can be used. Nonabsorbable skin sutures should be left in place for 10-14 days. Aftercare consists of daily exercise to reduce edema, and topical and systemic medications to prevent infection of the surgical site. Stallions require strict isolation from mares for 3-4 weeks following surgery. The extent of preputial resection that interferes with a stallion's reproductive performance has not been established. Certainly, variation exists among individual stallions. If possible, radical excision of preputial tissue should be avoided to preserve sexual function.

Congenital or Familial Diseases

Aplasia/Dysgenesis

Preputial aplasia/dysgenesis most commonly is encountered in connection with intersexuality (see Intersexuality). A malformed prepuce also has been observed in genotypic, gonadal and phenotypic stallions with a retroverted penis.[4] This condition is rare, and the cause is unknown.

Diseases with Physical Causes

Preputial Trauma

Preputial trauma, whether blunt or sharp, usually incites acute posthitis that is manifested clinically by rapid and profuse preputial swelling. Because of its dependent position, the prepuce is subject to accumulation of edema following injury. If left untreated, phimosis or paraphimosis may develop, with attendant complications. The edema can extend to the scrotum, disrupting spermatogenesis and epididymal function.

Treatment should be instituted immediately to reduce inflammation and curtail any possible complications. Guidelines for treatment follow those described for scrotal trauma (Chapter 7). Management of phimosis and paraphimosis also has been described previously.

Castration

Excessive preputial edema, phimosis and paraphimosis are possible complications of castration. Therapeutic guidelines are discussed in Chapter 5.

Inflammatory, Infectious and Immune Diseases

Acute Posthitis

Acute inflammation of the prepuce usually occurs with penile inflammation; inflammation of the penis and prepuce is called balanoposthitis. Infectious causes of balanoposthitis are few and include coital exanthema, dourine, microfilariasis (*Onchocerca* and *Setaria*) and possibly treponemiasis. More often, balanoposthitis occurs secondary to trauma, paraphimosis, phimosis, penile paralysis or priapism. These conditions were described previously. Pathogenic or potentially pathogenic organisms can accumulate on the surface of the prepuce and penis without inducing an inflammatory response. See the sections entitled Contagious Equine Metritis and Bacterial Colonization, in Chapter 14 for a full discussion.

Preputial Abscesses

Abscess formation in the prepuce is uncommon but may be a complication of penetrating injuries or a sequel to a systemic infection, especially with *Streptococcus equi* or *Corynebacterium pseudotuberculosis*. *Corynebacterium pseudotuberculosis* typically causes equine ulcerative lymphangitis of the distal limbs. In various parts of the country, however, the equine biotype of *C pseudotuberculosis* has been identified as the causative agent of large abscesses in the pectoral, ventral abdominal and inguinal regions.[5,7]

Abscessation caused by *C pseudotuberculosis* has no predisposition for sex, breed, or age, but horses less than one year of age are seldom affected.[5] The disease is most prevalent in California but is expanding to other parts of the country. The occurrence peaks in late summer, fall and early winter. The seasonal occurrence and geographic pattern indicate that an unidentified arthropod vector may be a factor in the disease. The highest annual occurrences of the disease follow winters of above-average rainfall. High rainfall in the winter may result in optimal breeding condition for insects during the subsequent summer and autumn. Abscessation caused by *C pseudotuberculosis* has been associated with cutaneous infestation of habronema larvae.[8] *Corynebacterium pseudotuberculosis* is thought to be an inhabitant of the soil; infection may be related to overcrowding of stock.[6]

Abscesses caused by *C pseudotuberculosis* swell extensively. The cavity of the abscess may be relatively small; most of the swelling is edema. Abscessation of the prepuce may cause extensive edema resulting in phimosis or paraphimosis (Fig 3). Abscessation is accompanied by considerable pain, but usually the horse displays no signs of systemic illness. Occasionally abscessation is accompanied by fever, weight loss and lameness. Most horses with marked or prolonged fever develop complications, such as multiple or internal abscesses. Though the disease is seldom fatal, death caused by bacteremia has been reported.[7]

Antibiotics are usually unsuccessful in halting the course of the disease, and exacerbations of the disease are more common following their use.[5,6] Hydrotherapy and hot-packing appears to facilitate maturation of the abscess. Surgical exploration of the swelling may be necessary to establish ventral drainage, which usually results in rapid recovery. Lancing is usually possible about 7-10 days after an abscess is first noticed. Some abscesses, particularly those in the inguinal area, may require up to 4 months to mature. When lanced, the abscess generally heals within 2 weeks.

Figure 3. Abscessation of the prepuce of a gelding, caused by *Corynebacterium pseudotuberculosis.*

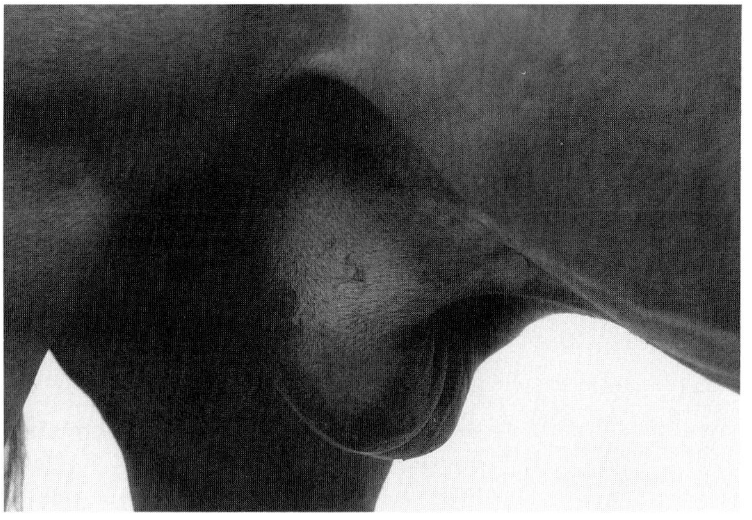

Chronic Dermatitis

The sebaceous and sweat glands of the preputial integument secrete products that combine with dirt and desquamated epithelial cells to form the malodorous substance called smegma, which accumulates on the surface of the penis and prepuce. This material may irritate the genital skin, causing a chronic inflammatory response (posthitis or balanoposthitis). Thickening and induration of the preputial lamina can develop if the tissue inflammation does not subside. Excessive glandular secretions can occur in longstanding cases, imparting a thick, greasy texture to the prepuce. Treatment consists of thoroughly cleansing the prepuce and penis to remove smegma from these areas (see Smegma Accumulation in Chapter 14). Frequent application of lotions or ointments containing a corticosteroid may help control persistent or recurrent posthitis. Some refractory cases require preputial resection (see Preputial Resection above).

Coital Exanthema

Coital exanthema is a herpetic genital disease transmitted venereally. Viral lesions generally are confined to the external genitalia. Chapter 14 contains a discussion of coital exanthema.

Dourine

Dourine is a venereally transmissible systemic disease caused by the protozoan *Trypanosoma equiperdum.* Preputial edema is a consistent manifestation of early stages of this disease. Dourine is discussed further in Chapter 2.

Microfilariasis

Migrating microfilariae of the genera *Onchocerca* and *Setaria* may induce swelling and dermatitis of the external genitalia of male horses, though the incidence of these conditions is unknown and difficult to document. Chapter 2 contains a discussion of onchocerchiasis.

Contagious Equine Metritis

Contagious equine metritis (CEM) is a venereal disease caused by the bacterium *Taylorella equigenitalis.* The stallion is an asymptomatic carrier of the disease. The causal organism resides on the surface of the penis and prepuce of affected horses for an indefinite period if untreated. See Chapter 14 for a discussion of this disease.

Cutaneous Habronemiasis (Summer Sores)

Cutaneous habronemiasis is a granulomatous skin condition caused by the infective larvae of the stomach worms *Draschia megastoma, Habronema muscae* and *Habronema microstoma.* The prepuce is a relatively common site for infestation. For a discussion of cutaneous habronemiasis, see Chapter 14.

Neoplasia

Squamous-Cell Carcinoma

Squamous-cell carcinoma is the most common neoplasm of the external genitalia of male horses. It is locally invasive and capable of metastasis. Squamous-cell carcinoma is discussed in Chapter 14.

Squamous Papilloma

Squamous papillomas can occur on the prepuce and penis of horses, though the incidence is very low. Genital papillomas generally are quite refractory to treatment. Chapter 14 contains a discussion of squamous papillomas.

Sarcoid

Sarcoids are nonmetastatic, locally proliferative cutaneous tumors peculiar to horses, donkeys and mules.[9,10] They are the most common tumors of horses but may occur more frequently on donkeys and mules than horses. There is no predilection for breed, color or sex.[11] Sarcoids have been reported in all ages of horses, but the tumor has a definite tendency to occur in younger horses (≤6 years of age).[12]

Sarcoids are most commonly located on the head, limbs and ventral midline but can appear anywhere on the body; the prepuce or scrotum are occasionally affected (Fig 4).[13] About one-third of affected horses have multiple lesions. Sarcoids often occur on wounds or sites of previous wounds.[14,15] Sites predisposed to trauma have a higher incidence for occurrence, as do areas that come in contact with existing sarcoids.[11,15] There is evidence that sarcoids can be transferred mechanically, such as by biting or scratching, from one part of the body to another. Epizootics have been observed in large herds.[13] A familial tendency to develop sarcoids has been reported.[16]

Though the cause is unknown, the causative agent may be a virus closely related to the bovine papilloma virus.[13] A retrovirus has been isolated from cells explanted from a tumor induced by intradermal inoculation of cells from a sarcoid into a foal with combined immunodeficiency;[17] however, retrovirus has also

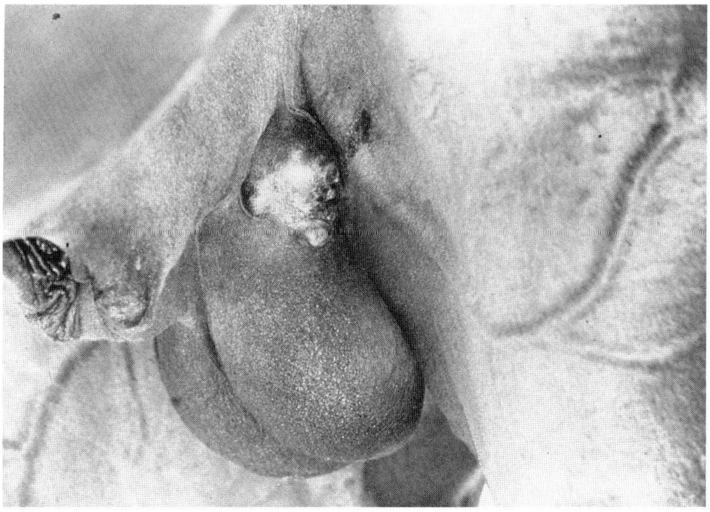

Figure 4. Sarcoid at the base of a stallion's scrotum. (Courtesy of Drs. R.M. Kenney and L.P. Tate)

been isolated from normal tissue, and injection of retrovirus alone does not appear to result in sarcoid formation.[18,19]

Morphologically, sarcoids are classified as verrucous or warty (Type I), fibroblastic (Type II) or mixed (Type III).[11-13] Each of these types of sarcoid may be sessile or pedunculated. Verrucous sarcoids are flat and dry, generally less than 6 cm in diameter, and relatively slow growing or static. If traumatized or partially excised, the wart-like verrucous sarcoid may transform into a fibroblastic type. The fibroblastic sarcoid resembles exuberant granulation tissue and may be found in granulating wounds. Fibroblastic sarcoids are the more aggressively growing type. They may appear initially or may spontaneously transform from the verrucous type. The mixed type of sarcoid is the least common and is most often seen when a verrucous sarcoid progresses into a fibroblastic sarcoid.

Histologically, the tumor may be mistaken for a sarcoma, as its histologic appearance resembles that of a sarcoma of moderate malignancy.[9,10] The term "sarcoid" was proposed to distinguish it from sarcomas, as well as fibrosarcomas, fibromas, granulomas and papillomas.[2] Distinguishing histologic features of sarcoids are: epidermal hyperkeratosis and hyperplasia, with formation of long rete-pegs that extend into the dermis; dermal fibropblasia, with irregularly arranged immature fibroblasts and fibrocytes (in a whorl or bundled formation) having increased mitotic figures and nuclei of variable size; and no invasion of underlying tissue.[11]

Though spontaneous regression of sarcoids has sometimes been recorded, sarcoids present for more than 6 months very rarely regress. Treatments have included excision, cryotherapy, intratumoral hyperthermia, chemotherapy, radiotherapy and immunotherapy.[11,19]

Conventional excision is followed by recurrence in almost 50% of cases within 3 years (most recurrent tumors appear within 6 months), and growth is frequently accelerated.[13,14] Cords of neoplastic cells extend into the adjacent dermis, and failure to excise all of these cords may explain the high rate of recurrence of sarcoids. Wide excision, including a 0.5- to 1-cm margin of normal tissue, occasionally eliminates the sarcoid.[20] Successful excision of sarcoids with a carbon dioxide laser has been reported.[21] This treatment has not been tested sufficiently to evaluate its efficacy, but it has the advantages of more precise dissection of the sarcoid, with minimal destruction to surrounding tissues and reduced scar formation at the excision site.[19,21] Improved cosmetic appearance following excision of sarcoids may be attained by applying split-thickness skin grafts to the excision site.[22] Considering the lack of metastasis and the possibility of recurrence with treatment, nonaggressive sarcoids may best be left untreated.

Cryotherapy is one of the most successful means of eliminating sarcoids. Larger sarcoids require debulking by excision and hemostasis by electrocoagulation before applying the cryogen.[23] The extreme cold causes cryonecrosis via direct damage by the cryogen and from anoxia caused by thrombosis of microvasculature. In addition, cryotherapy may have some immunotherapeutic effects. The mass is frozen throughout to -20 to -30 C, using liquid nitrogen or nitrous oxide. A thermocouple should be used to ensure adequate freezing. A double freeze-thaw cycle with a fast freeze and slow thaw causes the most cryonecrosis.

Intratumoral hyperthermia induced by radiofrequency current (2 mHz) has been successfully used in treatment of sarcoids.[24] The piercing probe of a hyperthermia unit is inserted into the tumor, and radiofrequency current is used to heat the tissue to 50 C for 30-60 seconds. Multiple insertions of the probe are recommended, and multiple treatments, administered at 7- to 10-day intervals, are usually necessary. The effect of the localized hyperthermia on thermoregulation of the testes must be determined before this treatment can be recommended for treatment of lesions near the scrotum.

Chemical cautery with escharotic agents has produced variable results.[20] Podophyllin, an irritant cathartic, is mixed with equal parts of tincture of benzoin (which acts as an adhesive to bind the podophyllin to the sarcoid) and applied daily to the sarcoid until a scab forms. Treatment is discontinued until the scab loosens and can be removed. After the scab is removed, daily treatment is again repeated until a new scab forms. The sarcoid reduces in size each time a scab is removed, so the process is repeated until the sarcoid is eliminated.

Flucytosine, which inhibits synthesis of nucleic acid by blocking synthesis of pyrimidine, may be effective in treatment of small sarcoids.[20] The sarcoid is excised, then flucytosine is applied to the wound daily for 30-90 days, or until the wound has healed. Prolonged use of the drug may cause inflammatory swelling of the prepuce and penis. Intralesional implants containing flucytosine or cisplatin are also available commercially.

These implants offer the advantage of maintaining high intralesional drug concentrations over an extended period.[19] Several implants, administered at 1- to 3-week intervals, may be required to eliminate a sarcoid, and resolution is not absolute.

Radiation therapy with radon or iridium implants has produced good results in treatment of sarcoids.[26-28] For best results, the tumor should be debulked before implantation of the radioactive material. Tumor regression may take several months and the procedure may be prohibitively expensive. Radiation therapy constitutes a health hazard, and can be performed only at a licensed facility. Ionizing radiation should not be used for treatment of sarcoids near the testes of breeding stallions because it is extremely toxic to the germinal epithelium of the seminiferous tubules.

Sarcoids have been successfully treated by intralesional injection with an attenuated strain of *Mycobacterium bovis*, *Bacillus* Calmette-Guerin (BCG) or nonviable immunotherapeutic agents isolated from the cell walls of the *Bacillus* organism.[29,30] It is thought that BCG stimulates an intense local reaction that causes activation and sensitization of macrophages, and perhaps T-lymphocytes against tumor-specific antigens, leading to cell-mediated killing of tumor cells. Response to treatment can be slow; several injections may be required. Use of this therapeutic approach has not been reported for sarcoids in the area of the prepuce.

Melanoma

Melanomas are potentially metastatic tumors arising from melanocytes. The tumors are most common in older gray horses. Increased melanoblastic activity in the skin of aging gray horses probably predisposes them to development of melanomas. About 80% of gray horses over 15 years of age develop melanomas. Primary melanotic tumors typically arise from the skin of the perianal area. The tumors are found occasionally on the prepuce or scrotum as dermal or subcutaneous lesions (Fig 5).

Melanomas vary in size, and may be firm or soft in texture. The overlying epidermis generally remains intact but may ulcerate. Melanomas are mostly seen in aged horses, typically grow slowly, and can remain benign. These tumors are rapidly fatal, however, following metastasis with vital organ involvement. Malignant melanomas initially spread by way of lymphatics, but

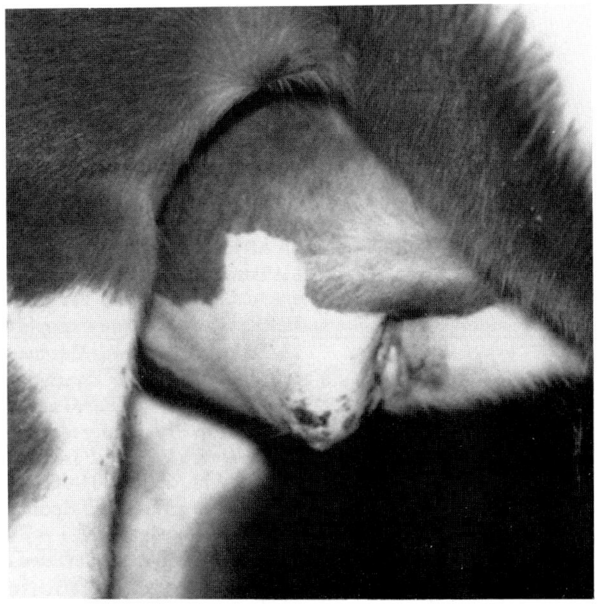

Figure 5. Melanoma involving the prepuce of a gelding.

the final involvement of the internal organs is mainly by hematogenous spread.

Diagnosis is based on gross and histologic appearance.[31-33] The neoplastic cells tend to be medium to large, round or oval, and often multinucleated (up to 20 nuclei). Large amounts of melanin in the cytoplasm of the neoplastic cells is common, but some melanomas are so amelanotic that the diagnosis must be made by use of special stains. Some melanomas contain numerous perivascular eosinophils and lymphocytes.

Melanomas often are not treated, as most melanomas grow slowly over several years without metastasis. Small tumors may be removed by excision or cryotherapy. Extensive melanomas have been treated with cimetidine (2.5 mg/kg PO once daily), but this drug is an androgen antagonist, and is known to impair testicular function in men.[34,35]

References

1. Ashdown RR and Done SH: *Colour Atlas of Veterinary Anatomy - The Horse.* Gower Medical Publishing, New York, 1987. pp 8.26-8.28.

2. O'Connor JJ: *Dollar's Veterinary Surgery.* Alexander Eger, Chicago, 1938. pp 716-723.

3. Frank ER: *Veterinary Surgery.* 7th ed. Burgess Publishing, Minneapolis, 1964. pp 267-270.

4. Walker DF and Vaughan JT: *Bovine and Equine Urogenital Surgery.* Lea & Febiger, Philadelphia, 1980. pp 105-182.

5. Knight HD: *Corynebacterium* infections in the horse: Problems of prevention. *JAVMA* 155:446-452, 1969.

During transport to the laboratory, semen must be shielded from natural and artificial light, and agitation of the sample should be avoided. The semen then is mixed gently with a suitable prewarmed (37-38 C) extender, preferably within 2-5 minutes after sample procurement (see Chapter 4 for formulations of semen extenders). Once semen is placed in a protective extender, the contained spermatozoa become tolerant of cold temperatures (at least temperatures down to 4-5 C). In fact, *in-vitro* preservation of cooled but unfrozen spermatozoa is optimized when extended equine semen is refrigerated (4-6 C).[2,7-10] Conversely, *in-vitro* maintenance of extended equine semen near body temperature results in rapid deterioration of spermatozoal viability (see Chapter 4).[2] Safeguards against agitation and light exposure should be provided when stored semen is transported.

Toxic Causes of Altered Semen

Ejaculated spermatozoa are sensitive to chemical toxins, just as they are susceptible to physical injury. Artificial vagina liners, semen-collection receptacles, or semen storage containers that are improperly selected or maintained contaminate the ejaculate with spermicidal products. Similarly, semen extenders with improper constituents can cause rapid destruction of spermatozoa. Precautions must be taken to avoid these circumstances. Most of these events can be circumvented by routine use of sterile disposable equipment proven to have no spermicidal activity for semen collection and storage (see Chapter 4). There is no substitute for quality control.

Hemospermia

Hemospermia refers to contamination of an ejaculate with blood, whether in minute or large quantities (Fig 1). Blood-laden ejaculates are easily detected by their pink to reddish color. Less obvious contamination is detected by microscopic analysis. A disproportionately elevated number of leukocytes (especially neutrophils) to erythrocytes in ejaculated semen suggests an internal genital infection. Stallions with overt hemorrhage into ejaculates are considered highly subfertile.[11] Erythrocytes, rather than serum, have been implicated for the marked disruption in spermatozoal fertilizing potential, though the precise factor(s) involved are unknown. A certain amount of blood contamination of ejaculates is compatible with fertility, especially if the semen is diluted properly with semen extender before insemination.[12] If only natural service is permitted for a horse with this disorder, semen extender can be placed in the mare's uterus before breeding to help dilute the erythrocyte concentration.

Specific causes of hemospermia have been discussed in previous chapters, and generally include lacerations on the exterior penis, cutaneous habronemiasis of the urethral process or glans penis, urethritis, urethral lacerations and infection/inflammation of the accessory genital glands. Diagnosis and treatment of these disorders have been addressed previously.

Urination During Ejaculation

(Urospermia)

Urospermia, or contamination of an ejaculate with urine, is an uncommon and perplexing disorder. Affected stallions generally exhibit normal libido and mating ability, but semen becomes contaminated with urine during the ejaculatory process (Fig 2). The problem may be incessant, or intermittent with an unpredictable patten. Urination can occur at any time or continuously during the process of ejaculation. The amount of urine contamination ranges from a few milliliters to quantities >250 ml.

Gross contamination of ejaculated semen with urine is easily detected by evaluation of the sample's color and odor. Elevated

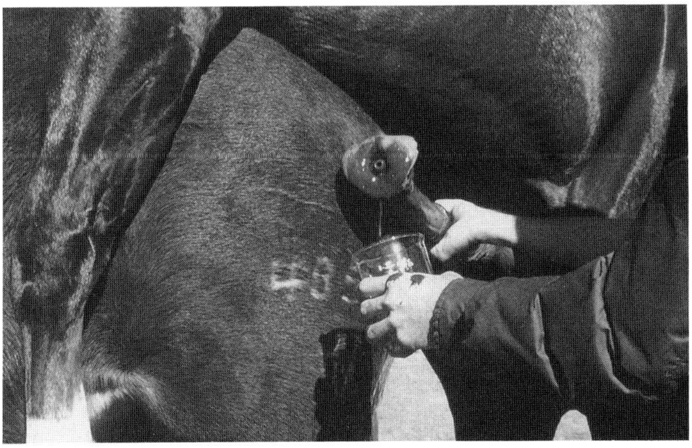

Figure 1. Profuse arterial hemorrhage from the corpus spongiosum penis at the time of breeding. The bleeding was associated with a rent in the mucosa of the pelvic urethra that communicated with the corpus spongiosum penis.

semen concentrations of urea nitrogen (>25-30 mg/dl) or creatinine (>2 mg/dl) are required to document urine contamination that may be imperceptible by evaluation of the sample's color or odor. Semen samples containing as little as 10% urine (v/v) can be readily confirmed in the field by using commercially available test strips for either urea nitrogen or nitrite.[13] To minimize false-positive or false-negative results, urea nitrogen test strips (Azostix: Miles Laboratory) should be fully immersed in the semen sample, then removed and held horizontally for 10 seconds before examination. Samples positive for urine turn the reagent pad from pale yellow to green. False-positive readings are likely if the reagent pad is evaluated for color change after the recommended 10-second exposure period. Nitrite reagent pads (Multistix: Miles Laboratory) can also be used in a similar manner. Best results with this test are achieved if the sample is evaluated 3.5 minutes after immersion in the suspect sample. The color change for urine contamination with this test is from yellow to a radiant orange.

Semen can be separated into fractions during collection to determine where urination is occurring during ejaculation.[14] An open-ended artificial vagina can be used to collect semen, as it permits exposure of the glans penis. Successive jets of semen are fractionated by covering the glans penis with a funnel system, which diverts semen jets into several receptacles.[13-15]

Minute amounts of urine are tolerable in ejaculated semen, but the adverse effects of urine contamination on spermatozoa

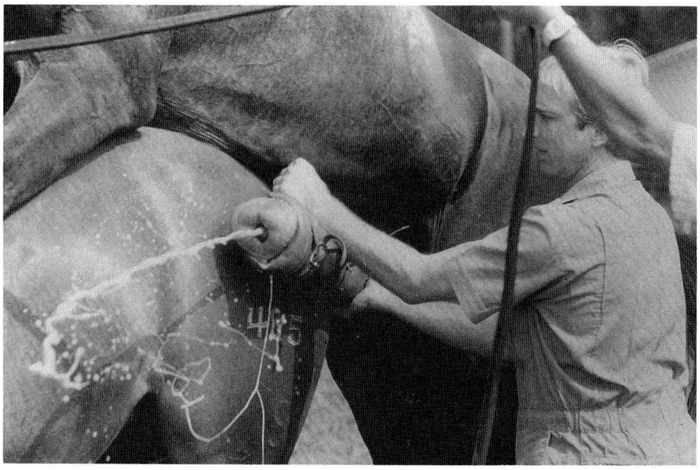

Figure 2. Excessive urination at the time of copulation, documented with the aid of an open-ended artificial vagina.

generally are evident by reduced motility and fertilizing capacity. The concentration of urine required to reduce semen quality has not been established but is presumed to be very low.

The underlying causes of urospermia are speculative, as this ejaculatory disturbance has not been adequately studied. Because closure of the bladder sphincter and semen emission are considered to be controlled by the alpha-adrenergic sympathetic nervous system, a disturbance in this nervous pathway might be involved in the pathogenesis of this disorder.[17] Similarly, neuropathies causing bladder paralysis, such as cauda equina neuritis, nerve damage secondary to EHV-1 infection, or sorghum/sudangrass poisoning, could create urinary incontinence during ejaculation.[18] Peculiarly, most stallions with urospermia do not exhibit signs of a neurologic deficit other than urinary incontinence at the time of breeding. However, we have observed recurrent and pronounced urospermia in a stallion that also dribbled urine from the penis when not sexually aroused.

Treatments for urospermia vary, and tend to be arduous and often unrewarding. Delaying semen collection (or breeding) until immediately after the stallion has urinated is helpful. Urination can be stimulated by diuretic administration, such as furosemide. Many stallions "reflexly" void urine when exposed to stallion fecal piles. Some stallions have been trained to urinate on command. Alternatively, the bladder can be catheterized to evacuate urine before ejaculation. Subsequent of urethritis/cystitis is an obvious drawback to routine catheterization.

Fractionation of ejaculates can be used alone or in combination with any of the above measures to obtain urine-free semen samples. This procedure generally is helpful only if the stallion tends to urinate in the final stages of the ejaculatory process. Dilution of semen in an appropriate extender may help protect the spermatozoa from urine-related damage if urine contamination is minimal. It also is advantageous to centrifuge contaminated semen samples after initial dilution in a semen extender, decant the supernatant, then resuspend the sperm pellet in more extender before insemination. This treatment can be used only in breeds in which artificial insemination is permitted. Bethanechol chloride or flavoxate hydrochloride have been used to correct urospermia in stallions, but the effectiveness of these products is questionable. Alpha-sympathomimetic drugs have been used to prevent retrograde ejaculation in men by stimulating bladder neck closure.[17] Results have been encouraging. Similar therapeutic regimens have not been reported for urospermia in stallions but are worthy of investigation.

Inflammatory, Infectious and Immune Causes of Altered Semen

Bacterial Contamination of Semen (Bacteriospermia)

See Chapters 12 and 14 for discussions regarding bacterial contamination of semen.

Equine Viral Arteritis

For a discussion of equine viral arteritis, see Chapters 2 and 12.

Dourine

See Chapter 2 for a discussion of this protozoal disease.

Multifactorial Causes of Altered Semen

Abnormal Spermatozoal Morphology

Though irrefutable proof of spermatozoal fertilizing capacity requires fertilization trials, assessment of spermatozoal morphology long has been considered a standard laboratory procedure for estimating the fertilizing potential of a semen sample. Unfortunately, the fertilizing capacity of spermatozoa with specific morphologic defects (*eg,* acrosomal defects or distal cytoplasmic droplets) is generally unknown, and the pathogenesis of spermatozoal morphologic abnormalities is poorly understood. Abnormal spermatozoal morphology may result from deranged spermatogenesis, impaired epididymal function, improper semen-handling techniques, or a combination of these factors.

Genetic and environmental factors affect spermatozoal morphology.[19] These 2 components are difficult to differentiate and may interact. Environmental conditions contributing to abnormal spermatozoal morphology include elevated scrotal temperature (*eg,* that associated with high ambient temperature, scrotal inflammation/insulation or fever), incomplete testicular descent, malnutrition, noxious agents (chemicals, drugs, irradiation), and hormonal imbalances. Aging also affects spermatozoal morphology.

Defective spermatozoal morphology may be temporary or permanent. Evaluation of semen from sequential ejaculates (at 1- to 2- month intervals), combined with an accurate and in-depth clinical history, usually is the only way to distinguish between temporary and permanent conditions. A time lag usually exists between gonadal insult and its effect on spermatozoal morphology. This effect typically persists long after the insult is removed (See Chapters 7 and 8).

No ejaculate is free of morphologically defective sperm; rather, spermatozoa with abnormal morphology constitute varying proportions of spermatozoal populations. Individual variation exists among stallions, and ejaculates of a single stallion vary. The effect of various morphologic defects on fertility is difficult to measure, primarily because prevalence of any one type of defect may be low or may fluctuate. Spermatozoa with abnormal morphology are present in stallions with excellent fertility. The upper limit of abnormal spermatozoa necessary to reduce fertility is difficult to determine and involves several factors. These include the type and incidence of each defect, as some defects are more detrimental to fertility than others. For instance, midpiece defects or proximal cytoplasmic droplets appear to hamper fertility more than distal cytoplasmic droplets.[20]

As a rule, fertile stallions have a minimum of 60% morphologically normal spermatozoa in their ejaculates and <10-15% incidence of any single morphologic defect. Morphologically abnormal spermatozoa do not seem to exert a negative influence on normal sperm. Therefore, the total number of morphologically normal sperm in ejaculates probably provides more information about fertility than the percentage or absolute number of morphologically abnormal spermatozoa.[21]

Methods for assessing spermatozoal morphology are described in Chapter 2. Accurate evaluation of spermatozoal morphology with light-microscopic techniques requires experience, good sperm-processing techniques, and a high-quality microscope. Numerous types of morphologic defects can be identified in equine spermatozoa, including acrosome defects (*eg,* degenerating or knobbed acrosomes), head defects (*eg,* crater defects, abnormal shapes or degenerative changes), midpiece defects (*eg,* absence or malformation of the mitochondrial sheath), retained cytoplasmic droplets (proximal and distal), tail defects (*eg,* absent or bent tails) and detached heads. Premature germ cells (spermatogonia, spermatocytes or spermatids) also may be observed in semen, indicating premature release from the spermatogenic epithelium. The type and incidence of all defects should be recorded. Abaxial midpieces are considered normal in equine spermatozoa.

Interpreting the findings is difficult and should be done on the basis of the findings described above. The incidence of abnormal midpiece and tail defects usually is reflected in the percentage of progressively motile spermatozoa in the sample. Spermatozoa are less susceptible to artifactual changes in morphology than in motility, so assessment of spermatozoal morphology is an integral part of a breeding soundness examination. Spermatozoal morphology, however, should not be used singularly to predict a stallion's fertility. One study indicated that abnormal heads, abnormal midpieces or proximal cytoplasmic droplets are most likely to interfere with stallion fertility.[22]

Clinicians unfamiliar with techniques for evaluating spermatozoal morphology are encouraged to use a reference laboratory with qualified personnel. An excellent reference text is available on evaluation of bovine spermatozoal morphology.[23] Much of the information provided in this text would be useful to individuals studying morphology of stallion spermatozoa.

Abnormal Spermatozoal Motility

Assessing spermatozoal motility is a traditional way to predict the fertilizing capacity of spermatozoa in all domestic animal species. Though spermatozoal motility may be a relatively sensitive indicator of fertility, the degree and type of motility depend on environmental conditions. Inappropriate handling of ejaculated semen before analysis of spermatozoal motility can adversely affect observer accuracy, unjustly discrediting a stallion's innate fertility. Precautions should be taken to protect sperm from such artifactual changes. It is important to note that spermatozoal motility, as morphology, does not correlate absolutely with fertility. For accuracy, these tests must be incorporated into a battery of tests, and the limitations of each test recognized.

Methods of estimating spermatozoal motility are described in the section entitled Semen Evaluation in Chapter 2. Causes of intrinsic reductions in spermatozoal motility are varied and numerous, and are similar to those described for abnormal spermatozoal morphology. Potential genetic and environmental causes must be explored if a depression in spermatozoal motility is observed. If artifactual damage to spermatozoal motility is avoided, the percentage of progressively motile spermatozoa in a semen sample seems to be inversely proportional to the percentage of spermatozoa with flagellar abnormalities in that sample.

Oligospermia/Azoospermia

Oligospermia is a deficiency of spermatozoa in an ejaculate, whereas azoospermia implies a complete absence of spermatozoa. The causes of these disorders are similar, the only difference being the magnitude of the problem. Causes include reduced spermatogenesis, obstruction of extragonadal duct lumina for spermatozoal passage, and sexual overuse. Testicular hypoplasia and degeneration are common causes of oligospermia/azoospermia, and are due to inadequate spermatozoal production by the seminiferous epithelium. Obstruction of the epididymal or deferent ducts can produce clinical signs similar to those of testicular degeneration/hypoplasia, so a careful physical examination is critical to differentiate these disorders.

Increased frequency of ejaculation reduces spermatozoal quantity per ejaculate. However, spermatozoal number is unlikely to drop below the critical number required for impregnation in a normal mature breeding stallion. The libido of a fertile stallion usually drops and the animal fails to copulate or ejaculate before the spermatozoal number in ejaculates drops to a level insufficient for impregnation.[24]

Accurate assessment of daily sperm output is of vital importance to a stallion fertility examination (Chapter 2) and is subject to several physiologic factors, including testicular size, age of the stallion, and season, as well as pathologic conditions (see Estimation of a Stallion Book in Chapter 3). Estimates of daily sperm production from only 1-2 semen samples are likely to be erroneous because of the variability in extragonadal spermatozoal storage capacity among different stallions.

Treatment of oligospermia/azoospermia varies with the underlying cause (see Testicular Degeneration, Testicular Hypoplasia, Spermiostasis and Ejaculatory Failure in appropriate chapters).

References

1. Cooper WC: The effect of rapid temperature changes on oxygen uptake by and motility of stallion spermatozoa. *Proc Ann Mtg Soc Theriogenol,* 1979. pp 10-13.

2. Varner DD *et al:* Effects of cooling rate and storage temperature on equine spermatozoal motility parameters. *Theriogenology* 29:1043-1054, 1988.

3. Bogart R and Mayer DT: The effects of egg yolk on the various physical and chemical factors detrimental to spermatozoan viability. *J Anim Sci* 9:143-152, 1950.

4. Nishikawa Y and Shinomiya S: Studies on the resistance of horse spermatozoa. II. Resistance to temperature. *Jpn J Zootech Sci* 29:116-122, 1949.

5. Watson PF *et al:* Quantitative assessment of membrane damage in cold-shocked spermatozoa of stallions. *J Reprod Fertil* (Suppl) 35:651-653, 1987.

6. Amann RP and Pickett BW: Principles of cryopreservation and a review of cryopreservation of stallion spermatozoa. *J Equine Vet Sci* 7:145-173, 1987.

7. Householder DD *et al:* Effect of extender, number of spermatozoa and hCG on equine fertility. *J Equine Vet Sci* 1:9-13, 1981.

8. Palmer E: Factors affecting stallion survival and fertility. *Proc Intl Cong Anim Reprod Artif Insem,* 1984. pp 377-379.

9. Squires EL *et al:* Fertility of equine spermatozoa cooled to 5 or 20°C. *Proc Intl Cong Anim Reprod Artif Insem,* 1988. Abstr #297.

10. Varner DD *et al:* Fertilizing capacity of equine spermatozoa stored for 24 hours at 5 or 20°C. *Theriogenology* 32:515-525, 1989.

11. Voss JL *et al: Proc Intl Cong Anim Reprod Artif Insem,* 1976. pp 1093-1095.

12. Blanchard TL *et al:* Use of a semen extender containing antibiotic to improve the fertility of a stallion with seminal vesiculitis due to *Pseudomonas aeruginosa. Theriogenology* 28:541-546, 1987.

13. Althouse GC *et al:* Diagnostic aids for the detection of urine in the equine ejaculate. *Theriogenology* 31:1141-1148, 1989.

14. Nash WO *et al:* Urination during ejaculation in a stallion. *JAVMA* 176:224-227, 1980.

15. Tischner M *et al:* Analysis of the pattern of ejaculation in stallions. *J Reprod Fertil* 41:329-335, 1974.

16. Kosiniak K: Characteristics of the successive jets of ejaculated semen of stallions. *J Reprod Fertil* (Suppl) 23:59-61, 1975.

17. Kaufman DG and Nagler HM, in Howards SS and Lipshultz LI: Male infertility. *Urol Clin No Am* 16:489-498, 1987.

18. Hackett RP *et al,* in Mansmann RA *et al: Equine Medicine and Surgery.* 3rd ed. American Veterinary Publications, Goleta, CA, 1982. pp 907-922.

19. Foote RH: Factors influencing the quantity and quality of semen harvested from bulls, rams, boars and stallions. *J Anim Sci* 47:1-11, 1978.

20. Hurtgen JP, in Robinson NE: *Current Therapy in Equine Medicine 2.* Saunders, Philadelphia, 1987. pp 558-563.

21. Kenney RM *et al: Manual for Clinical Fertility Evaluation of the Stallion.* Soc for Theriogenol, Hastings, NE, 1983.

22. Jasko DJ *et al:* Determination of the relationship between sperm morphologic classification and fertility in stallions: 66 cases (1987-1988). *JAVMA* 197:389-395, 1990.

23. Barth AD and Oko RJ: *Abnormal Morphology of Bovine Spermatozoa.* Iowa State Univ Press, Ames, 1989.

24. Squires EL *et al:* Effect of successive ejaculation on stallion seminal characteristics. *J Reprod Fertil* 27:7-12, 1979.

Index

A

B

C

R

S

T

U

V

W